AF572702

Human Nutrition

Human Nutrition

MURRAY M. TUCKERMAN, Ph.D.
Professor of Pharmaceutical Chemistry
Temple University School of Pharmacy
Philadelphia, PA

and

SALVATORE J. TURCO, Pharm.D.
Professor of Pharmacy
Temple University School of Pharmacy
Philadelphia, PA

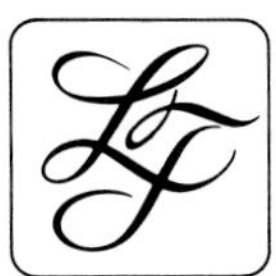

Lea & Febiger • *1983* • *Philadelphia*

Lea & Febiger
600 Washington Square
Philadelphia, PA 19106
U.S.A.

Library of Congress Cataloging in Publication Data

Tuckerman, Murray M.
Human Nutrition

Bibliography: p.
Includes index.
1. Parenteral feeding. 2. Nutrition.
I. Turco, Salvatore. I. Title
RM224.T8 1982 613.2 82-13033
ISBN 0-8121-0853-1

PRINTED IN THE UNITED STATES OF AMERICA

Print No. 3 2 1

Preface

This text was written to fill a specific need in the education of human health specialists, particularly clinical pharmacists. It presupposes a knowledge of biochemistry and physiology. It presumes a need for knowledge of nutrition for counseling healthy people who may seek advice about nutritional supplements. To this end, nutritional interactions, the effects of nutrients on each other, and the effects of drugs on the absorption or utilization of nutrients are presented. Information is also provided to aid in understanding the needs of patients with inherited metabolic disorders or acquired diseases that necessitate the administration of large quantities of nutrients. A foundation is provided for understanding the needs of the hospitalized patient and the ways in which those needs can be met.

As an aid to counseling, a discussion of the problem of obesity and analyses of the many diet plans that have been published in the popular literature are included. As a basis for diet planning, there is an exposition of the exchange lists. No attempt has been made to discuss diet therapy, menus, or recipes used as adjuncts in the treatment of various pathologic conditions.

All of the information has been taken from the literature. The correlations, interpretations, and evaluations, however, are the sole responsibility of the author. Particular reliance has been placed on the following sources.

1. Vitamin and Mineral Drug Products for Over-the-Counter Human Use. Federal Register, *44*:16126-16201 (March 16, 1979).
2. Committee on Dietary Allowances, Food and Nutrition Board, National Research Council: Recommended Dietary Allowances, 9th Ed. Washington, DC, National Academy of Sciences, 1980.
3. Watt, B.K., and Merrill, A.L.: Composition of Foods. Agriculture Handbook No. 8, Consumer and Food Economics Research Division, Agricultural Research Service, U.S. Dept. of Agriculture, Washington, DC, 1963.
4. Goodhart, R.S., and Shils, M.E. (eds.): Modern Nutrition in Health and Disease, 6th Ed. Philadelphia, Lea & Febiger, 1980.

The chapter on drug–food interactions has been prepared especially for this volume by Margherita LaFranco, Pharm.D., and contains an exhaustive bibliography.

The section on parenteral and enteral nutrition consists of reprints of articles published in the American Journal of Intravenous Therapy & Clinical Nutrition, edited by Salvatore J. Turco, Pharm.D.

Philadelphia, PA

Murray M. Tuckerman
Salvatore J. Turco

Acknowledgment

The contribution of Barbara H. Grissani in drawing the figures and careful typing of the manuscript from hand-written copy is recognized with thanks and gratitude.

Contents

Part I

Nutritional Elements

MURRAY M. TUCKERMAN, PH.D.

Chapter 1

Human Nutritional Patterns and U.S. Recommended Dietary Allowances

An adequate diet is the prime requisite for attaining and maintaining optimum health. The search for an optimum diet for humans is made difficult by the inadequacy of animal models, the large differences in requirements between individual humans, and the changing requirements of each human with changes in age, environment, and physical condition.

The basic concern in human nutrition today is to obtain a balanced diet from natural food sources, insofar as our present level of knowledge about optimum human nutrition will permit. In order to evaluate such a diet, it is convenient to refer to the individual essential nutrients. These nutrients may be divided into the following groups:

- I. Macronutrients
  - A. Water and electrolytes
    1. Sodium
    2. Potassium
    3. Calcium
    4. Magnesium
    5. Chloride
    6. Phosphate
  - B. Protein
  - C. Carbohydrate and fiber
  - D. Fats and cholesterol
- II. Micronutrients
  - A. Fat soluble vitamins
    1. Vitamin A
    2. Vitamin D
    3. Vitamin E
    4. Vitamin K
  - B. Water soluble vitamins
    1. Vitamin C
    2. Thiamin
    3. Riboflavin
    4. Niacin
    5. Pantothenic acid
    6. Vitamin B_6
    7. Folacin
    8. Cobalamin
    9. Biotin
  - C. Trace elements
    1. Iron
    2. Fluoride
    3. Iodide
    4. Zinc
    5. Copper
    6. Manganese
    7. Selenium
    8. Chromium
    9. Molybdenum

For ordinary living, it is generally not necessary to analyze diet in detail. The planning of meals, however, must be based on sound nutritional principles rather than on hearsay, food advertising, the many different philosophies of groups advocating extensive use of particular foods or food supplements, and diets designed to treat specific medical problems rather than for the general maintenance of health.

Good nutrition is defined as the overall balance of the food intake and not the consumption of any particular nutrient or group of nutrients.

If one looks at what is purchased in the supermarket and health food stores, there can be little doubt that people as a group are ignorant of good dietary practices. They consume too many calories, too much fat, too much sugar, too much protein, and spend too much money on nutritional supplements which, instead of improving nutrition, in many cases displace natural foods, promote poor dietary practices, and further unbalance the nutrient intake. In the search for good nutrition, some people have abandoned the "standard American diet" for "natural" and "organically grown" products, thereby nearly doubling the cost while attaining no better nutrition. Some have turned to vegetarian diets, robbing themselves of essential nutrients because of their lack of knowledge in constructing an adequate vegetarian diet. Some have turned to special foods, such as wheat germ or bran fiber, to be sprinkled over every dish as a kind of magic which immediately confers extraordinary nutrient value on the foods, without the least understanding of the amounts of nutrients added or the interrelationships between the various nutrients. In the search for proper weight maintenance many choose fad diets, which promise marvelous short-term results but are hazardous for long-term use. For the average person, attempts at improving nutrition are made more difficult by ignorance of proven nutritional principles, acceptance of sweeping generalities, acceptance of partial and misinterpreted data, prejudice, superstition, and the frequently misleading advertising of food companies.

TABLE 1-1. Basic Four Food Groups

Food	A Serving Is	Servings Per Day
I. Milk Group		
Milk, whole or skim	8 ounces	Children 0- 9: 2 to 3
Yogurt, plain	8 ounces	Children 9-12: 3
Hard cheese	1¼ ounces	Teenagers: 4
Cheese spreads	2 ounces	Adults: 2
Cottage cheese	16 ounces (2 cups)	Pregnant: 3
Ice cream	12 ounces (1½ cups)	Nursing: 4
This serving provides the amount of calcium in 8 ounces of milk.		
II. Meat Group		
Meat, lean part	2 to 3 ounces	2
Poultry	2 to 3 ounces	If only vegetable protein is used, it must be of adequate nutritional quality as explained in the section on protein
Fish	2 to 3 ounces	
Eggs	2 to 3	
Beans and peas, cooked	1 to 1½ cups	
Nuts and seeds	½ to ¾ cups	
Peanut butter	4 tablespoons	
Hard cheese	2 to 3 ounces	
Cottage cheese	½ cup	
Cheese can be counted in both the milk and meat groups; thus ½ cup of cottage cheese is 1 meat serving and ¼ milk serving.		
III. Vegetable and Fruit Group		
Vegetables, cut up	½ cup	1 vitamin C source, such as orange, grapefruit, or equivalent amount of juice
Fruit, cut up	½ cup	1 vitamin A source, a deep yellow or dark green vegetable
Grapefruit	½ medium	2 other choices to give a total of 4 servings
Orange	1	
Melon	½ medium	
Potato	1 medium	
Salad	1 bowl	
Lettuce	1 wedge (⅛ head)	
IV. Bread and Cereal Group		
Bread	1 slice (1 ounce)	1 whole grain
Cooked cereal	½ to ¾ cup	3 whole grain or enriched to give a total of 4 servings
Pasta, cooked	½ to ¾ cup	
Rice, cooked	½ to ¾ cup	
Dry cereal	1 ounce	

Obtaining detailed knowledge of human nutritional needs can be a long and tedious process. Good eating, however, can be reduced to two basic principles: variety and moderation. This simply means eating a wide variety of foods in amounts that are not too large. Even the venerable Weight Watchers organization has finally recognized that a proper diet can contain any food, provided that only a moderate amount is eaten.

A simple approach to adequate nutrition is to use the "Basic Four" food groups (replacing the older "Basic Seven") established by the U.S. Department of Agriculture. The "Basic Four" food groups are described in Table 1-1.

A modification of the Basic Four has been developed by the Center for Science in the Public Interest (1755 S. Street, N.W., Washington, DC 20009), which takes into account recommendations made in 1977 by the Senate Select Committee on Nutrition and Human Needs, in setting dietary goals for the United States to modify current diet in the direction of lowered fat, cholesterol, salt, and added sugars, and increased fiber, starches (complex carbohydrate), and natural vitamins and minerals. It permits variety without unbalancing the total nutrient intake by indicating foods that can be used daily, foods that can be used in moderation several times a week, and foods that should be used only occasionally (Table 1-2). For people requiring dietary modification because of medical conditions, the guide also indicates, by number, foods high in unsaturated fat (1), saturated fat (2), cholesterol (3), and sodium (4).

Generally, "anytime" foods have less than 30% of their calories as fat and are usually low in sugar and salt. The "moderate use" group have medium amounts of fat, with a low or medium proportion as saturated fat or larger amounts of mostly polyunsaturated fat. The "occasional use" group have about 50% of their calories as fat, with a substantial portion of this as saturated fat. Some are high in sugar or salt.

To provide more sophisticated criteria for

TABLE 1-2. New American Eating Guide

Anytime	Moderate Use	Occasional Use
I. Milk Group		
Buttermilk from skim milk	Cocoa with skim milk	Cheesecake (2)
Low-fat cottage cheese	Regular 4% cottage cheese	Cheese fondue (2, 4)
Low-fat (1%) milk	Frozen yogurt	Cheese souffle (2, 3, 4)
Nonfat dry milk	Low-fat (2%) milk	Eggnog (3)
Skim milk	Sweetened low-fat yogurt	Hard cheeses (2, 4) blue, brick, Camembert, cheddar, Muenster, Swiss
	Part-skim mozzarella	Ice cream (2)
		Process cheeses (2, 4)
		Whole milk (2)
		Whole milk yogurt (2)
II. Meat Group		
Cod	Fried fish (4)	Commercial fried chicken
Flounder	Herring (1, 4)	Cheese omelet (2, 3)
Gefilte fish (4)	Canned mackerel (4)	Whole egg or egg yolk (1, 3) (limit to 3 a week)
Haddock	Canned salmon (4)	Bacon (2, 4)
Halibut	Sardines (4)	Fried beef liver (3)
Perch	Shrimp (3)	Bologna, salami, hot dogs, sausage (2, 4)
Pollock	Canned tuna, oil pack (4)	Corned beef (2, 4)
Rockfish	Chicken liver (3)	Ground beef (2, 4)
Shellfish, except shrimp	Homemade fried chicken (1)	Spareribs (2)
Sole	Chicken or turkey with skin	Untrimmed red meat (4)
Canned tuna, water packed	Beef, pork, lamb, veal—lean	
Chicken or turkey without skin		

TABLE 1-2. (continued)

Anytime	Moderate Use	Occasional Use
III. Vegetable and Fruits Group		
All fruits and vegetables except those listed in other columns	Avocado (1)	Coconut (2)
Unsweetened applesauce	Cole slaw (1)	Pickles (4)
Unsweetened fruit juices	Cranberry sauce	
Unsalted vegetable juices	Dried fruit	
Potatoes	French fries	
Sweet potatoes	Fried egg plant	
Canned fruits, packed in unsweetened fruit juice	Fruits canned in syrup	
	Gazpacho (4)	
	Glazed carrots (4)	
	Guacamole (1)	
	Au gratin potatoes (4)	
	Salted vegetable juices (4)	
	Sweetened fruit juices	
	Vegetables canned with salt (4)	
IV. Bread and Cereal Group (beans, grains, and nuts)		
Bread and rolls, whole grain	Cornbread	Croissant (2)
Dried beans and peas	Flour tortilla	Doughnut (1, 2)
Lentils	Granola cereals	Presweetened cereal
Oatmeal	Hominy grits	Sticky buns
Pasta, whole wheat	Macaroni and cheese (4)	Stuffing (2, 4)
Rice, brown	Matzoh	
Sprouts	Nuts (1)	
Hot and cold cereals, whole grain	Peanut butter (1)	
Matzoh, whole grain	Pizza (4)	
	Refried beans	
	Seeds (1)	
	Soybeans	
	Tofu	
	Waffles or pancakes with syrup	
	White bread and rolls	
	Pasta, white flour	
	Rice, white	
	Unsweetened cereal	

evaluating diet on a quantitative basis, the guidelines of Recommended Dietary Allowances have been developed by the Food and Nutrition Board of the National Research Council/ National Academy of Sciences. It is unfortunate that these values, derived from consideration of nutrients contained in natural foods and ingested at the concentrations in natural foods, and based on long-term intakes but expressed as average amounts per day, have been taken over by the Food and Drug Administration for the labelling of food supplements (vitamin and mineral tablets) and enriched foods under the heading of Recommended *Daily* Allowances. There is a reasonable amount of evidence to show that many of these added nutrients, either because of their abnormal concentration or abnormal chemical form, are not utilized by the body in the same manner as the naturally occurring substances in their original unconcentrated form.

RECOMMENDED DIETARY ALLOWANCES

The National Academy of Sciences, Washington, DC, defines Recommended Dietary Allowances as follows:

The "Recommended Dietary Allowances (RDA) are the levels of intake of essential nutrients considered, in the judgment of the Committee on Dietary Allowances of the Food and Nutrition Board, on the basis of available scientific knowledge, to be adequate to meet the known nutritional needs of practically all healthy persons" (Table 1-3).

The RDA are the nutritional needs, over a long period of time, of population groups, expressed as a daily average. They should not be misinterpreted as a daily minimum or as a requirement for any specific individual. The daily values (except for energy) are thought to exceed the requirements for most individuals, although they represent a safe level of excess. All nutrients are potentially toxic in large doses. RDA values, even though known to be excessive for at least 80% of the population, are also known to be safe for 100% of the healthy population. Intakes below the recommended level, either on a daily or a long-term basis, are not necessarily inadequate.

The RDA is meant for healthy populations. A special need for nutrients may exist in cases of inherited metabolic disorders, infections, chronic disease, use of some medications, premature births, and absorption problems.

The RDA is based on the assumption that it will be met by a diet containing a wide variety of foods rather than by nutritional supplements (vitamin/mineral tablets) or by extensive fortification of single foods. The RDA is based on *intake* and has included within it allowances for less than 100% availability and less than 100% absorption of the various nutrients from a normal, varied diet.

In determining the RDA, it is necessary to start with the concept of a minimum daily requirement (MDR). Immediately, a conceptual problem arises in defining this minimum. It seems appealing to define the MDR for adults as the minimum intake that will maintain body weight, normal function, and health and to define MDR for children as the minimum intake that will maintain "satisfactory" growth. Another definition is the amount that will just prevent failure of a specific function or will just prevent a specific sign or deficiency. A third definition is the amount needed to maintain "acceptable" blood and tissue concentrations and to prevent depletion of body stores as judged by balance studies. A fourth definition is the amount needed to maintain maximum body stores (although this may be toxic levels for vitamin A, vitamin D, and iron). With the initial disagreement about proper definition of an MDR, it can be seen why the concept had to be abandoned and replaced by the RDA concept. It is not that the definitions are poor or invalid, but rather that the range of variability in humans is so great that it is difficult to establish minimum values quantitatively.

For all requirements except energy, the RDA is based on a variety of considerations.

1. Estimating the average requirement of a population for a nutrient and estimating the variability of the requirement within that population arrives at an amount sufficient to meet the needs of nearly everyone in that population. This estimate of average and variance is obtained from a variety of sources, some of which are as follows:
   a. The amount of each nutrient present in the food supply of apparently normal, healthy people.
   b. Epidemiologic evidence, when clinical symptoms of nutrient deficiency can be corrected by dietary improvement.
   c. Chemical analyses to determine the degree of tissue saturation.
   d. Biochemical measurement for adequacy of molecular function or relationship of specific enzyme activity to nutritional status.
   e. Balance studies that measure nutritional status as a function of nutrient intake.
   f. Rarely, when risk is minimal, human studies with nutritionally deficient diets to produce clinical symptoms, followed by correction of the deficit with measured amounts of nutrients.
   g. When information on a nutrient requirement is inadequate, extrapolation from data available. Some of

TABLE 1-3. Recommended Daily Dietary Allowances,[a] Revised 1980

Food and Nutrition Board, National Academy of Sciences—National Research Council.
Designed for the maintenance of good nutrition of practically all healthy people in the U.S.A.

							Fat-Soluble Vitamins			Water-Soluble Vitamins							Minerals					
	Age (years)	Weight (kg)	Weight (lbs)	Height (cm)	Height (in)	Protein (g)	Vitamin A (μg R E)[b]	Vitamin D (μg)[c]	Vitamin E (mg α T E)[d]	Vitamin C (mg)	Thiamin (mg)	Riboflavin (mg)	Niacin (mg N E)[e]	Vitamin B_6 (mg)	Folacin[f] (μg)	Vitamin B_{12} (μg)[g]	Calcium (mg)	Phosphorus (mg)	Magnesium (mg)	Iron (mg)[h]	Zinc (mg)	Iodine (μg)
Infants	0.0-0.5	6	13	60	24	kg × 2.2	420	10	3	35	0.3	0.4	6	0.3	30	0.5	360	240	50	10	3	40
	0.5-1.0	9	20	71	28	kg × 2.0	400	10	4	35	0.5	0.6	8	0.6	45	1.5	540	360	70	15	5	50
Children	1-3	13	29	90	35	23	400	10	5	45	0.7	0.8	9	0.9	100	2.0	800	800	150	15	10	70
	4-6	20	44	112	44	30	500	10	6	45	0.9	1.0	11	1.3	200	2.5	800	800	200	10	10	90
	7-10	28	62	132	52	34	700	10	7	45	1.2	1.4	16	1.6	300	3.0	800	800	250	10	10	120
Males	11-14	45	99	157	62	45	1000	10	8	50	1.4	1.6	18	1.8	400	3.0	1200	1200	350	18	15	150
	15-18	66	145	176	69	56	1000	10	10	60	1.4	1.7	18	2.0	400	3.0	1200	1200	400	18	15	150
	19-22	70	154	177	70	56	1000	7.5	10	60	1.5	1.7	19	2.2	400	3.0	800	800	350	10	15	150
	23-50	70	154	178	70	56	1000	5	10	60	1.4	1.6	18	2.2	400	3.0	800	800	350	10	15	150
	51+	70	154	178	70	56	1000	5	10	60	1.2	1.4	16	2.2	400	3.0	800	800	350	10	15	150
Females	11-14	46	101	157	62	46	800	10	8	50	1.1	1.3	15	1.8	400	3.0	1200	1200	300	18	15	150
	15-18	55	120	163	64	46	800	10	8	60	1.1	1.3	14	2.0	400	3.0	1200	1200	300	18	15	150
	19-22	55	120	163	64	44	800	7.5	8	60	1.1	1.3	14	2.0	400	3.0	800	800	300	18	15	150
	23-50	55	120	163	64	44	800	5	8	60	1.0	1.2	13	2.0	400	3.0	800	800	300	18	15	150
	51+	55	120	163	64	44	800	5	8	60	1.0	1.2	13	2.0	400	3.0	800	800	300	10	15	150
Pregnant						+30	+200	+5	+2	+20	+0.4	+0.3	+2	+0.6	+400	+1.0	+400	+400	+150	[h]	+5	+25
Lactating						+20	+400	+5	+3	+40	+0.5	+0.5	+5	+0.5	+100	+1.0	+400	+400	+150	[h]	+10	+50

[a] The allowances are intended to provide for individual variations among most normal persons as they live in the United Sates under usual environmental stresses.
[b] Retinol equivalents. 1 retinol equivalent = 1 μg retinol or 6 μg beta-carotene.
[c] As cholecalciferol. 10 μg cholecalciferol = 400 IU of vitamin D.
[d] Alpha-tocopherol equivalents. 1 mg d-alpha-tocopherol = 1 α-TE.
[e] 1 NE (niacin equivalent) is equal to 1 mg of niacin or 60 mg of dietary tryptophan.
[f] The folacin allowances refer to dietary sources as determined by *Lactobacillus casei* assay after treatment with enzymes (conjugases) to make polyglutamyl forms of the vitamin available to the test organism.
[g] The recommended dietary allowance for vitamin B_{12} in infants is based on average concentration of the vitamin in human milk. The allowances after weaning are based on energy intake, as recommended by the American Academy of Pediatrics, and consideration of other factors, such as intestinal absorption.
[h] The increased requirement during pregnancy may not be met by the iron content of habitual American diets nor by the existing stores of many women; therefore, the use of 30 to 60 mg of supplemental iron is recommended. Iron needs during lactation are not substantially different from those of nonpregnant women, but continued supplementation of the mother for 2 to 3 months after parturition is advisable in order to replenish stores depleted by pregnancy.

TABLE 1-3. (continued)

	Age (years)	Vitamins			Trace Elements[b]						Electrolytes		
		Vitamin K (µg)	Biotin (µg)	Pantothenic Acid (mg)	Copper (mg)	Manganese (mg)	Fluoride (mg)	Chromium (mg)	Selenium (mg)	Molybdenum (mg)	Sodium (mg)	Potassium (mg)	Chloride (mg)
Infants	0-0.5	12	35	2	0.5-0.7	0.5-0.7	0.1-0.5	0.01-0.04	0.01-0.04	0.03-0.06	115-350	350-925	275-700
	0.5-1	10-20	50	3	0.7-1.0	0.7-1.0	0.2-1.0	0.02-0.06	0.02-0.06	0.04-0.08	250-750	425-1275	400-1200
Children	1-3	15-30	65	3	1.0-1.5	1.0-1.5	0.5-1.5	0.02-0.08	0.02-0.08	0.05-0.1	325-975	550-1650	500-1500
and	4-6	20-40	85	3-4	1.5-2.0	1.5-2.0	1.0-2.5	0.03-0.12	0.03-0.12	0.06-0.15	450-1350	775-2325	700-2100
Adolescents	7-10	30-60	120	4-5	2.0-2.5	2.0-3.0	1.5-2.5	0.05-0.2	0.05-0.2	0.1-0.3	600-1800	1000-3000	925-2775
	11+	50-100	100-200	4-7	2.0-3.0	2.5-5.0	1.5-2.5	0.05-0.2	0.05-0.2	0.15-0.5	900-2700	1525-4575	1400-4200
Adults		70-140	100-200	4-7	2.0-3.0	2.5-5.0	1.5-4.0	0.05-0.2	0.05-0.2	0.15-0.5	1100-3300	1875-5625	1700-5100

[a] Because there is less information on which to base allowances, these figures are provided in the form of ranges of recommended intakes.
[b] Since the toxic levels for many trace elements may be only several times usual intakes, the upper levels for the trace elements given in the table should not be habitually exceeded.

this data is from animal experiments in which deficiency is produced by exclusion of a single nutrient. Extrapolation of data from animal experiments to human needs is highly controversial.

2. Increasing the calculated value to account for inefficient utilization of the nutrient as ingested includes the efficiency of the conversion of precursors to active forms and less than complete absorption.
3. For infants up to 6 months old, the starting point is the average amount consumed by thriving infants breastfed by a healthy, well-nourished mother. Since there is uncertainty about the utilization of some nutrients in synthetic milk formulas, the recommendation is to supply these nutrients in somewhat larger quantities than found in human milk in order to provide a safety factor (Table 1-4).
4. For infants from 6 months to one year, the recommendation is based on a diet of synthetic milk and an increasing amount of varied solid foods.

For energy, guidelines based on averages by age and sex are given, but not as recommended allowances. No recommendations can be made because any surplus of energy is stored as fat; therefore, continued surpluses lead to obesity, which may be detrimental to health. On the other side, there must be sufficient energy intake to balance expenditures and assure efficient functioning of the body systems.

Recommended Dietary Allowances have been set for protein, vitamins A, D, E, C, thiamin, riboflavin, niacin equivalent, vitamin B_6, folacin, vitamin B_{12}, calcium, phosphorus, magnesium, iron, zinc, and iodine. In addition, estimated “safe and adequate” intakes have been set for vitamin K, pantothenic acid, biotin, copper, chromium, fluoride, manganese, molybdenum, and selenium. These are generally given as a range of intake because available information does

TABLE 1-3 (continued)

Mean Heights and Weights and Recommended Energy Intake[a]
Recommended Dietary Allowances Revised 1980

Category	Age (years)	Weight (kg)	Weight (lb)	Height (cm)	Height (in)	Energy Needs (with range) (kcal)	(MJ)
Infants	0.0-0.5	6	13	60	24	kg × 115 (95-145)	kg × .48
	0.5-1.0	9	20	71	28	kg × 105 (80-135)	kg × .44
Children	1-3	13	29	90	35	1300 (900-1800)	5.5
	4-6	20	44	112	44	1700 (1300-2300)	7.1
	7-10	28	62	132	52	2400 (1650-3300)	10.1
Males	11-14	45	99	157	62	2700 (2000-3700)	11.3
	15-18	66	145	176	69	2800 (2100-3900)	11.8
	19-22	70	154	177	70	2900 (2500-3300)	12.2
	23-50	70	154	178	70	2700 (2300-3100)	11.3
	51-75	70	154	178	70	2400 (2000-2800)	10.1
	76+	70	154	178	70	2050 (1650-2450)	8.6
Females	11-14	46	101	157	62	2200 (1500-3000)	9.2
	15-18	55	120	163	64	2100 (1200-3000)	8.8
	19-22	55	120	163	64	2100 (1700-2500)	8.8
	23-50	55	120	163	64	2000 (1600-2400)	8.4
	51-75	55	120	163	64	1800 (1400-2200)	7.6
	76+	55	120	163	64	1600 (1200-2000)	6.7
Pregnancy						+300	
Lactation						+500	

[a] The data in these tables have been assembled from the observed median heights and weights of children and from desirable weights for adults, for mean heights of men (70 inches) and women (64 inches), between the ages of 18 and 34 years, as surveyed in the United States population (HEW/NCHS data).

The energy allowances for the young adults are for men and women doing light work. The allowances for the two older groups represent mean energy needs over these age spans, allowing for a 2% decrease in basal metabolic rate per decade and a reduction in activity of 200 kcal/day for men and women between 51 and 75 years, 500 kcal for men over 75 years, and 400 kcal for women over 75. The customary range of daily energy output is shown in parentheses, emphasizing the wide range of energy intakes appropriate for any group of people.

Energy allowances for children through age 18 are based on mean energy intakes of children of those ages followed in longitudinal growth studies. The values in parentheses are the tenth and ninetieth percentiles to indicate the range of energy consumption among children of those ages.

not allow the establishment of a recommended single value.

Another concept which has been found useful in nutrition is that of "nutrient density," the amount of a nutrient per 1000 kcal of a food. For nutrients that are largely used in the metabolism of food, nutrient density calculations can ascertain whether there is enough of the nutrient to assure efficient food utilization. When energy intake is high, such as for active children or for people engaged in strenuous work, the nutrient density of a diet may be low and still provide optimum nutrient intake. When energy intake is low, for example, in the elderly or when anorexia is present, such as in the hospitalized patient, special care must be given to provide a diet with high nutrient density.

Despite the many claims for special benefits, and despite the numerous loud voices and advertising encouraging the ingestion of excessive amounts of individual nutrients or combinations of nutrients, there is no scientifically acceptable evidence of any unique nutritional benefits from such a regimen. Large doses of individual nutrients have been recommended as exerting some specific pharmacologic action. Although there is some evidence of pharmacologic action of some nutrients, the effect is extremely weak, even when taken in megadoses. At high dosage levels of some nutrients, such as vitamins A, D, and C, toxic effects may be seen. In any event, the pharmacologic effects of a nutrient are not related to its nutritional functions.

Because of consumer concern about nutri-

TABLE 1-4. Human Milk-Substitute Formulas for Infant Nutrition

Based on a report of the Committee on Nutrition, American Academy of Pediatrics (Pediatrics 57:278, 1976), the Food and Drug Administration has established the following standard for infant formula, under the Infant Formula Act of 1980. Per 100 kcal:

Nutrients	Units	Minimum	Notes
Protein	g	1.8	4.5 g maximum
Fat	g	3.3	6.0 g maximum
Percent of total calories	%	30	
Essential fatty acids (linoleate)	g	0.3	
Percent of total calories	%	3	
Vitamins			
A (retinol equivalents)	μg	75.0	225.0 μg maximum
D	IU	40.0	100.0 IU maximum
K	μg	4.0	
E	IU	0.3	0.7 IU/g linoleic acid
C	mg	8.0	
Thiamin (B_1)	μg	40.0	
Riboflavin (B_2)	μg	60.0	
Pyridoxine (B_6)	μg	35.0	15μg/g protein
Cyanocobalamin (B_{12})	μg	0.15	
Niacin	μg	250.0	
Folic acid	μg	4.0	
Pantothenic acid	μg	300.0	
Biotin	μg	1.5	
Choline	mg	7.0	
Inositol	mg	4.0	
Minerals			
Calcium	mg	50.0	Calcium/phosphorus
Phosphorus	mg	25.0	ratio 1.1 to 2.0
Magnesium	mg	6.0	
Iron	mg	0.15	
Iodine	μg	5.0	
Zinc	mg	0.5	
Copper	μg	60.0	
Manganese	μg	5.0	
Sodium	mEq/L	6.0	17 mEq/L maximum
Potassium	mEq/L	14.0	34 mEq/L maximum
Chloride	mEq/L	11.0	29 mEq/L maximum

Notes: 1. Folic acid plus tryptophan in protein provide about 800 μg equivalents of folate.
2. The osmolarity of human milk is about 300 mOsm/L. Prepared synthetic milk should not exceed 400 mOsm/L.

tion in a diet in which new food products and foods formulated from highly refined or purified ingredients have replaced more traditional foods, the FDA requires "nutritional labeling" on all food products which make nutritional claims or to which nutrients have been added (Table 1-5). In using nutritional labeling, the following observations are offered for guidance.

1. Individual foods are not nutritionally complete. Adequate nutrition is assured by grouping foods according to patterns of nutrient distribution, then assuring nutritional adequacy by using a wide variety of foods with complementary patterns of nutrients.
2. Except for food replacement and therapeutic purposes, it is neither necessary nor advantageous to make any food nutritionally balanced or complete.
3. In looking at new products that displace more traditional foods in the diet, it is more appropriate that the

TABLE 1-5. Nutritional Labeling

Nutritional Label

Name of Food
Manufacturer or Distributor
Serving Size (ounces) or number of servings per package/package weight

Nutritional Information per Serving

Required	**Percent of RDA**
Calories	Protein
Protein (g)	Vitamin A
Carbohydrate (g)	Vitamin C
Fat (g)	Thiamin
	Riboflavin
	Niacin
	Calcium
	Iron
Optional	
Polyunsaturated fat (g)	Vitamin D
Saturated fat (g)	Vitamin E
Cholesterol mg/serving	Vitamin B_6
Cholesterol mg/100 g	Folacin
Sodium mg/serving	Vitamin B_{12}
Sodium mg/100 g	Phosphorus
	Iodine
	Magnesium
	Zinc
	Copper
	Biotin
	Pantothenic Acid

new product have the nutrient composition of the food it displaces than that it meet a standard derived from the RDA.

4. For new products that are primarily energy sources and are unrelated to traditional foods, the nutrient density expressed a percent of RDA/1000 kcal is probably a reasonable measure of the nutritional value.
5. There is no nutritional advantage to nutrient intakes greater than the RDA. If the diet as a whole meets the RDA test for nutritional adequacy, there is no reason for eliminating so-called "junk foods" or "empty calories," that is, foods in which the nutrient density is low. No foods in themselves are either "healthy" or "unhealthy." The dietary intake must be considered as a whole. It is only when "empty calories" displace food with needed nutrients from the diet that there should be any cause for concern.

RDA labeling is expressed in increments of 2% for values up to 10%, in 5% increments from 10 to 50%, and in 10% increments above 50%. Claims prohibited by the FDA are as follows:

1. That a food is a significant source of a nutrient, unless a serving contains at least 10% of the RDA.
2. That one food is a better source of a nutrient than another, unless it contains at least 10% more of the RDA than the other food.
3. That a lack of optimal nutritive quality of a food, because of the soil on which that food was grown, is or may be responsible for an inadequacy or deficiency in the daily diet.
4. That storage, transportation, processing, or cooking of a food is or may be responsible for an inadequacy or deficiency in the daily diet.
5. That a natural vitamin is superior to an added or synthetic vitamin.
6. That a food contains certain nutrients when such substances are of no known need or significant value in human nutrition. This prohibition is aimed at rutin, other bioflavonoids, para-aminobenzoic acid, inositol, and similar substances. These items have been promoted in the past as having nutritional properties. They have not been proven to be essential in human nutrition, and therefore, FDA would prefer them not to be mixed with other vitamins or minerals or mentioned on a label. They may be sold separately if no nutritional, dietary, or therapeutic claim is stated or implied. This last prohibited claim has been challenged in the courts, which have held that the FDA does not have the authority to enforce this prohibition.

REFERENCE

Committee on Dietary Allowances, Food and Nutrition Board, National Research Council: Recommended Dietary Allowances. 9th Revised Ed. Washington, DC, National Academy of Sciences, 1980.

Chapter 2

Water and Electrolytes As Nutrients

WATER

Water constitutes one half to three quarters of total body weight and is the medium in which most of the biochemical processes of the body take place. Excesses or deficits in water of more than 5% of the optimal value produce measurable effects and large deficits may lead to death.[1] The usual turnover rate for water ranges from 15% in infants to 6% in adults (Table 2-1). There are several homeostatic mechanisms for the maintenance of total water and for water/electrolyte balance.[2,3]

An estimate of water needs may be made from knowledge of obligatory water losses and sweat losses. For adults, per day, these include the following:

1. Urinary loss. At maximal concentration of 1400 mOsm/kg, ranges are from 200 to 900 ml, depending on solute load (urea, sodium, potassium, chloride).
2. Stool loss. About 100 ml.
3. Insensible loss from lungs and nonsweating skin. This is about 1300 ml, and is proportional to the metabolic rate.
4. Sweat losses. Highly variable, from 1 L for sedentary workers in a temperate climate to more than 10 L for workers in a hot, dry environment.

Under the most favorable conditions for water conservation (diet low in excretable solutes, little physical activity, no sweating), water loss is about 1.5 L per day. The usual need is about 2.8 L.

For infants, the picture is somewhat changed. The maximum urinary concentration is about 700 mOsm/kg, and since the

TABLE 2-1. Average Daily Water Turnover of An Adult Weighing 70 kg[4]

	Water Intake (g)			Water Output (g)	
	Obligatory	Facultative		Obligatory	Facultative
Drink	650	1000	Urine	700	1000
Food	750		Skin	500	
Oxidative	350		Lungs	400	
			Feces	150	
Subtotal	1750	1000	Subtotal	1750	1000
Total	2750		Total	2750	

TABLE 2-2. Daily Water Requirements in Milliliters per Kilogram of Body Weight at Various Ages Under Normal Conditions[5,6]

Age	Average Body Weight kg	Estimated Water Requirement ml/kg
3 days	3.0	80-100*
10 days	3.2	125-150*
3 months	5.4	140-160
6 months	7.3	130-155
9 months	8.6	125-145
1 year	9.5	120-135
2 years	11.8	115-125
4 years	16.2	100-110
6 years	20.0	90-100
10 years	28.7	70-85
14 years	45.0	50-60
18 years	54.0	40-50
Adults	70.0	21-43

In adults, the daily water, electrolyte, and calorie requirements can be calculated with sufficient accuracy from the body weight. In spite of the greater accuracy of values derived from body surface area, this method offers no advantage since the actual requirements are also subject to other factors like age, sex, the functional state of the heart, kidneys and lungs, fever, disease, nutritional status, and calorie consumption. In newborn as well as older children, however, the requirements should be calculated from the body surface area or the daily calorie turnover (Tables 2-3 or 2-4).

* Average value for breast-fed infants.

surface/weight ratio is larger, there is more insensible moisture loss on a weight basis. Stool loss is about 50 ml. For a 7 kg infant, the minimal need is about 700 ml; the actual need is about 1000 ml. Daily water requirements at various ages under normal conditions are listed in Table 2-2.

Another way to estimate water need is to base it on caloric intake. Values of 1 ml/kcal for adults and 1.5 ml/kcal for infants is generally adequate with the usual mixed diet.

TABLE 2-3. Daily Water Requirements per Square Meter of Body Surface Area[6]

Minimum requirement	870 ml/m^2
Average requirement	1500 ml/m^2
Maximum tolerance	2730 ml/m^2

TABLE 2-4. Average Daily Water Turnover per 100 kcal[7]

Water intake	80-110 ml/100 kcal
Urine	50-70 ml/100 kcal
Insensible water loss (see also Table 2-5)	40-60 ml/100 kcal
Water of oxidation (see also Table 2-6)	10-20 ml/100 kcal

Additional quantities are needed for high-protein diets, especially in infants, because of high urea excretion. Other conditions requiring increased water are coma, fever, vomiting, diarrhea, polyuria, and use of diuretics. Other methods of calculating water requirements are shown in Tables 2-3, 2-4, and 2-5.

Water Intoxication

This condition is rare, occurring mainly in patients overloaded with intravenous fluids, particularly if renal function is impaired, and occasionally, in pregnant patients given posterior pituitary extract to induce labor and then overloaded with fluid, either intravenously or orally. The symptoms are headache, nausea, lack of coordination, and hypertension.

Water Depletion

Water depletion usually occurs as a result of prolonged sweating or during starvation

TABLE 2-5. Average Daily Insensible Water Loss at Different Ages[7]

Age	ml/m^2	ml/100 kcal
0-3 years	1150	59
3-8 years	950	49
8-16 years	700	45
Adults	550	40

At body temperatures above normal, the insensible water loss increases by about 13% for each degree Centigrade (7% for each degree Farenheit). In resting infants under 12 months, the pulmonary water loss amounts to about 1 g/kg body weight per hour.[5]

With normal bodily activity, 25% of the total heat loss of the body is accounted for by evaporation of water (insensible water loss).[8]

TABLE 2-6. Water of Oxidation[7]

Metabolic Breakdown Of	Gives Rise To
100 g fat	107 ml water of oxidation
100 g protein	41 ml water of oxidation
100 g carbohydrate	55 ml water of oxidation
100 g nonfatty tissue	15 ml water of oxidation

That the proteins of nonfatty tissue are not fully oxidized is shown by the presence of a nonoxidized carbon atom in the urea excreted in the urine. The breakdown of nonfatty tissue not only gives rise to water of oxidation but also releases the intracellular water (73 ml/100 g). Fatty tissue contains practically no water.[9] See also Table 2-7.

TABLE 2-7. Water Arising from Metabolic Breakdown of Body Tissue

Metabolic Breakdown Of	Gives Rise To	
500 g fatty tissue	535 ml water of oxidation	—
500 g nonfatty tissue	75 ml water of oxidation	365 ml intracellular water
1000 g fatty and nonfatty tissue together	610 ml water of oxidation	365 ml intracellular water
		Total: 975 ml water

The breakdown of 1 kg of the body's own tissue, assuming it is made up of equal parts of fatty and nonfatty tissue, thus gives rise to about 1 L of endogenous, practically sodium-free water. It is important that this should be allowed for in patients with a limited caloric consumption whose water excretion is low (e.g., after operations), since otherwise, they may easily become waterlogged. A patient given only electrolytes and 5% glucose solution after an uncomplicated abdominal operation should therefore lose 100 to 400 g of weight per day.[9]

when proteins are being broken down and when there is no access to water. The body will normally prevent water depletion through the thirst reflex, if water is available. Symptoms are thirst, fatigue, vertigo, oliguria, and fever, followed by delirium, coma, and death.

A special case is heat exhaustion, which is caused by depletion of both water and electrolytes. When a person does unaccustomed work in a hot climate, both water and salt are lost. If the work is continued over a period of time, the salt content of the sweat decreases and stabilizes at a low value as the body becomes acclimated, in about 14 days. Early in this acclimatization period, both water and salt are needed, but the need for salt steadily decreases until the supply in the usual diet is enough to meet the need.

In addition to the water needs, heavy work in a hot environment may lead to heat hyperpyrexia (heat stroke) and heat syncope (fainting) due to a failure of temperature homeostasis. Upset of the water and/or electrolyte balance due to large water intake without adequate salt may produce heat cramps, usually toward the end of the work day. Cramps are merely painful, but heat stroke has a mortality of about 20%.

REFERENCES—Water

1. Adolph, E.F., et al.: Physiology of Man in the Desert. NY, Interscience, 1947.
2. Buskirk, E.R., and Mendez, J.: Fed. Proc., *26:*1760, 1967.
3. Gamble, J.L.: Harvey Lect., *42:*247, 1946-47.
4. Wolf, A.V.: Thirst. Springfield, IL, Charles C Thomas, 1958.
5. Bland, J.H.: Clinical Recognition and Management of Disturbances of Body Fluids. Philadelphia, W.B. Saunders, 1956.
6. Balbot, N.B., et al.: N. Engl. J. Med., *248:*1100, 1953 and *252:*896, 1955.
7. Elkinton, J.R., and Danowski, T.S.: The Body Fluids. Baltimore, Williams & Wilkins, 1955.
8. Newburgh, L.H., Wiley, F.H., and Lashmet, F.H.: J. Clin. Invest., *10:*703, 1931.
9. Moore, F.D.: Metabolic Care of the Surgical Patient. Philadelphia, W.B. Saunders, 1959.

ELECTROLYTES

Electrolytes are ionized substances dissolved in body water, which contribute to osmotic pressure inside and outside the body cells. Three major compartments can be identified as follows:

1. Intracellular fluid: within the cells, characterized by a sodium:potassium ratio of about 1:16 mEq/L (Figure 2-1).

2. Plasma: characterized by a sodium: potassium ratio of about 33:1 mEq/L.

3. Interstitial fluid: differing from plasma in that it has a low protein content (Figure 2-2).

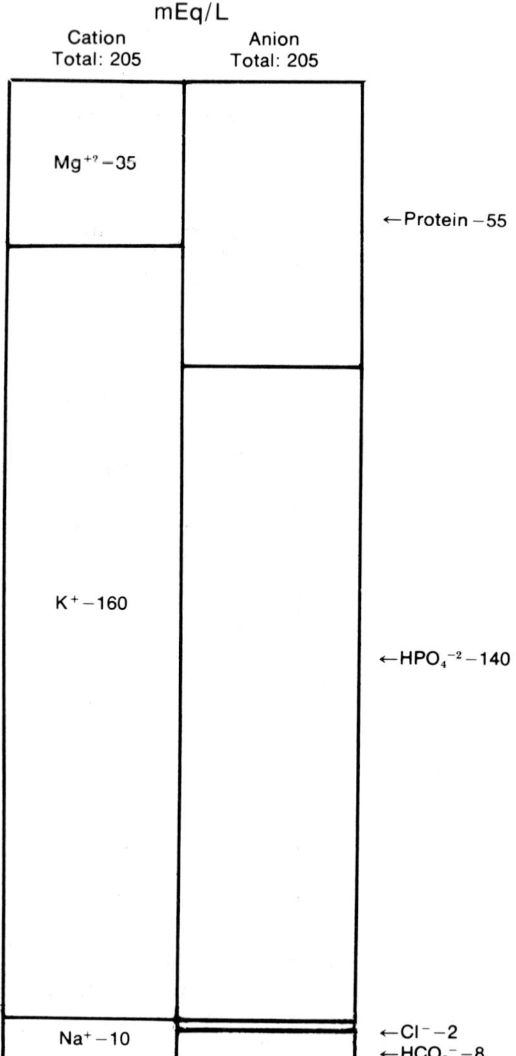

Figure 2-1. Electrolytes in Intracellular Fluid

TABLE 2-8. Products for Water and Electrolyte Replacement

Product **Manufacturer**	Lytren Mead Johnson	Pedialyte Ross
Electrolytes (mEq/L as diluted)		
sodium	25	30
potassium	25	20
calcium	4	4
magnesium	4	4
chloride	30	30
sulfate	4	0
phosphate	5	0
citrate	32	0
lactate	4	28
Dextrose (g/L)	74	50
Kcal per fluidounce	9	6

The intracellular fluid has about 205 mEq/L each of anions and cations, whereas plasma and interstitial fluid contain about 154 mEq/L. When living membranes are involved, the osmolarity of the solutions within and without the cells is not as important as their tonicity. Isotonicity refers to the situation in which cells surrounded by a given medium neither gain nor lose water. Tonicity of body cells is maintained by changes in permeability of the semipermeable membrane and by active transport of various ions across the membrane. These processes which maintain cell tonicity are not well understood. Disturbances in electrolyte balance, however, cause physiologic problems because of the upset of osmotic relationships in addition to the specific pharmacologic effects due to alterations in concentrations and concentration ratios.

Water and Electrolyte Replacement

When food and liquid intake is discontinued or markedly reduced, such as post-operatively, or there is risk of dehydration, as in diarrhea in infants or young children, oral replacement of water and electrolytes should be considered. The products listed in Table 2-8 are balanced in terms of electrolyte concentrations in water. They should

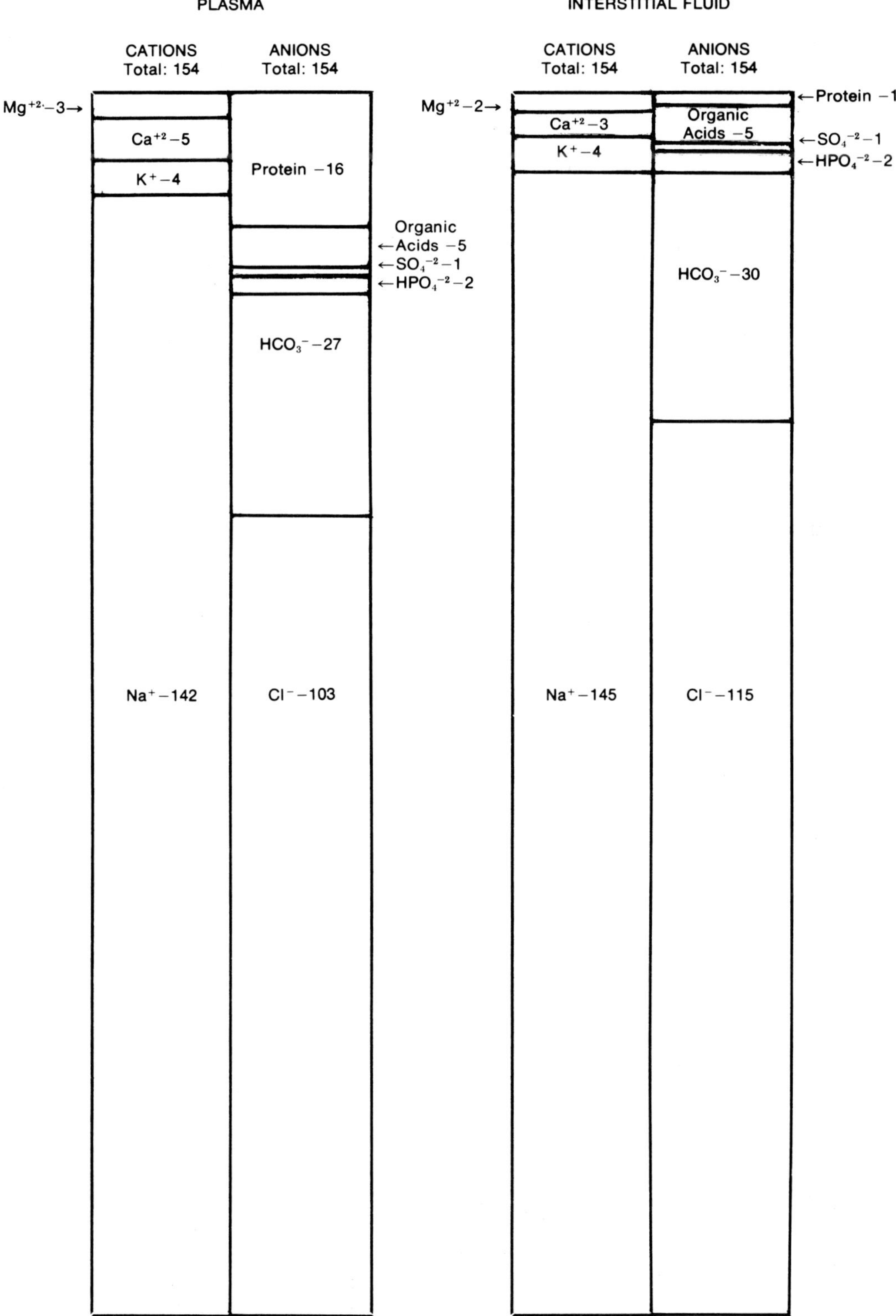

Figure 2-2. Normal Electrolyte Concentrations (mEq/L)

not be given with other electrolyte-containing liquids such as milk or juices. They may be used as an adjunct to parenteral administration of water and electrolytes, but should not be used instead of the parenteral route in cases of severe electrolyte loss such as found in severe continuing diarrhea, severe vomiting, or intestinal obstruction. Their correct use requires medical supervision even though the products are available without prescription, because of their classification as nutritional supplements. The dose of supplement must be reduced when other sources of electrolytes, such as food, become part of the diet. The volume to be administered as a replacement is calculated on the requirement of the patient for water. If this volume does not relieve thirst, plain water should be used to obtain this relief.

SODIUM

Sodium is usually available as sodium chloride (NaCl).

Safe and Adequate Intake

Maintenance of sodium balance in the adult body can be estimated from the following daily losses:[1]

1. Minimal fecal loss, 23 mg (1 mEq).
2. Minimal urinary loss, 23 mg (1 mEq).
3. Sodium in insensible loss, 46 to 92 mg (2 to 4 mEq).
4. Maximum sweat loss, 8 g (350 mEq).

Note: during acclimatization, loss drops from 7 g/L of sweat to 2 g/L.[2]

Active adults in temperate climates need about 1 g (43 mEq) per day of sodium, equivalent to 2.5 g of salt. A restricted salt diet would be below this level. Note that diets containing less than 300 mg of sodium per day are unpalatable.

The usual daily intake is 2.3 to 6.9 g (100 to 300 mEq)[3] equal to 6 to 18 g of salt.

In infants, sodium needs are based on growth as well as on losses. Needs are estimated to be met by intakes of 90 to 185 mg per day (4 to 8 mEq). Human milk contains 161 mg (7 mEq)/L. Infant formula contains 161 to 391 (7 to 17 mEq)/L. Cow's milk contains 483 mg (21 mEq)/L. The average intake ranges from about 300 mg (13 mEq) per day at 2 months to 1.4 g (60 mEq) per day at 12 months.[4]

In pregnancy, the rate of glomerular filtration increases by about 50%. In addition, the increasing progesterone level decreases sodium resorption. To compensate, if there is a functioning renin-angiotensin-aldosterone system, plasma aldosterone levels increase. In late pregnancy, the increased volume of extracellular fluid and the decreased ability to concentrate protein produces a decrease in osmotic pressure, which causes increase in renin and finally of aldosterone. These increases increase tubule resorption and conserve sodium.

The average *total* need for sodium during pregnancy has been estimated as 17.25 g (760 mEq), based on an average weight gain of 11 kg, 70% of which is water. This translates to about 69 mg (3 mEq) per day over nonpregnant needs. This is easily supplied by diet.

If sodium is restricted during pregnancy, the sodium conservation mechanisms may become exhausted. Osmoregulation will be

TABLE 2-9. Products for Sodium Chloride Replacement

	Sodium Chloride		
	Brand	Manufacturer	Strength
Tablets	Generic	Various	0.65, 1.0, 2.25 g/tablet
Tablets—enteric coated	Generic	Lilly	1 g/tablet
Tablets—slow release	Slo-Salt	Mission	600 mg/tablet

sacrificed in order to maintain volume. The resulting hyponatremia is deleterious to mother and fetus.[5]

Distribution

Sodium is the chief cation in the extracellular fluid. It participates in osmoregulation and water balance.

Excretion

The homeostatic mechanism of the renin-angiotensin-aldosterone system causes prompt excretion of excessive intakes and conservation during periods of low intake.

Laboratory Values

The normal laboratory values for plasma are 130 to 150 mEq/L (310 to 345 mg/dl).

Deficiency Symptoms

1. Dehydration
2. Nausea, anorexia
3. Fatigue
4. Muscle cramps

Toxicity

1. Some adult humans live normal lives with intakes of 40 g of salt per day (700 mEq). Nevertheless, feeding high salt levels in infancy to animals, especially those genetically selected for salt sensitivity, produced hypertension, and there is evidence that chronic high-level salt intake is one of the factors associated with hypertension in humans, although there is no causal relationship.[6]

2. Since there is no known benefit of large sodium intakes, a low-salt intake is recommended beginning early in life and continuing, in the hope of providing some protection for the 15% of the population who will later develop hypertension.

3. Sodium should be used cautiously in
   a. congestive heart failure
   b. circulatory insufficiency
   c. kidney dysfunction
   d. hypoproteinemia

Uses in Therapy

Prophylaxis of dehydration and heat cramps: 0.5 to 1 g/250 ml of water, 5 to 10 times a day. Products for sodium chloride replacement are listed in Table 2-9.

REFERENCES—Sodium

1. Dole, V.P., et al.: J. Clin. Invest., *29:*1189, 1952.
2. Lee, D.H.K.: Terrestrial Animals in Dry Heat: Man in the Desert, *In* Handbook of Physiology, Sect. 4, D.B. Dill, sect. ed. Baltimore, Williams & Wilkins, 1964.
3. Dahl, L.K.: Am. J. Clin. Nutr., *25:*231, 1972.
4. Committee on Nutrition, American Academy of Pediatrics: Pediatrics, *53:*115, 1974.
5. Pike, R.L., and Smiciklas, H.A.: Int. J. Gynecol. Obstet., *10:*1, 1972.
6. Kirkendall, W.M., et al.: *In* International Symposium on Renin-Angiotensin-Aldosterone-Sodium in Hypertension, J. Genest and E. Koiw, eds. New York, Springer-Verlag, 1972, pp. 360-73. ex Recommended Dietary Allowances, 9th Ed. Washington, DC, National Academy of Sciences, 1980, p. 172.

POTASSIUM

Potassium is widely available in fruits and vegetables. It is available as a drug in the form of potassium chloride and potassium gluconate.

Safe and Adequate Intake[1]

The usual adult intake is 1950 to 5900 mg (50 to 150 mEq) per day. Although homeostasis for potassium is not as good as for sodium, equilibrium can be maintained on as little as 1 g per day. Because of the availability of potassium in both plants and animals, a normal diet which is calorically adequate will provide a surplus of potassium for the normal, healthy person.

In infants, potassium is needed for the expansion of intracellular fluid due to growth. This amounts to about 2.73 g (70 mEq)/kg of lean body mass.[2] Considering this plus all body losses, the minimal requirement is about 90 mg (2.3 mEq) per day. Human milk contains 500 mg (13 mEq)/L; cow's milk, 1365 mg (35 mEq)/L. Thus, a surplus of potassium is available in the diet.

Absorption

Absorption is efficient (90%) in the jejunum and ileum when the concentration is above 200 to 300 mg (5 to 6 mEq)/ml of intestinal contents. In humans, absorption is not influenced by the presence of sodium or the direction of water movement.[3]

Distribution

Potassium is the principal intracellular cation. The average 70-kg man contains about 140 g (3500 mEq) of potassium, of which only 2.6 g (65 mEq) is in the extracellular fluid. Muscle accounts for 120 g (3000 mEq); liver, 8 g (200 mEq); and red cells, 10 g (235 mEq).

Excretion

About 90% of the daily loss appears in the urine. Smaller amounts (200 to 400 mg, 5 to 10 mEq) appear in the sweat. Sweat losses of potassium in the tropics can be significant before acclimatization and may approach the sweat loss of sodium.

Potassium filtered in the renal tubules is almost completely resorbed in the proximal portion of the convoluted tubules. In the distal portion, it is re-excreted under the influence of aldosterone in exchange for sodium. Thus, a low-sodium diet enhances potassium conservation, whereas a high-sodium diet promotes potassium excretion.[4]

Deficiency

Because normal mixed diet provides an excess of potassium, deficiency is associated with excessive renal losses or substantial extrarenal loss rather than with inadequate intake.

SYMPTOMS

1. Lethargy
2. Irritability
3. Decrease in deep tendon reflex
4. Tetany
5. Paresthesia
6. Muscle weakness
7. Paralytic ileus
8. Abnormal electrocardiogram (ectopic beats)
   a. depression of ST segment
   b. prolongation of QRS interval
   c. U-waves
9. Increased sensitivity of myocardium to digitalis alkaloids

Note: Deficiency of potassium is usually accompanied by deficiency of chloride.

POPULATIONS AT RISK

1. Anorexic, comatose, and alcoholic patients:[5] obligatory losses coupled with low intake.
2. Excessive gastrointestinal losses[3]
   a. vomiting
   b. laxative abuse
   c. prolonged nasogastric suction
   d. fistula
   e. diarrhea, especially in children
3. Excessive renal loss
   a. diuretics
   b. diabetic ketoacidosis
   c. renal tubular acidosis (This is accompanied by hyperchloremia. Treatment with potassium salts other than the chloride is required.)
   d. metabolic alkalosis
   e. excessive adrenal corticosteroids
   f. hyperaldosteronism
   g. surgery accompanied by nitrogen loss
   h. some uremic patients
   i. consumption of more than 100 g per day of licorice
4. Redistribution of serum potassium due to alkalosis or insulin administration.

Toxicity

1. Hyperkalemia is defined as plasma levels above 4 mEq/L. This is unlikely in normal patients ingesting less than 18 g per day.
2. Single doses of 40 mg (1 mEq)/kg elevate serum potassium by about 1 mEq/L. Doses of 80 to 100 mg (2 to 2.5 mEq)/kg may produce plasma levels of 6 to 8 mEq/L.[4]
3. Ingestion of concentrated preparations of potassium salts causes irritation of the gastrointestional tract and may cause tissue destruction.

TABLE 2-10. Chemical Sources of Potassium

Name	Formula	Mol. Wt.	mg/mEq	mEq/mg
Potassium acetate	$C_2H_3KO_2$	98.14	98.14	0.010190
Potassium bicarbonate	$KHCO_3$	100.12	100.12	0.009988
Potassium carbonate, anhydrous	K_2CO_3	138.21	69.16	0.014471
Potassium chloride	KCl	74.55	74.55	0.013414
Potassium citrate	$C_6H_5K_3O_7H_2O$	324.41	108.14	0.009248
Potassium gluconate	$C_6H_{11}KO_7$	234.25	234.25	0.004269

SYMPTOMS

1. Severe muscle weakness
2. Muscle pain
3. Abnormal electrocardiogram
   a. prolongation of PR interval
   b. prolongation of QRS interval
   c. peaking of T-waves
4. Cardiac arrest

TREATMENT

1. 10 to 25% dextrose containing 0.5 U of insulin/g of dextrose given intravenously at 300 to 500 mg per hour.
2. Sodium form of cation exchange resins may be given orally and by retention enema. Ammonium form may also be used, except in patients with cirrhosis.
3. Dialysis (peritoneal dialysis and hemodialysis) may be indicated.

TABLE 2-10a. USP Official Preparations

Potassium Acetate Injection
Potassium Chloride Elixir
Potassium Chloride Injection
Potassium Chloride Oral Solution
Potassium Chloride for Oral Solution
Potassium Citrate and Citric Acid Oral Solution
Potassium Gluconate Elixir
Potassium Gluconate Tablets

TABLE 2-11. Potassium Products
(Nearly all are by prescription only)

Brand	Manufacturer	Strength
Potassium Chloride		
Oral Solution (Note: 1% = 2 mEq/15 ml)		
Generic	Various	5%, 10%, 20%
Cena-K	Century	10%, 20%
Klor-10%	Upsher-Smith	10%
Klor-Con	Upsher-Smith	20%
Rum-K	Fleming	15%
Elixir		
Kaochlor 10%	Adria	10%
Kaochlor S-F	Adria	10%
Kaon-CL-20%	Adria	20%
Kay Ciel	Berlex	10%
Kloride	Amfre-Grant	10%
Klorvess 10%	Dorsey	10%
Pan-Kloride	Panray	10%
Potasalan	Lannett	10%
Powders for Oral Solution (unit dose packet)		
Generic	Various	20 mEq
Kato	Syntex	20 mEq
Kay Ciel	Berlex	20 mEq
K-Lor	Abbott	15, 20 mEq
Klor-Con	Upsher-Smith	20 mEq
K-Lyte Cl	Mead Johnson	25 mEq (also in 30-dose cans)

TABLE 2-11. (continued)

Brand	Manufacturer	Strength
Tablets (enteric coated)		
Potassium Cl	Various	325 mg (4 mEq), 650 mg (8.7 mEq), 1000 mg (13.4 mEq)
Tablets (wax matrix)		
Kaon-CL	Adria	500 mg (6.7 mEq)
Slow-K	Ciba	600 mg (8 mEq)
Potassium Gluconate		
Tablets		
Generic	Various	486 mg (2 mEq)
Kao-Nor*	North American	595 mg (2.5 mEq)
Kaon	Adria	1.2 g (5 mEq)
Elixir		
Generic	Various	20 mEq/15 ml
Kaon	Adria	20 mEq/15 ml
Kao-Nor	North American	20 mEq/15 ml
Kaylixir	Lannett	20 mEq/15 ml
K-G	Geneva	20 mEq/15 ml

Mixed Potassium Salts

Brand	Manufacturer	Strength	Potassium Salts
Liquid			
Twin-K	Boots	20 mEq/15 ml	gluconate, citrate
Duo-K	Various	20 mEq/15 ml	gluconate, chloride
Kolyum	Pennwalt	20 mEq/15 ml	gluconate, chloride
Powder (unit dose packet)			
Kolyum	Pennwalt	20 mEq	gluconate, chloride
Powder, effervescent (unit dose packet)			
Klorvess	Dorsey	20 mEq	chloride, bicarbonate
Tablets			
Osto-K*	Parthenon	39 mg (1 mEq)	chloride, citrate, gluconate
Tablets, effervescent			
Kaochlor-Eff	Adria	20 mEq	chloride, citrate, bicarbonate
KEFF	Lemmon	20 mEq	chloride, carbonate, bicarbonate
Klorvess	Dorsey	20 mEq	chloride, bicarbonate
K-Lyte	Mead Johnson	25 mEq	chloride, bicarbonate
K-Lyte/Cl	Mead Johnson	25 mEq	chloride, bicarbonate
K-Lyte/Cl 50	Mead Johnson	50 mEq	chloride, bicarbonate
K-Lyte DS	Mead Johnson	50 mEq	bicarbonate, citrate
Potassium Citrate and Citric Acid Oral Solution (systemic alkalyzer)			
Polycitra K	Willen	2 mEq/ml	

* Available **WITHOUT** prescription.

TABLE 2-12. Dietary Instruction Sheet

Your high blood pressure is being treated with a diuretic. This drug increases the amount of salt or sodium that is washed out of your body. Diuretics may also cause a decrease in the body stores of another mineral called potassium. Most of the time, an adequate diet will prevent excess loss of potassium. In some cases, especially in older people or in patients taking a medicine called digitalis, it may be necessary to give extra potassium as a tablet or liquid. This may also be necessary in patients with kidney disease or when symptoms of weakness or muscle cramps occur.

The following lists may give you an idea of which foods to eat or stay away from in order to keep your potassium intake high and your salt or sodium intake low.

1. Foods high in potassium but also high in sodium or salt. These foods should be avoided if possible.

Tomato juice, canned	Peas, frozen
Clams, raw	Peas, canned
Sardines	Spinach, canned
Lima beans, frozen	Carrots, canned

2. Foods high in potassium and low in sodium. Extra amounts of these foods will prevent a potassium deficiency.

Fruits	*Vegetables*
Apples, raw, whole	Asparagus, frozen
Apricots, canned	Beans, white, cooked
Apricots, dried	Beans, green, cooked
Avocado	Brussel sprouts, fresh or frozen
*Banana	Cabbage
Cantaloupe	Cauliflower, fresh or frozen
Dates, dried, pitted	Corn on the cob
Grapefruit	Lima beans, fresh, cooked
Nectarine, raw	Peas, fresh, cooked
Prunes, dried, cooked	Peppers, green, raw
*Raisins, dried, seeded	*Potato, baked
Watermelon	Potato, boiled, no skin
	Radish, red, raw
	Squash, frozen, cooked

Fruit Juices

Apple, fresh or canned	Grapefruit, canned
Prune, canned	* Orange, fresh, canned or frozen
Tomato, canned, low sodium	

* Especially helpful.

4. Acidosis, if present, should be corrected with sodium bicarbonate.
5. Cardiotoxicity of potassium may be antagonized with calcium ion, given intravenously.
6. As serum potassium drops, digitalis toxicity may appear in patients receiving digitalis.

Uses in Therapy

Therapy requires monitoring of serum potassium values (*Normal Serum Value:* 3.5 to 5.0 mEq/L) and individualization of dose. Because of the possibility of ulceration with solid dosage forms, liquids are preferred. Dosage is usually 20 mEq/day for prevention of depletion; 40 to 100 mEq/day for treatment of depletion. Potassium is also used for treatment of digitalis intoxication. Chemical sources of potassium are listed in Tables 2-10 and 2-10a; potassium products are shown in Table 2-11.

CONTRAINDICATIONS

1. Severe renal impairment (oliguria, anuria, or azotemia).
2. Untreated Addison's disease (failure of adrenal corticosteroid production).
3. Patients taking potassium-sparing diuretics (triameterene, spironolactone).

WARNINGS

1. Patients with renal impairment who are given potassium, especially intravenously, may develop hyperkalemia with no symptoms except cardiac arrest.
2. Gastrointestinal stenosis, ulcerative lesions, and death have been produced by potassium chloride tablets. Incidence of lesions is about 40 to 50/100,000 patient years for enteric coated tablets, about 1/100,000 patient years for slow-release wax matrix tablets. The wax matrix tablets are not enteric coated and may produce bleeding in the upper gastrointestinal tract.
3. Hypokalemia with metabolic acidosis

requires an alkalizing salt such as bicarbonate, citrate, acetate, or gluconate.
4. Patients receiving aldosterone antagonists (which impair potassium excretion) should be treated with extreme care.

PRECAUTIONS

1. Note that acute alkalosis reduces serum potassium and acute acidosis may bring serum values into the normal range even if there is a total body deficit.
2. Frequent monitoring of serum level and electrocardiogram is suggested.
3. Watch for atrioventricular (AV) disturbance when therapy is for digitalis intoxication.

PATIENT EDUCATION

A sample of instructions to patients for whom extra dietary potassium is recommended because of treatment with diuretics causing potassium loss is shown in Table 2-12.

REFERENCES—Potassium

1. Schultze, R.G., and Nissenson, A.R.: Potassium: Physiology and Pathophysiology, *In* Clinical Disorders of Fluid and Electrolyte Metabolism, 3rd Ed. M.H. Maxwell and C.R. Kleeman, eds. New York, McGraw-Hill, 1980.
2. Forbes, G.B.: Pediatrics, *29:*477, 1962.
3. Soffer, A. (ed.): Potassium Therapy: A Seminar. Springfield, IL, Charles C Thomas, 1968.
4. Schwartz, W.B.: N. Engl. J. Med., *253:*601, 1955.
5. Shaw, S., and Lieber, C.S.: Nutrition and Alcoholism, *In* Modern Nutrition in Health and Disease, 6th Ed. R.S. Goodhart and M.E. Shils, eds. Philadelphia, Lea & Febiger, 1980.

CHLORIDE

Chloride is usually available as sodium chloride.

Safe and Adequate Intake

Since the major source of chloride is salt, chloride intake parallels that of sodium. The daily turnover is 3 to 9 g.

Human milk contains about 390 mg (11 mEq)/L. This gives a sodium-plus-potassium:chloride milliequivalents ratio of close to 2. Good acid-base balance in infants is maintained on ratios of 1.5 to 2.0.[1] Dietary sources of chloride are shown in Table 2-13.

Deficiency

Deficiency of chloride alone is rare. It may be produced when hydrochloric acid is removed from the stomach by prolonged gastric aspiration or severe vomiting.

SYMPTOMS

1. Loss of weight
2. Poor water retention
3. Poor digestion
4. Achlorhydria
5. Convulsions
6. Retardation of growth (children)
7. Hypochloremic metabolic alkalosis[2]

POPULATIONS AT RISK

1. Loss of gastric juice in severe vomiting.
2. Lack of intake on salt-restricted diets.

REFERENCES—Chloride

1. Committee on Nutrition, American Academy of Pediatrics: Pediatrics, *57:*278, 1976.
2. Kassirer, J.P., et al.: Am. J. Med., *38:*172, 1965.

TABLE 2-13. Dietary Sources of Chloride*

Food	mg/100 g	Food	mg/100 g
Bacon	1250	Flounder	151
Bread, white	621	Flour, whole wheat	177
Cabbage	108	Kale	122
Celery	137	Milk	106
Corn meal	146	Olives	1877
Dates	283	Oysters	628
Eggs	120	Turkey	123
Figs, dried	105	Watercress	109

* Chloride generally parallels both sodium and potassium in foods.

MAGNESIUM

Magnesium is the fourth most abundant cation in the human body. It is available commercially as various salts. The sulfate is used as a source of magnesium ion for intravenous therapy. The gluconate and a protein complex are used in tablets for prophylaxis of magnesium deficiency. The citrate and sulfate are used as laxatives. The carbonate, hydroxide, oxide, and trisilicate are used as antacids. Magnesium salts of pharmacologically active anions, such as the ascorbate, nicotinate, para-aminobenzoate, and salicylate, are not significant sources of magnesium ion.

Recommended Dietary Allowance

1. Magnesium content of the average American diet is about 120 mg/1000 kcal.
2. Estimates of requirements based on balance studies range from 200 mg per day (3.0 mg/kg per day) up to 700/mg per day.[1,2]

After examining the evidence, the RDA was set at 350 mg per day for adult males and 300 mg per day for adult females.

Little information is available about requirements during pregnancy and lactation. An additional allowance of 150 mg per day (total = 450 mg) is recommended.

Human milk contains about 40 mg/L, infant formulas about 50 mg/L, cow's milk about 120 mg/L. These concentrations are adequate for growth and health of all infants, even those with low birth weights. The RDA was set at 50 mg per day for young infants and 70 mg per day for older infants.

Allowances for children and adolescents are estimates, but are intended to provide for increased magnesium needs due to bone growth.

Absorption

Magnesium is probably actively absorbed in the ileum. Absorption from rectal enemas shows, however, that absorption can occur in the colon. At normal dietary intakes of 250 to 300 mg (21 to 25 mEq), about 44% is absorbed. The fraction absorbed decreases with dose.[3] Calcium competes with magnesium for a common absorptive pathway.[4] Fecal magnesium falls if dietary calcium is reduced.

Distribution

The adult body contains 20 to 28 g (approximately 2000 mEq). Only about half of this is freely exchangeable. About 55% is present in bone, combined with calcium and phosphorus. About 27% is present in the musculature. The rest is found in soft tissues and body fluids, especially the intracellular fluids. In plasma, 55% is free, 13% is complexed, and 32% is protein-bound. Parathormone controls serum levels of magnesium (similarly to calcium).

Excretion[3]

The kidney is able to excrete 40 to 60 mEq per day. Nevertheless, the kidney is highly efficient in conserving magnesium. If magnesium is restricted in the diet, in a few days, urinary excretion falls to less than 12 mg (1 mEq) per day. Renal clearance of magnesium is increased by aldosterone (similarly to potassium). Resorption of magnesium in the kidney varies inversely with resorption of calcium.

Pharmacology

A. Magnesium is a cofactor for all enzymes involved in phosphate transfer reactions (phosphokinase) that utilize adenosine triphosphate (ATP) and the other nucleotide phosphates as substrates. Magnesium is involved in the following:
   1. Phosphorylation of glucose in anaerobic metabolism.
   2. Oxidative decarboxylation of glucose as cofactor for thiamin pyrophosphate (citric acid cycle).
   3. Cofactor in alkaline phosphatase activity.
   4. Cofactor in cyclic AMP reactions.
   5. Cofactor in protein synthesis
      a. ribosomal aggregation.

TABLE 2-14. Dietary Sources of Magnesium

Food	mg/100	Food	mg/100
Grains		*Fruit*	
Barley, pearled	37	Bananas	33
Bread, white or whole wheat	23	Blackberries	30
Corn meal	47	Cantaloupe	20
Graham crackers	51	Dates	58
Oat cereals (Cheerios)	112	Figs, dried	92
Oatmeal, dry	144	Raisins, dried	35
Fish	20 to 35	*Nuts*	
Shellfish	22 to 45	Almonds	270
Shrimp, cooked	51	Brazil nuts	225
		Hazel nuts	184
		Peanuts	206
		Walnuts	131
Meat		*Vegetables*	5 to 25
Bacon, fried	25	Lima beans, frozen	48
Beef	15 to 29	Parsnips	33
Chicken	23 to 30	Spinach	59
Lamb	17 to 30	Swiss chard, raw	65
Pork	18 to 32		
Turkey	28		
Veal	15 to 20		
		Miscellaneous	
		Chocolate	131
		Salt, table	260 to 310
		Molasses	
		light	46
		medium	81
		blackstrap	258
		Peanut butter	360

b. binding of messenger RNA to 70-S ribosomes.
c. synthesis and degradation of DNA.

B. Magnesium is involved in neuromuscular transmission and activity, but little is known about the movement of magnesium across membranes. It may act either synergistically or antagonistically with calcium, thus producing a complex interaction.

Deficiency

Deficiency of magnesium is extremely rare because the ion is efficiently absorbed and highly conserved. Deficiency is defined as serum levels below 0.45 mEq/L (0.55 mg/dl). Dietary sources of magnesium are shown in Table 2-14; magnesium products are listed in Table 2-15.

SYMPTOMS

1. Neuromuscular disturbances[5]
   a. tetany
   b. convulsions
   c. ataxia
   d. tremors
2. Behavior disturbances[3]
   a. depression
   b. irritability
   c. psychosis
3. Cardiac disturbances
   a. characterized by hypocalcemia or hypokalemia

POPULATIONS AT RISK

1. Genetic renal magnesium-wasting syndrome.[6]
2. Conditions decreasing magnesium absorption[3,6,7]
   a. malabsorption syndrome

TABLE 2-15. Magnesium Products*

	Brand	Manufacturer	Strength
Magnesium Gluconate			
Tablets			
	Generic	Various	30 mg, 500 mg
	Almora	O'Neal, Jones & Feldman	500 mg
	GYN	Amfre-Grant	500 mg
	Pangyn	Panray	500 mg
Magnesium-Protein Complex			
Tablets			
	Mg-Plus	Miller	60 mg
Magnesium Sulfate Injection	Generic	Various	9.86, 24.65, 49.30 mg/ml (10%, 25%, 50% $MgSO_4 \cdot 7H_2O$) (0.81, 2.03, 4.06 mEq/ml)

* Only those products used as a source of magnesium ion for maintenance of serum magnesium levels are listed.

b. steatorrhea
c. kwashiorkor

3. Conditions increasing magnesium elimination[7]
   a. diuretics
   b. alcohol[3]

Toxicity

Hypermagnesemia is rare except in renal failure. It is defined as serum levels above 2.5 mEq/L (3.0 mg/dl).

SYMPTOMS

1. Loss of patellar (knee jerk) reflex (used to monitor therapy).
2. Depression of deep tendon reflexes (flaccid paralysis) (plasma level: 4 to 10 mEq/L).
3. Depression of respiration (due to profound CNS-depression), leading to death. It may occur when intravenous magnesium is given in the treatment of eclampsia. The respiratory rate must be monitored and should be at least 16 per minute (plasma level: 10 mEq/L).
4. Heart block leading to death (plasma level: 12 mEq/L).

Toxicity due to oral doses is rare because ingestion of large amounts of magnesium ion causes an osmotic diarrhea.

TREATMENT

Toxicity is treated by intravenous administration of 10 to 20 ml of 10% calcium gluconate. Intravenous administration of furosemide or ethacrynic acid plus continuous and adequate hydration increases urinary excretion of magnesium.

In extreme cases, peritoneal dialysis or hemodialysis may be required.

Uses in Therapy

Magnesium Sulfate Injection, USP, is the sole agent used.

1. As an anticonvulsant in the prevention and control of seizures in
   a. pre-eclampsia
   b. eclampsia
2. In control of convulsions in conditions associated with low plasma levels of magnesium, although generally, other agents should be tried first.
   a. epilepsy
   b. glomerulonephritis
   c. hypothyroidism
3. In hypertension, because it acts peripherally as a vasodilator.
4. To treat acute magnesium deficiency.
5. As an antidote to the intense muscle stimulation of barium poisoning, intravenously (1 to 2 g of $MgSO_4 \cdot 7H_2O$)

and as a gastric lavage with a 2 to 5% solution. (The sulfate ion precipitates any barium remaining in the gastrointestinal tract and causes laxation.)

The dose is usually administered intravenously because therapy should be controlled by monitoring serum levels. Intramuscular injection is also possible, but the onset of action is delayed by about one hour and necrosis occurs at the injection site. Nevertheless, because of the prolonged action, intramuscular injection is sometimes used as an adjunct to intravenous therapy.

The intravenous dose should have a concentration of not more than 200 mg $MgSO_4 \cdot 7H_2O$/ml (20%) and should not be administered at a rate greater than 150 mg of $MgSO_4 \cdot 7H_2O$/minute. For intramuscular use in adults, solutions of 25 and 50% $MgSO_4 \cdot 7H_2O$ have been used.

Several different regimens have been used for initiating therapy. One of these is 0.17 g of magnesium sulfate heptahydrate/kg. Of this, 4 g are given intravenously in 250 ml of 5% dextrose injection, the rest is given intramuscularly. Thereafter, additional dosing is based on blood levels and urinary excretion. Subsequent doses are usually designed to replace the amount lost by urinary excretion. Care should be taken not to exceed the urinary excretion capacity of 30 to 40 g/24 hours. In renal insufficiency, the maximum dose may be only 10 g/24 hours.

EXPERIMENTAL

Magnesium has been used as an experimental therapy in the following:

1. Uterine tetany associated with use of oxytocic agents.
2. Cerebral edema (as an osmotic agent).
3. Paroxysmal atrial tachycardia (only when everything else has failed and there is no evidence of damage to the myocardium).
4. Tetanus.

CAUTIONS

1. Calcium gluconate injection should be available as an antidote before the start of therapy.
2. Changes in calcium and phosphorus balance should be anticipated, including hypocalcemic tetany.
3. Magnesium ion is a central nervous system (CNS) depressant. Its effect is additive to other CNS depressants such as barbiturates, general anesthetics, and narcotics.
4. It depresses neuromuscular action. Its effect is additive to neuromuscular blocking agents.
5. Extreme caution should be used in magnesium therapy of patients who are receiving digitalis. Use of calcium ion as an antidote for overdosage of magnesium ion may cause changes in cardiac conduction, leading to conduction blockage.
6. Continuous intravenous infusion of magnesium into the maternal circulation for treatment of toxemia of pregnancy (especially for more than 24 hours before delivery) may cause hypermagnesemia in the newborn. Magnesium administration should be stopped about 2 hours before delivery, and the need for resuscitation of the neonate should be anticipated. These measures include intravenous calcium and assisted ventilation by endotracheal intubation or intermittent positive pressure ventilation.

REFERENCES—Magnesium

1. Seelig, M.S.: Am. J. Clin. Nutr., *14*:342, 1964.
2. Jones, J.E., Manalo, R., and Flink, E.B.: Am. J. Clin. Nutr., *20*:632, 1967.
3. Wacker, W.E.C., and Parisi, A.F.: N. Engl. J. Med., *278*:658, 1968.
4. Alcock, N., and MacIntyre, I.: Clin. Sci., *22*:185, 1968.
5. Wong, H.B., and Teh, Y.F.: Lancet, *2*:18, 1968.
6. Gitelman, H.J., and Welt, L.G.: Ann. Rev. Med., *20*:233, 1969.
7. Martin, H.E.: Ann. NY Acad. Sci., *162*:891, 1969.

CALCIUM

Calcium is found in milk, cheese, nuts, green leafy vegetables, and bones. It is available commercially as calcium caseinate, citrate, glubionate, gluconate, lactate, dibasic phosphate, sulfate, and precipitated carbonate.

Recommended Dietary Allowance

The views on calcium requirements in man are changing with new evidence. The following are considerations.

1. The calcium:phosphorus ratio. The range over which absorption is maximized and loss of calcium from bone is minimized appears to be wider in humans than in most animals. Acceptable Ca:P ratios vary from 2:1 to 1:2;[1] there is even some evidence that calcium absorption is not affected by this ratio.[2] In setting the RDA for both calcium and phosphorus, a ratio of 1:1 was maintained, even though the ratio in the average American diet is 1:1.5 to 1.6.[3]
2. Urinary calcium excretion, while varying widely among individuals, remains relatively constant for any given person. Fecal calcium excretion correlates with calcium intake.[4]
3. Average daily loss in sweat is about 15 mg.
4. If an adult accustomed to a dietary intake of calcium greatly in excess of needs has the intake suddenly reduced, the relative absorption remains low for a period of time, leading to a temporary condition of nonequilibrium.[5] Prolonged fasting reduces absorption efficiency.
5. Adults can maintain calcium balance on intakes of 200 to 400 mg per day, but there are no ill effects from intakes as high as 1500 mg per day. Intakes above 1500 mg per day do not prevent development of osteoporosis, nor are intakes below 300 mg per day associated with osteoporosis.[6]
6. Although the efficiency of absorption varies inversely with the dose, the amount retained increases with the dose.[7]
7. Calcium losses may be large when protein intake is high.[8]
8. Efficiency of calcium absorption decreases with advanced age.[9]

On examining all the evidence, the RDA was set at 800 mg for adults, with the recognition that people on diets involving a lower protein intake than the average American diet will be in calcium balance at much lower intakes.

In pregnancy, the fetal skeleton accumulates about 30 g of calcium in the third trimester.[10] Efficiency of calcium absorption increases and excretion decreases in pregnancy.[11] Even though calcium storage in pregnancy is not known to take place, the recommendation is an increase of 400 mg per day (for a total of 1200 mg) *throughout* pregnancy.

Human milk has an average calcium content of 300 mg/L. To meet the 250 mg/850 ml daily loss during lactation, an increase of 400 mg per day (a total of 1200 mg) is recommended to prevent maternal demineralization.[12]

An infant retains about two thirds of the calcium in human milk. In contrast, only about 25 to 30% of the 650 mg/L present in cow's milk is retained. The RDA is set at 60 mg/kg.

For ages 1 to 10, the RDA of 800 mg allows for growth and is about 4 times the adult allowance based on weight. During the period of rapid growth between 10 to 18 years of age, the RDA is 1200 mg per day.

Absorption

1. Calcium absorption is an active process, taking place primarily in the duodenum and proximal jejunum, with lesser absorption in the more distal portions of the small intestine.

2. Calcium absorption is never complete. It is dependent on:

   a. calcium in soluble ionized form (acid pH).
   b. presence of vitamin D.[13]
   c. adequate parathyroid hormone.

Calcium absorption is retarded by alkaline pH, precipitation or complexation of calcium by oxalates, phytates, sulfates, fatty acids, low serum calcitonin levels, and corticosteroids.

3. Calcium absorption may also be decreased by
   a. decreased gastrointestinal transit time (diarrhea).
   b. stress.
   c. immobilization.
   d. thyroid hormone.

4. Calcium absorption is increased by some antibiotics (penicillin, neomycin, chloramphenicol).

Distribution

After absorption, calcium enters the extracellular fluid and is rapidly deposited in the skeleton (which contains about 99% of the 1200 g of calcium in the standard male). Note, however, that calcium does not stimulate bone formation.

Normal serum calcium levels are 9 to 10.4 mg/dl (4.5 to 5.2 mEq/L). About 50% is ionized, about 45% is protein-bound, and about 5% is complexed with phosphate, citrate, or other anions.

Excretion

Excretion is primarily in the feces, representing unabsorbed calcium and secretion of bile and pancreatic juice.

Most of the calcium filtered in the glomeruli is reabsorbed in Henle's loop and the convoluted tubules. Urinary excretion is decreased by thiazide diuretics, parathyroid hormone, and vitamin D. Urinary excretion is proportional to plasma concentrations.

Pharmacology

Calcium functions in the following processes:

1. Blood coagulation.
2. Neuromuscular excitability.
3. Contraction of smooth, skeletal, and cardiac muscle.
4. Cellular adhesiveness.
5. Storage and release of neurotransmitters.
6. Storage and release of hormones.
7. Uptake and binding of amino acids.
8. Regulation of cyanocobalamin (B_{12}) absorption.
9. Regulation of gastrin secretion.
10. Respiration.
11. Conversion of thrombin to prothrombin.
12. Maintenance of osmotic balance.
13. Activation of enzyme systems.

Deficiency

Symptoms of calcium deficiency may be caused by the following:

1. Inadequate parathyroid hormone.
2. Inadequate vitamin D.
3. Insufficient availability of dietary calcium.
4. Chronic impairment of absorption.

SYMPTOMS

1. Osteoporosis (in adults).
2. Rickets or osteomalacia.
3. Poor development of teeth and bones.
4. Delayed coagulation.
5. Muscle tetany (low serum calcium).
6. Loss of intestinal tone and inflammation of the mucosa.
7. Hypertrophy of parathyroid glands.

POPULATIONS AT RISK

Persons with the following conditions generally require treatment for the underlying condition as well as calcium replenishment.

1. Hyperparathyroidism.
2. Achlorhydria.
3. Chronic diarrhea.
4. Vitamin D deficiency.
5. Steatorrhea.
6. Sprue.
7. Menopause.
8. Pancreatitis.
9. Renal failure.

Toxicity

1. Elevated serum levels of calcium affect the following:
   a. cognitive functions
   b. cardiac rhythmicity
   c. renal function (polyuria, nocturia, thirst)

d. gastrointestinal tract (nausea, vomiting, diarrhea, anorexia)
2. Deposition of calcium in soft tissue affects the function of
   a. kidneys (stones)
   b. blood vessels
   c. heart

Uses in Therapy

1. Treatment or prevention of calcium depletion: orally, 1 g Ca per day, in divided doses.
2. Hypocalcemic tetany is usually secondary to hypoparathyroidism, renal failure, and, in neonates, prematurity or maternal diabetes mellitus.
   Adults: intravenously, 4.5 to 16 mEq.
   Children: 0.5 to 0.7 mEq/kg, 3 to 4 times a day, intravenously.
   Neonates: 2.4 mg/kg per day in divided doses, intravenously.
   Continue therapy until tetany is controlled.
3. Administration with citrated blood.
   Adults: 1.35 mEq, intravenously, concomitantly with each 100 ml of blood.
   Neonates (blood exchange): intravenously, 0.45 mEq after every 100 ml of blood.
4. Antagonism of hyperkalemia.
   Adult: intravenously, 2.25 to 14 mEq with continuous EKG monitoring.
5. Cardiac arrest not responsive to isoproterenol or epinephrine: intravenously or by direct injection into the ventricular cavity.
   Adult: 3 to 6 mEq.
   Children and infants: 0.3 mEq/kg.
6. Poisoning with magnesium, oxalates, carbon tetrachloride, fluoride, phosphate (including radioactive phosphate), strontium, or radium: intravenously, 7 mEq initially, additional doses dependent on response.
7. Emergency elevation of serum calcium.
   Adults: intravenously, 7 to 14 mEq.
   Children: intravenously, 1 to 7 mEq.
   Infants: intravenously, less than 1 mEq.
   Repeat every 1 to 3 days, depending on patient response.

INTRAVENOUS ADMINISTRATION

The chloride, gluceptate, gluconate, or levulinate salt may be used for intravenous administration.

Rate: 0.7 to 1.5 mEq/min. Stop if patient complains of discomfort. Keep patient lying down for a short time after completion of therapy.

Scalp veins in children should not be used for intravenous administration of calcium.

If intravenous route is not possible, the gluceptate, gluconate, and levulinate may be given intramuscularly in the gluteal region, in volumes of less than 5 ml. Local reactions include burning sensation, necrosis, cellulitis, and soft tissue calcification. Oral administration or foods with high calcium content should replace parenteral therapy as soon as possible (Tables 2-16 and 2-17).

CAUTIONS

1. Intravenous administration should be through a small needle into a large vein to prevent extravasation. Too rapid injections may cause the following problems:
   a. vasodilation
   b. bradycardia
   c. cardiac arrhythmia
   d. fainting
   e. cardiac arrest
2. Intracardial administration must be into the ventricular space. Injection into the myocardium may produce laceration of coronary arteries, cardiac tamponade, and intractable ventricular fibrillation.
3. Hypercalcemia may be more dangerous than hypocalcemia. Frequent determinations of serum levels should be made to adjust range to 9 to 10.4 mg/dl

TABLE 2-16. Dietary Sources of Calcium

Food	mg/100 g	Food	mg/100 g
Almonds	235	Collards	180
Anchovies	168	Cornbread	110
Brazil nuts	186	Dandelion greens	140
Bread, whole wheat	254	Herring, canned	147
Buttermilk	121	Ice cream	123
Bok Choy	148	Ice milk	156
Chocolate milk	228	Kale	134
Cheese, blue	315	Milk, cow's	118
brick	730	Milk, goat's	129
Camembert	105	Molasses, light	165
cheddar	750	blackstrap	684
cottage	94	Mustard greens	104
parmesan	1140	Salmon, canned	150 to 250
Swiss	925	Sardines, canned	303
American	697	Syrup, sorghum	172
Pasteurized process cheese food	570	maple	104
Pasteurized process cheese spread	565	Soybean curd (tofu)	128
		Turnip greens	174
		Yogurt	117

TABLE 2-17. Calcium Products

Note: Calcium carbonate products promoted as antacids can also be used as sources of calcium.

Brand	Manufacturer	Strength	Calcium	
		g	mg	mEq
Precipitated Calcium Carbonate, USP				
$CaCO_3$, 40.04% Ca, 19.98 mEq/g, 1 mEq = 50.05 mg				
Tablets, USP				
Generic	Various	0.65	260	
Os-Cal 500	Marion	1.25	500	
Tablets, chewable, USP				
Alka-2	Miles	0.50	200	
Amitone	Norcliff Thayer	0.35	140	
Calcilac	Schein	0.42	168	
Calglycine	Rugby	0.42	168	
El-Da-Mint	Elder	0.35	140	
Equilet	Mission	0.50	200	
Mallamint	Mallard	0.42	168	
P.H.	Scrip	0.42	168	
Spentacid	Spencer-Mead	0.42	168	
Titracid	Trimen	0.42	168	
Titralac	Riker	0.42	168	
Trialka	Commerce	0.33	132	
Tums	Norcliff Thayer	0.42	168	
Suspension, oral				
Titralac	Riker	1.0/5 ml	410	
Calcium Chloride, USP				
$CaCl_2 \cdot 2H_2O$, 27.26% Ca, 13.60 mEq/g, 1 mEq = 73.5 mg				
Injection, USP*				
Generic	Various	50/L	13.63/ml	0.68
Generic	Various	100/L	27.26/ml	1.36

TABLE 2-17. (continued)

Brand	Manufacturer	Strength g	Calcium mg	Calcium mEq
Calcium Glubionate				
$C_{18}H_{32}CaO_{19} \cdot H_2O$, 6.56% Ca, 3.276 mEq/g, 1 mEq = 305.3 mg				
Oral solution				
Neo-Calglucon Syrup	Dorsey	1.8/5 ml	23/ml	
Calcium Gluceptate, USP				
$C_{14}H_{26}CaO_{16}$, 8.17% Ca, 4.078 mEq/g, 1 mEq = 245.2 mg				
Injection, USP*				
Generic	Various	220/L	18.04/ml	0.9/ml
Calcium Gluconate, USP				
$C_{12}H_{22}CaO_{14}$, 9.31% Ca, 4.647 mEq/g, 1 mEq = 215.2 mg				
Injection, USP*				
Generic	Various	100/L	9.32/ml	0.465**/ml
Kalcinate	Kay	100/L	9.32/ml	0.465**/ml
Tablets, USP				
Generic	Various	0.5, 0.65, 1.00	45, 58.5, 90	
Calcium Lactate, USP				
$C_6H_{10}CaO_6 \cdot 5H_2O$, 13.00% Ca, 6.487 mEq/g, 1 mEq = 154.2 mg				
Tablets, USP				
Generic	Various	0.325, 0.65	42.3, 84.5	0.84, 1.69
Dibasic Calcium Phosphate, USP				
$CaHPO_4 \cdot 2H_2O$, 23.29% Ca, 11.62 mEq/g, 1 mEq = 86.05 mg				
Tablets, USP				
Various	Generic	0.5	116.45	
Calcium Protein Complex, Tablets				
Ca-Plus	Miller	—	280	

* By prescription only.
** Contains small amounts of other calcium salts.

(4.5 to 5.2 mEq/L). Slightly lower values are preferred by some clinicians.

4. Dibasic calcium phosphate should not be used for hypocalcemia-hyperphosphatemia of hypoparathyroidism.
5. Some clinicians prefer to use calcium carbonate in the treatment of renal failure because it removes phosphate from the intestine and lowers serum phosphate levels, thus partially correcting the metabolic acidosis of chronic renal failure.
6. Calcium chloride is an acidifier and produces diuresis. It is the most irritating of the calcium salts. It should be used cautiously in the presence of
   a. cor pulmonale.
   b. respiratory acidosis.
   c. renal disease.
   d. respiratory failure.
7. Calcium salts are contraindicated in ventricular fibrillation.
8. Calcium inotropic and toxic effects are synergistic with those of cardiac glycosides.

Interference with Laboratory Tests

Intravenous calcium can produce false low results for magnesium in urine and plasma when determination is made by the Titan yellow method.

Drug Interactions

Tetracyline antibiotics are inactivated through the formation of a calcium complex.

REFERENCES—Calcium

1. Life Sciences Research Office: Evaluation of the Health Aspects of Phosphates as Food Ingredients. SCOGS-32. Bethesda, MD, Federation of American Societies for Experimental Biology, 1975, 37 pp. ex Recommended Dietary Allowances, 9th Ed., Washington, DC, National Academy of Sciences, 1980, p. 132.
2. McBean, L.D., and Speckmann, E.: Am. J. Clin. Nutr., *27:*603, 1974.
3. Page, L., and Friend, B.: BioScience, *28:*192, 1978.
4. Alvioli, L.V.: Calcium and Phosphorus, *In* Modern Nutrition in Health and Disease, 6th Ed. R.S. Goodhart and M.E. Shils, eds. Philadelphia, Lea & Febiger, 1980.
5. Wilkinson, R.: Absorption of Calcium, Phosphorus and Magnesium, *In* Calcium, Phosphate and Magnesium Metabolism, B.E.C. Nordin, ed. Edinburgh, Churchill Livingstone, 1976.
6. Garn, S.M., Rohmann, C.G., and Wagner, B.: Fed. Proc., *26:*1729, 1967.
7. Coulston, A., and Lutwak, L.: Fed. Proc., *31:*721, 1972, Abstr. 2845.
8. Johnson, N.E., Alcantara, E.N., and Linkswiler, H.: J. Nutr., *100:*1425, 1970.
9. Bullamore, J.R., et al.: Lancet, *2:*535, 1970.
10. Pitkin, R.M.: Am. J. Obstet. Gynecol., *121:*724, 1975.
11. Duggin, G.G., et al.: Lancet, *2:*926, 1974.
12. Goldsmith, N.F., and Johnson, J.O.: J. Bone Joint Surg., *A57:*657, 1975.
13. Neer, R.M.: Nature, *229:*255, 1971.

PHOSPHORUS

Phosphorus is widely available in foods. Therapeutically, dibasic calcium phosphate is used orally.

Recommended Dietary Allowance

The average daily intake of phosphorus is estimated as 800 to 1500 μg. The primary source is milk. Other sources are poultry, fish, and meat. Soft drinks containing phosphoric acid may be an important source for some people.[1]

The relatively greater availability of phosphorus as compared with calcium may produce a Ca:P dietary ratio lower than that thought necessary to maintain the skeleton. Diets with low Ca:P ratios have led to bone loss in rats, dogs, and horses.

The RDA is set generally at the same level as calcium to give a Ca:P ratio of 1:1. For infants, it is set at 1.5:1.0.

Absorption

The efficiency of phosphate absorption depends on the source and on total intake. At usual levels, 60 to 70% is absorbed from food. At low intakes, up to 90% is absorbed.[2] Phosphate in organic phosphate esters is not available to humans because they lack intestinal phytase.

Effects of various substances on phosphorus absorption in humans is unknown.

Excretion

There is no known physiologic regulatory mechanism for the absorption of phosphorus. Control of plasma levels is primarily by renal excretion. Fecal phosphorus represents unabsorbed phosphorus and secreted phosphorus. On intakes of 100 to 1500 mg per day, secretion is about 3 mg/kg per day.[2]

Urinary excretion is generally cyclic and mediated by adrenal secretions (cortisone, cortisol).[3] It is related to physical activity, being lowest a few hours after awakening.

Phosphate excreted by the glomeruli is 85 to 95% reabsorbed in the tubules. Reabsorption is rate-limited, with a capacity of 4 to 8 mg per minute. Reabsorption is increased by cortisol at physiologic levels and by growth hormone. Reabsorption is decreased by digoxin, estrogen, parathyroid hormone, and pharmacologic levels of cortisone and its analogs,[4] as well as by elevations in serum calcium.

Distribution

The normal adult contains 11 to 14 g of phosphate per kg of lean body mass. About 85% is in the skeleton as inorganic ortho-

TABLE 2-18. Dietary Sources of Phosphorus*

Food	mg/100 g	Food	mg/100 g
Abalone, canned	128	Haddock	200
Almonds	504	Hake	142
Anchovies	210	Halibut	248
		Herring, canned	297
Barley	189	Ice cream	115
Bluefish	287		
Bran flakes (40%)	495	Lamb	147
Bread, cracked wheat	128	Lentils, cooked	119
whole wheat	271	Liver, fried	500
rye	147	Lobster, cooked	192
pumpernickle	229		
enriched	100	Mackerel, canned	274
Buckwheat, whole	282	Milk, cow's	93
		Milk, goat's	106
Chocolate, semisweet	284	Oysters	150
milk	231		
Cashew nuts	373	Peanuts, roasted	407
Caviar	355	Peanut butter	395
		Perch, ocean	226
Cheese, American	771	Pistachio nuts	604
blue	339	Popcorn	216
brick	455	Pork	200
Camembert	184	Potatoes, baked in skin	65
cheddar	478	peeled	53
cottage	152	from fresh french fried	111
parmesan	781	reconstituted	53
Swiss	563	frozen	50
Cheese food, pasteurized		Potato chips	178
process	754		
Cheese spread, pasteurized		Salmon, canned	288
process	875	Sausage, liver	245
		bologna	128
Chicken	120	frankfurters	133
Chile con carne, canned	126	pork sausage	200
Clams	137	Scallops	338
Cod	270	Shad	313
Cornbread	211	Shrimp	263
Crab	175	Soybeans	191
Crayfish	160	Soybean curd (tofu)	126
		Swordfish, broiled	275
Doughnuts, cake type	190		
Duck	175	Tuna, canned, drained solids	234
Frog legs	147	Turkey	251
		Wheat germ	1118
		Whitefish	270

* Phosphorus in nuts, legumes, and outer coats of cereal grains is present mostly as phytic acid, which combined with calcium, magnesium, or iron, is then eliminated without being absorbed.

phosphate. The phosphorus in soft tissues and cell membranes is mostly in the form of organic esters. Plasma phosphate is in equilibrium with skeletal and tissue inorganic phosphate and also with organic phosphate compounds resulting from cellular metabolism. Serum inorganic phosphate levels for normal adults are 2.5 to 4.4 mg/dl (mean = 3.5 mg/dl). Levels in children are 5 to 6 mg/dl. Variability in fasting serum levels is produced by dietary intake, stage of growth, age, time of day, hormonal levels, and renal function. About 88% of the plasma phosphate is ultrafilterable. About 8% of this is HPO_4^{-2}, most of the rest is $H_2PO_4^-$.

Pharmacology

1. Phosphorus is found in enzymes involved in lipid, protein, and carbohydrate metabolism and in energy transfer.
   a. carboxylase
   b. flavoprotein
   c. DPN
   d. TPN
   e. adenosine diphosphate
   f. adenosine triphosphate
   g. lecithin
   h. cephalin
2. It is needed for normal bone and tooth structure.

Deficiency

Phosphorus deficiency can occur during prolonged and excessive use of nonabsorbable antacids (aluminum and magnesium compounds).

SYMPTOMS

1. Weakness
2. Anorexia
3. Malaise
4. Skeletal aches
5. Hemolytic anemia[5]
6. Granulocyte dysfunction[6]
7. Erythrocyte glycolysis[7]

Symptoms are reversible when medication is discontinued and dietary phosphorus is adequate. Dietary sources of phosphorus are listed in Table 2-18.

Toxicity

1. Hyperphosphatemia is rare in the absence of severe chronic renal disease with filtration rates below 20 mg per minute.
2. Hyperphosphatemia may be produced in hypoparathyroidism and pseudohypoparathyroidism.

SYMPTOMS

No specific symptoms are associated with hyperphosphatemia. Symptoms are produced by the hypocalcemia which usually accompanies hyperphosphatemia.

REFERENCES—Phosphorus

1. Moon, W.-H., Malzer, J.L., and Clark, H.E.: J. Am. Diet. Assoc., *64:*386, 1974.
2. Nordin, B.E.C., and Smith, D.A.: Diagnostic Procedures in Disorders of Calcium Metabolism. Boston, Little, Brown and Co., 1965.
3. Goldsmith, R.S., et al.: J. Clin. Endocrinol. Metab., *25:*1649, 1965.
4. Massry, S.G., Friedler, R.M., and Coburn, J.W.: Arch. Intern. Med., *131:*828, 1973.
5. Craddock, P.R., et al.: N. Engl. J. Med., *290:*1403, 1974.
6. Jacob, H.S., and Amsden, T.: N. Engl. J. Med., *285:*1446, 1971.
7. Sheldon, G.F.: J. Trauma, *13:*971, 1973.

Chapter 3

Energy (Caloric) Requirements

In the utilization of foods, meeting the need for energy takes precedence over all other needs. Unless caloric intake from carbohydrates and fats is adequate, dietary protein will be diverted from use in maintenance and growth in order to become an energy source. At low caloric intakes, therefore, the problem of inadequate dietary protein which usually accompanies a starvation diet is exacerbated.

There is no RDA for energy because of the high variability in energy requirements. Even within a homogeneous group of normal people, the difference between the highest and lowest requirement is a factor of two.[1]

The dominant variable in energy requirements is the amount of physical activity, with greater exertion and longer exertion times requiring more energy (Table 3-1). Another variable is body mass, since exertion frequently involves moving the body mass through a distance. A third variable is the individual basal metabolism (Table 3-2).

Basal metabolism is defined as the "resting metabolism" of a person in a normal life situation, while at rest, in a thermally neutral environment, and includes the specific dynamic action of meals. It is usually measured on awakening and represents an average minimal metabolism for the night, with no exercise and no exposure to cold. Specific dynamic action of meals refers to the amount of energy expended in digestion.

If body weight is maintained, the body composition changes with age by replacement of lean body mass with fat.[2] Since the resting metabolism of fat cells requires less energy than that of muscle cells, the basal metabolic rate at a given body weight must decrease with age, and therefore, the energy needs must decrease. In children, energy requirements reflect both their rate of growth and amount of activity. Recommended energy intake is shown in Table 3-3.

The need for energy is increased by environmental temperature in two ways. First, the energy cost of work increases slightly with a decrease in temperature, being about 5% higher below 15°C. In addition, there is about a 3% increase due to the weight of warmer clothing worn at lower temperatures. Second, at high temperatures (above 30°C), energy requirements increase about 0.5%/°C, primarily due to an increase in metabolic rate necessary to maintain the thermal balance of the body.[3,4]

In pregnancy, extra energy needs are associated with the building of tissue for the placenta and fetus, expressed as an increase in the resting metabolic rate, and the increased work load associated with moving

TABLE 3-1. Energy Expenditure[11]

Activity	Men (70 kg) kcal/minute	Women (58 kg) kcal/minute	kcal/kg/hour
Sleeping, reclining	1.0-1.2	0.9-1.1	—
Very light activity Seated and standing activities, painting, driving, typing, sewing, laboratory work, ironing	1.2-2.5	1.1-2.0	1.4
Light activity Walking on level at 2.5 to 3 mph, ironing (pressing), garage mechanic, electrician, carpenter, restaurant work, cannery work, washing clothes, golf, sailing, ping-pong, volley ball	2.5-4.9	2.0-3.9	2.7
Moderate activity Walking at 3.5 to 4 mph, plastering, weeding, stacking bales, scrubbing floors, bicycling, skiing, tennis, dancing	5.0-7.4	4.0-5.9	4.2
Heavy activity Uphill walking with a load, pick-and-shovel work, wood chopping, basketball, football, swimming	7.5-12.0	6.0-10.00	8.2

the increased weight. Although the energy required for the pregnancy itself may be calculated, the figure is only of academic interest since it does not take into account variations in physical activity and mean ambient temperature during pregnancy nor the growth needs of young mothers. A useful statement, however, is that energy in-

TABLE 3-2. Typical Basal Metabolic Rates at Age 25

	MEN		WOMEN	
Height cm	Weight kg	BMR kcal/day	Weight kg	BMR kcal/day
145			47.0	1140
150			51.5	1220
155	56.0	1400	52.5	1260
160	59.0	1470	54.0	1300
165	62.0	1530	59.5	1390
170	65.5	1600	63.5	1460
175	70.0	1690	67.0	1520
180	73.5	1760		
185	77.5	1830		
190	82.0	1910		

Calculated from data obtained from Altman, P.L., and Dittmer, D.S., eds.: Metabolism. Bethesda, MD, Federation of American Societies for Experimental Biology, 1968.

TABLE 3-3. Recommended Energy Intake[12]

Category	Age (years)	Weight kg (U.S. median)	Height cm (U.S. median)	Energy Needs Light Work	(kcal/day) Range Percentiles 10th	90th
Infants	0.0-0.5	6	60	kg × 115	95	145
	0.5-1.0	9	71	kg × 105	80	135
Children	1-3	13	90	1300	900	1800
	4-6	20	112	1700	1300	2300
	7-10	28	132	2400	1650	3300
Females	11-14	46	157	2200	1500	3000
	15-18	55	163	2100	1200	3000
	19-22	55	163	2100	1700	2500
	23-50	55	163	2000	1600	2400
	51-75	55	163	1800	1400	2200
	75+	55	163	1600	1200	2000
Pregnancy				+300		
Lactation				+500		
Males	11-14	45	156	2700	2000	3700
	15-18	66	176	2800	2100	3900
	19-22	70	177	2900	2500	3300
	23-50	70	178	2700	2300	3100
	51-75	70	178	2400	2000	2800
	75+	70	178	2050	1650	2450

take should not be reduced below 36 kcal/kg of pregnant body weight, since this value represents an optimum for protein utilization.[5]

Lactation increases energy requirements due to production of the milk and the energy content of the milk (0.72 kcal/ml). Lactation requires about 0.9 kcal/ml of milk produced or about 750 kcal/day to produce the average 850 ml/day during the first 3 months.[6] During pregnancy, the normal weight gain of 11 to 12.5 kg[7] represents an increase in body fat of 2 to 4 kg. This fat can provide about one third of the energy requirements for milk production during the first 3 months after parturition, or about 250 kcal per day. During lactation, therefore, only an extra 500 kcal per day, on the average, is necessary. Again, for young mothers, allowance must also be made for maternal growth needs.

Energy available from food can be roughly estimated from the following factors:[8,9,10]

Carbohydrates and sugars	4 kcal/g
Proteins	4 kcal/g
Fats	9 kcal/g
Alcohol (200 proof)	7 kcal/g (5.6 kcal/ml)

WEIGHT CHANGES

Caloric Equivalents[13]

Weight loss taking place in periods of negative energy balance is more complex than

TABLE 3-4. Conversion Table

kcal/kg to kcal/lb								
kcal/kg	'	kcal/lb	kcal/kg	'	kcal/lb	kcal/kg	'	kcal/lb
9100	'	4128	6500	'	2948	3400	'	1542
8000	'	3629	6000	'	2722	2596	'	1178
7043	'	3195	3610	'	1637	2160	'	980

simple loss of fat. A simplistic approach is to assume that the figure of 9100 kcal of animal fat shown by calorimetric experiments means a deficit of 9100 kcal would produce a 1 kg weight loss or that a 9100 kcal excess would produce a 1 kg weight gain. Data on human adipose tissue suggest a figure of 8000 kcal. "Obesity tissue," that actually lost or gained in weight change, suggests the figure of 6000 to 6500 kcal.

The fact is that weight loss is complicated. During the first few days on a reduction diet, the major loss is water. The actual values observed in human women cycled between deficient and excess diets showed figures of 2160 to 3510 kcal. Other studies show similar values for men. As dieting continues, however, the caloric value of weight change increases. In an experiment, the average values initially were 2596 kcal/kg, but between days 11 and 13 they were 7043 kcal/kg. Note also that as body weight de-

TABLE 3-5. Desirable Weights for Adults[15]

Reproduced from DOCUMENTA GEIGY Scientific Tables, 8th Ed.
With kind permission of CIBA-GEIGY Limited, Basle (Switzerland).

Weights of Insured Persons in the United States
Associated with the Lowest Mortality (Age 25 and over)

Height in Shoes 2.5 cm Heel cm	MEN Weight (in indoor clothing; for nude weight, deduct 2.2 to 3.2 kg) Small Frame Range kg		Medium Frame Range kg		Large Frame Range kg	
158	50.8	54.4	53.5	58.5	57.3	64.0
160	52.2	55.8	54.9	60.3	58.5	65.3
163	53.3	57.2	56.2	61.7	59.9	67.1
165	54.9	58.5	57.6	63.0	61.2	68.9
168	56.2	60.3	59.0	64.9	62.6	70.8
170	58.1	62.1	60.8	66.7	64.4	73.0
173	59.9	64.0	62.6	68.9	66.7	75.3
175	61.7	65.8	64.4	70.8	68.5	77.1
178	63.5	68.0	66.2	72.6	70.3	78.9
180	65.3	69.9	68.0	74.8	72.1	81.2
183	67.1	71.7	69.9	77.1	74.4	83.5
185	68.9	73.5	71.7	79.4	76.2	85.7
188	70.8	75.7	73.5	81.6	78.5	88.0
191	72.6	77.6	75.7	83.5	80.7	90.3
193	74.4	79.4	78.1	86.2	82.7	92.5
5 cm Heel	WOMEN Weight (in indoor clothing; for nude weight, deduct 0.9 to 1.8 kg)					
147	41.7	44.5	43.5	48.5	47.2	54.0
150	42.6	45.8	44.5	49.9	48.1	55.3
152	43.5	47.2	45.8	51.3	49.4	56.7
155	44.9	48.5	47.2	52.6	50.8	58.1
158	46.3	49.9	48.5	54.0	52.2	59.4
160	47.6	51.3	49.5	55.3	53.5	60.8
163	49.0	52.6	51.3	57.2	54.9	62.6
165	50.3	54.0	49.0	59.0	49.4	64.4
168	51.7	55.8	54.4	61.2	58.5	66.2
170	53.5	57.6	56.2	63.0	60.3	68.0
173	55.3	59.4	58.1	64.9	62.1	69.9
175	57.2	61.2	59.9	66.7	64.0	71.7
178	59.0	65.3	61.7	68.5	65.8	73.9
180	60.8	65.3	63.5	70.3	67.6	76.2
183	62.6	67.1	65.3	72.1	69.4	78.5

creases, the metabolic need for energy, which is a function of body mass, also decreases, so that at any caloric intake the body will come into energy equilibrium, thus average daily weight loss decreases with time at constant caloric intake. Table 3-4 shows the conversion from kcal/kg to kcal/lb.

On 10-day starvation (no food) diets, the average value was 3400 kcal/kg. In people who are starving, water loss is important, and protein as well as fat loss occurs.

In the same way, diets for weight gain show a rapid increase in the first few days due to water retention, then a slow tapering off of weight gain until the body is in equilibrium at the new increased weight level. Desirable weights for adults are shown in Table 3-5. Percentiles for weight and height from 0 to 18 years of age are available in the literature.[14]

Specific Dynamic Action[16]

Many weight-loss diets are planned in terms of specific dynamic action. This term refers to the percent of ingested energy that is required for the conversion of the food into a useable energy source. When single nutrients are ingested under laboratory conditions, the following are observed:

Substance	Specific Dynamic Action (calories used for digestion)
Proteins	12 to 30%
Carbohydrates	6 to 10%
Fats	2 to 6%

Results are highly variable between individuals and between experiments and are highly dependent on the exact conditions of measurement. Relative standard deviations of more than 40% have been observed.

The specific dynamic action of a meal, however, is *not* the sum of the specific dynamic action of the carbohydrates, fats, and proteins contained in the meal, but rather 25 to 50% less. The specific dynamic action of meals varies between the very narrow limits of 9% for meals high in carbohydrates to 17% for meals high in protein as extreme values for individuals. Since the specific dynamic actions of different diets differ at most by 8% (17% minus 9%) and this difference does not represent an appreciable change in the fraction of calories available, consideration of specific dynamic action has little or no value in constructing diets for weight reduction.

REFERENCES—Energy

1. Garrow, J.S.: Energy Balance and Obesity in Man, 2nd Ed. New York, Elsevier/North Holland Medical Press, 1978, ex Recommended Dietary Allowances, 9th Ed., Washington, DC, National Academy of Sciences, 1980, p. 29.
2. Forbes, G.B., and Reina, J.C.: Metabolism, *19:*653, 1970.
3. Johnson, R.E.: Fed. Proc., *22:*1439, 1963.
4. Consolazio, C.F., et al.: J. Nutr., *73:*126, 1961.
5. Oldham, H., and Sheft, B.B.: J. Am. Diet. Assoc., *27:*847, 1951.
6. Thomson, A.M., Hytten, F.E., and Billewicz, W.Z.: Br. J. Nutr., *24:*565, 1970.
7. Pitken, R.M., et al.: Obstet. Gynecol., *40:*773, 1972.
8. Merrill, A.L., and Watts, B.K.: Energy Value of Foods, Basis and Derivation. Agriculture Handbook No. 74, Human Nutrition Research Branch, Agricultural Research Service, U.S. Dept. of Agriculture. Washington, DC, U.S. Government Printing Office, 1973 (Stock No. 0100-02770).
9. Bernstein, L.M., et al.: Comparison of Various Methods for Determination of Metabolizable Energy Value of Mixed Diets in Humans (U.S. Army Medical Nutrition Lab. Rept. No. 168) Fitzsimons Army Hospital, Denver, CO, 1955, ex Recommended Dietary Allowances, 9th Ed. Washington, DC, National Academy of Sciences, 1980, p. 28.
10. Southgate, D.A.T., and Durnin, J.V.G.A.: Br. J. Nutr., *24:*517, 1970.
11. Durnin, J.V.G.A., and Passmore, R.: Energy, Work and Leisure. London, Heinemann Educational Books, 1967.
12. Committee on Dietary Allowances, Food and Nutrition Board, National Research Council: Recommended Dietary Allowances, 9th Ed. Washington, DC, National Academy of Sciences, 1980, p. 23.
13. Grande, F., and Keys, A.: Body Weight, Body Composition, and Calorie Status, *In* Modern Nutrition in Health and Disease. 6th Ed. R.S. Goodhart and M.E. Shils, eds. Philadelphia, Lea & Febiger, 1980.
14. Hamill, P.V.V., et al.: Am. J. Clin. Nutr., *32:*607, 1979.
15. Statistical Bulletin of the Metropolitan Life Insurance Company: *40:* (Nov.-Dec.) 1959, ex Scientific Tables, K. Diem and C. Lintner, eds. Ardsley, NY, Geigy Pharmaceuticals, 1970, p. 712.
16. Bradford, R.D., and Jourdan, M.H.: Lancet, *2:*640, 1973.

Chapter 4
Carbohydrates and Fiber

Carbohydrates and fiber are chemically related. The difference between them nutritionally is that simple sugars, starches, and some complex carbohydrates are converted into absorbable monosaccharides in the digestive tract, whereas in humans, fiber is not converted or only poorly converted to monosaccharides.

CARBOHYDRATES

Carbohydrates are divided into
1. Simple sugars
   a. monosaccharides
   b. disaccharides
2. Starches
   a. polysaccharides
3. Complex carbohydrates
   a. hemicellulose
   b. cellulose
   c. oligosaccharides
   d. gums
   e. fibrous matter

Carbohydrates can be made in the human body from some amino acids and the glycerol portion of fats. Since they can be synthesized in the body, there is no specific requirement for carbohydrates. Nevertheless, it is desirable to have some preformed carbohydrate to prevent ketosis (presence of ketone bodies from metabolism of fat and protein), excessive loss of body protein, and the accompanying load on the kidneys in the excretion of nitrogen-containing compounds. These require a concomitant loss of water and an accompanying loss of sodium, which may lead to dehydration and electrolyte imbalance. This undesirable metabolic response can be avoided by ingestion of 50 to 100 g/day of digestible carbohydrate; daily intake of 150 to 200 g will probably meet all requirements.[1]

It should be noted that in some reducing diets fat is replaced by carbohydrate. In some susceptible people, the relative increase in carbohydrate, especially if it is in the form of sugar, may produce high serum triglyceride levels, high enough to have a toxic effect. Diets high in simple sugars that are not removed promptly from the mouth have been implicated in dental caries. Since the proportion of carbohydrate to fat can vary enormously in diets of people in apparently good health, it seems sensible to replace reduced intake of fat with complex carbohydrate (starch, not sugar) to obtain the necessary calories.

Carbohydrate in the body is in the form of glucose, circulating in blood plasma, and glycogen, a storage form, in the liver. The total available energy from both these sources in normal humans is only about 1800 kcal from glycogen and about 16 kcal from glucose. All body tissues can derive energy from the metabolism either of fat or carbohydrate, except erythrocytes and the brain, which require glucose. Thus, some preformed carbohydrate is desirable in the diet, but no RDA can be set.

Because carbohydrates are so widely distributed, no list of dietary sources is given. Oral carbohydrate supplements are listed in Table 4-1.

Genetic Disorders[2]

Some people have genetic deficiencies in the metabolism of galactose, fructose, or glucose. The absence of insulin production, which prevents metabolism of glucose, is known as "juvenile diabetes" and will not be treated further here, as there is an extensive literature and ongoing research in this problem.

Fructosuria is common in many people after ingestion of foods containing large amounts of fructose or sucrose. Excretion of large amounts of fructose, however, is due to metabolic error. Essential fructosuria is an autosomal recessive, causing a deficiency in the production of fructokinase by the liver. It requires no treatment. Hereditary fructose intolerance is caused by a decrease in or the absence of activity of aldolase produced by the liver. In early infancy, the symptoms, in addition to fructosuria, are the following:

1. Anorexia
2. Vomiting
3. Failure to thrive
4. Retarded growth
5. Hepatomegaly
6. Aminoaciduria
7. Hypoglycemic convulsions
8. Splenomegaly
9. Ascites
10. Jaundice
11. Death

TABLE 4-1. Oral Carbohydrate Supplements

Brand	Manufacturer	Calories/ 100 ml
Liquids*		
Hycal Liquid	Beecham	295
Polycose Liquid	Ross	200
Sumacal	Organon	200
Powders		
Polycose Powder	Ross	376/100 g

* Liquids are usually hyperosmotic and may cause stomach upset at first. This may be avoided by initially diluting until iso-osmotic, then gradually increasing the concentration.

If the condition is mild, it may not be seen until later in life, with the only manifestations being hypoglycemia and an aversion to sweets.

Treatment is to restrict intake (complete elimination is not usually necessary) of fructose and sucrose (which is hydrolyzed to glucose and fructose). In the infant, administration of glucose to relieve the hypoglycemia and of electrolytes may be necessary. Foods high in sucrose or fructose should be avoided. These include most fruit, meats cured with sugar, peas, beans (including soy beans and soy milk formulas), sugar-containing breakfast cereals, honey, maple syrup, molasses, sugar syrups, and sweet chocolate.

Genetic deficiencies of two of the three enzymes involved in the major metabolic pathway for galactose have been identified. Galactokinase deficiency may be diagnosed on the basis of galactosuria and galactosemia and confirmed by erythrocyte galactokinase assay. If untreated, cataracts are produced. The treatment is elimination of galactose from the diet.

Classic galactosemia is caused by a deficiency of galactose-1-phosphate uridyl transferase. The incidence of this condition is about 1 in 60,000. The normal-at-birth infant shows symptoms only after galactose is introduced into the diet. The symptoms are as follows:

1. Anorexia
2. Vomiting
3. Diarrhea (occasionally)
4. Lethargy
5. Hypotonia
6. Jaundice
7. Hepatomegaly

8. Albuminuria
9. Failure to thrive
10. Mental retardation
11. Cataracts
12. Death

Since galactose is not an essential nutrient, treatment consists of simply removing galactose from the diet. The major source of dietary galactose is the disaccharide lactose. Milk and milk products, including whey protein which contains about 85% lactose, casein, and skim milk solids are to be avoided. Rigid exclusion of galactose is necessary during the early years, but small amounts of milk products are tolerated from about 6 years of age onward.

REFERENCES—Carbohydrates

1. Calloway, D.H.: Environ. Biol. Med., *1*:175, 1971.
2. Donnell, G.N.: Inborn Errors of Galactose and Fructose Metabolism, *In* Pediatric Nutrition Handbook, American Academy of Pediatrics, P.O. Box 1034, Evanston, IL 60204, 1980.

FIBER

Fiber is defined as nondigestible or poorly digestible carbohydrate and carbohydrate-like substances in the diet. It includes cellulose, lignin, hemicelluloses, pentosans, gums, and pectin. It should be clearly distinguished from "crude fiber," a value reported in food analysis which measures part of the cellulose and lignin in food. Ingested fiber aids in elimination by adding bulk and water retention to the feces.

Since 1900, the consumption of dietary fiber has decreased in industrialized countries. It has been hypothesized on the basis of statistical studies of selected populations, but not experimentally shown, that there is an inverse relationship between consumption of fiber and diverticulosis, cardiovascular disease, colonic cancer, and diabetes.[1–4]

Because of the possibility of reducing absorption of minerals by high intakes of fiber (particularly phytates in brans)[5] a marked

TABLE 4-2. Dietary Sources of "Crude Fiber"[6]

mg/100 g of Edible Portion					
FRUIT					
Apple, with skin	1.0	Currants, black	2.4	Peach	0.6
Apricot	0.6	Dates	2.3	Pear	1.4
Avocado	1.5	Figs, dried	5.6	Pineapple	0.4
Banana	0.5	Grapes	0.6	Plum	0.4
Blackberries	4.1	Grapefruit pulp	0.2	Quince, raw	1.7
Canteloupe	0.3	Loganberries	3.0	Raisins	0.9
Cherries	0.4	Nectarine	0.4	Raspberries	3.0
Cranberries	1.4	Olives	1.3	Strawberries	1.3
sauce	0.2	Orange	0.5	Tangerine	0.5
Currants	3.4			Watermelon	0.3
VEGETABLES					
Artichoke	2.4	Celery	0.6	Potato	0.5
Asparagus	0.7	Swiss chard	0.7	chips	1.6
Beans		Cucumber	0.6	Pumpkin	0.6
kidney	4.0	Eggplant	0.9	Radish	0.7
lima	1.8	Kale	1.3	Rhubarb	0.7
string	1.0	Beet greens	1.1	Rutabaga	1.1
Beets	0.8	Turnip greens	0.8	Sauerkraut	0.7
Broccoli	1.5	Lentils, dried	3.9	Soybeans,	
Brussel		Lettuce	0.5	cooked	1.4
sprouts	1.6	Corn	0.7	Spinach	0.6
Cabbage, raw		Parsnip	2.0	Squash	
red	1.0	Peas, green	2.0	(zucchini)	0.6
white	0.8	dried, split	1.2	Sweet potato	0.7
Carrot	1.0	Peas, podded	1.5	Tomato	0.5
Cauliflower	1.0	Peppers	1.4	Turnip	0.7

TABLE 4-2. (continued)

mg/100 g of Edible Portion					
NUTS					
Almonds	2.6	Coconut	4.0	Pecans	2.3
Brazil	3.1	Hazelnut	3.0	Pine	1.1
Cashew	1.4	Peanuts, roasted	2.7	Pistachio	1.9
Chestnut	1.1			Walnut	2.1

CEREALS			
Barley, pearled	0.6	Wheat germ, toasted	1.7
Bread		Flour	
white	0.2	buckwheat	2.6
whole wheat	1.6	farina	0.4
pumpernickel	1.1	corn	0.7
rye, American	0.4	light rye	0.4
Cornflakes	0.7	medium rye	1.0
Oats, puffed	1.1	whole wheat	2.3
Popcorn, plain	2.2	white wheat	0.3
Rice, cooked		soybean	2.4
polished	0.1		
brown	0.6		

increase in fiber intake is to be avoided for American diets. A moderate increase in consumption of vegetables, fruits, and whole-grain cereal products is recommended. Dietary sources of "crude fiber" are listed in Table 4-2.

For comparison with the values for "crude fiber" given in Table 4-2, the values

TABLE 4-3. Dietary Sources of Fiber

mg/100 g

Food	Serving		Food	Serving	
Bread					
Rye bread	4 slices	8.0	Graham crackers	14	10.5
Whole wheat bread	4 slices	9.6	Rye crackers	15	11.5
Cereal					
All-Bran	1½ cup	34.5	Grape Nuts	¾ cup	11.0
100% Bran	1½ cup	34.5	Grits, dry	½ cup	11.8
Bran Buds	1¼ cup	30.0	Rolled oats, dry	1 cup	9.0
Bulgur, dry	⅔ cup	11.2	Shredded wheat	4 bis	12.2
Fruit					
Apple	1 small	3.4	Peach, raw	1 med	2.3
sauce	½ cup	1.4	canned	½ cup	1.1
Banana	1 medium	1.8	Pear, raw	1 med	2.3
Cantaloupe	¾ cup	1.2	canned	½ cup	1.1
Cherries, raw	14	1.1	Plum, raw	2 small	1.8
Grapefruit	¼	1.3	Strawberries	½ cup	2.1
Grapes, raw	26	0.7	Tangerine	1 med	2.1
Orange	1 small	2.0			

TABLE 4-3. (continued)

		mg/100 g			
		Vegetables			
Kidney beans	1⅓ cup	4.8	Cucumber, 7 inch	½	1.5
Green beans	1 cup	2.4	Kale, cooked	½ cup	2.0
Beets, cooked	⅔ cup	2.1	Lentils, cooked	½ cup	4.0
Broccoli, cooked	1 cup	2.1	Lettuce	2 cups	1.6
Cabbage, raw	1⅓ cup	2.8	Parsnip, cooked	6 oz	4.9
cooked	¾ cup	2.2	Peas, cooked	1¾ cup	5.0
Cauliflower, raw	1 cup	1.8	Potato, cooked	¾ cup	3.5
cooked	½ cup	1.2	Rice, brown	1½ cup	1.7
Celery, raw	2½ stalks	3.0	white, cooked	1½ cup	0.6
cooked	½ cup	2.4	Spinach	4 leaf	3.6
Corn kernels	⅔ cup	4.2	Turnip, raw	1 cup	2.2

in Table 4-3 have been calculated from data given by J.E. Brody, *Jane Brody's Nutrition Book,* W.W. Norton, NY, 1981, pp. 146-7, and attributed to James W. Anderson, M.D., Professor of Medicine and Clinical Nutrition, University of Kentucky Medical Center, Lexington, KY. The values do not reflect all dietary fiber, but do include most of the pectins, gums, and mucilages as well as the "crude fiber." Each serving is about 100 g.

REFERENCES—Fiber

1. Burkitt, D.P., and Trowell, H.C.: Refined Carbohydrate Foods and Disease. New York, Academic Press, 1975.
2. Reilly, R.W., and Kirsner, J.B.: Fiber Deficiency and Colonic Disorders. New York, Plenum Publishing Corp., 1975.
3. Spiller, G.A., and Amen, R.J.: Fiber in Human Nutrition. New York, Plenum Publishing Corp., 1976.
4. Roth, H.P., and Mehlman, M.A., chmn.: Am. J. Clin. Nutr., *31:*S1-S291, 1978. (Symposium on role of dietary fiber in health.)
5. Reinhold, J.G., et al.: J. Nutr., *106:*493, 1976.
6. Watt, B.K., and Merrill, A.L.: Composition of Foods (Agriculture Handbook No. 8). Consumer and Food Economics Research Division, Agricultural Research Service, U.S. Dept. of Agriculture, Washington, DC, U.S. Government Printing Office, 1963.

Chapter 5

Fats, Fatty Acids, and Cholesterol

FATS AND FATTY ACIDS

All the cells of the body except the red blood cells can use fatty acids directly as a source of energy.[1] Cells of the nervous system can utilize ketone bodies only after adaptation to total starvation. Indeed, the body fat is mobile, part of it being converted to fatty acids and metabolized, while newly ingested fatty acids are resynthesized into fat and deposited. Note that any energy intake in excess of body need, irrespective of the dietary source (alcohol, protein, carbohydrate, or fat), is stored as adipose tissue.

Dietary fat acts as a carrier for the fat-soluble vitamins, and 15 to 25 g a day are needed for this purpose. Beyond this, there is no specific requirement for fat in the diet. It has been recommended by the Committee on Dietary Allowances[2] that fat not supply more than 35% of the calories in the diet, particularly if the daily intake is below 2000 kcal.

Most naturally occurring fat is triglyceride, that is, chemically formed from one molecule of glycerin and three molecules of fatty acid. (A fatty acid is composed of carbon atoms joined to each other to form a long straight chain, and also containing atoms of hydrogen and oxygen.) Derived from the triglycerides by chemical treatment to remove one or more of the fatty acid portions are the diglycerides and monoglycerides used as emulsifiers in foods.

The type of fatty acid present in fat is important for good nutrition and good health. Triglycerides are nearly tasteless, but they absorb and retain flavors. They generally enhance palatability of food. Because they delay gastric emptying time, they prevent premature feelings of hunger. (Most people are familiar with the experience of feeling hungry within 2 hours after eating meals that are very low in fat.) Most food fats, irrespective of vegetable or animal origin, are easily digested by healthy people.

Body fat is the major form of energy storage. It is derived from all dietary sources of energy: fat, carbohydrate, alcohol, and protein. The adipose tissue also cushions the body and its organs and serves as a heat insulator.

The primary essential fatty acid in man is linoleic acid (*cis* 9, *cis* 12-octadecadienoic acid), which can be converted into longer-chain fatty acids with three, four, or five double bonds. Linolenic acid (9, 12, 15-octadecatrienoic acid) is an essential acid in many animals, including one species of monkey,[3,4] but has an unclear role in humans.

Most vegetables and meats, and the vegetable oils, which are the major source of linoleic acid, also contain small amounts of linolenic acid. Since no specific symptoms due to linolenic acid deficiency have been reported in humans, it is assumed that either humans have no requirement for linolenic acid or that diets adequate in linoleic acid are also adequate in linolenic acid.

Animal studies showed the following deficiency symptoms:[5]

1. Scaling of epidermis over dorsa of feet and tail (rats).
2. Elevation of basal metabolism.
3. Lowered growth rate.
4. Increased water consumption with no increase in urinary output.
5. Disturbed ovulation.
6. Resorption of fetus.
7. Difficult labor.
8. Macroscopic testicular atrophy.

Fatty acid deficiency is not seen in the general population in the United States because general diet contains about 23 g of linoleic acid,[6] or about 6% of calories, as compared with a recommended[7] intake of 1 to 2% of calories for adults (1.2 to 2.4 g/1000 kcal) and 3% of calories for people on low-fat (less than 25% of calories) diets. For infants on infant formulas, the recommendation[8] is 3% of calories.

TABLE 5-1. Chief Dietary Sources of Unsaturated Fatty Acids*

Food	% Linoleic Acid	% Saturated Fatty Acid	%Oleic Acid
Oils and Fats			
Butter	2	46**	27
Corn	53	10	28
Cottonseed	50	25	21
Lard	10	38	46
Olive	7	11	76
Peanut	29	18	47
Safflower	72	8	15
Sesame	42	14	38
Soybean	52	15	20
Nuts			
Almonds	11	4	36
Brazil nuts	17	13	32
Filberts	10	3	34
Peanuts	14	11	21
Pecans	14	5	45
Pistachio	10	5	35
Walnut	40	4	10
Miscellaneous			
Chicken	5	7	9
Chick peas	2	0	2
Corn meal	2	0	1
Margarine, liquid oil	29	13	31
Margarine, hydrogenated oil	14	18	47
Peanut butter	14	9	25
Sesame seed	21	7	19
Sunflower seeds	30	6	9
Wheat germ	5	2	3

* Linoleic acid constitutes nearly all of the polyunsaturated fatty acid present. Oleic acid is mono-unsaturated.

** About 40% of this is in the form of short-chain fatty acids which are incorporated into human phospholipid.

TABLE 5-2. Oral Fat Supplements

Brand	Manufacturer	Fat, g	Calories
Lipomul Oral (corn oil)	Upjohn	30/45 ml 667/L	270/45 ml 6000/L
Microlipid (safflower oil)	Organon	500/L	4500/L
MCT*	Mead-Johnson		115/15 ml

* Medium-chain triglycerides (MCT) are C-8 and C-10 triglycerides from coconut oil. They have the following advantages: 1. more rapidly hydrolyzed than fat; 2. do not need to be emulsified by bile salts in order to be absorbed; 3. are not dependent upon formation of chylomicrons for transport in the lymph.

Infants fed formulas deficient in essential fatty acids showed drying and flaking of the skin (eczema) as the primary symptom.[9] Hospitalized patients, both infants and adults, fed exclusively by intravenous fluids not containing fats showed the following conditions:[10–12]

1. Dermatitis.
2. Impaired fat storage.
3. Alopecia (loss of hair, baldness).
4. Hyperkeratosis.

Since these risks are now known, care is taken to include adequate fatty acids in infant formula and in total parenteral nutrition (TPN).

The essential fatty acids, found in the body as phospholipids, have the following functions:

1. Maintain the integrity and function of cellular and subcellular membranes.
2. Regulate cholesterol metabolism.
3. Precursors of substances that have physiologic regulatory functions[13]
   a. prostaglandins.
   b. thromboxans.
   c. prostacyclins.
4. Required for some actions of pyridoxine (B_6) and pantothenic acid (B_5).
5. Required for infant growth and development.

It should be noted that requirements for vitamin E increase with increasing intake of essential fatty acids. The chief dietary sources of unsaturated fatty acids are shown in Table 5-1; oral supplements are listed in Table 5-2.

REFERENCES—Fats

1. Cahill, G.F., Jr., et al.: J. Clin. Invest., *45:*1751, 1966.
2. Committee on Dietary Allowances, Food and Nutrition Board, National Research Council: Recommended Dietary Allowances, 9th Ed. Washington, DC, National Academy of Sciences, 1980, p. 36.
3. Lampty, M.S., and Walker, B.L.: J. Nutr., *106:*86, 1976.
4. Fiennes, R.N.T.-W., Sinclair, A.J., and Crawford, M.A.: J. Med. Primatol., *2:*155, 1973.
5. Alfin-Slater, R.B., and Aftergood, L.: Physiol. Rev., *48:*758, 1968.
6. Rizek, R.L., Friend, B., and Page, L.: J. Am. Oil Chem. Soc., *51:*244, 1974.
7. Holman, R.T.: JAMA, *178:*930, 1961.
8. Committee on Nutrition, American Academy of Pediatrics: Pediatrics, *57:*278, 1976.
9. Wiese, H.F., Hansen, A.E., and Adam, D.J.D.: J. Nutr., *66:*345, 1958.
10. Collins, F.D., et al.: Nutr. Metab., *13:*150, 1971.
11. Paulsrud, J.R., et al.: Am. J. Clin. Nutr., *25:*897, 1972.
12. Richardson, T.J., and Sgoutas, D.: Am. J. Clin. Nutr., *28:*258, 1975.
13. Kadowitz, P.J., Joiner, P.D., and Lyman, A.L.: Ann. Rev. Pharmacol., *15:*285, 1975.

CHOLESTEROL

Cholesterol, a sterol, is present in all human cells. It is synthesized by humans, and has essential functions as a constituent of cell membranes and the myelin sheath of nerves and as a precursor of bile acids, steroid hormones, and vitamin D. It is not an essential part of the diet since the normal adult synthesizes enough to meet body needs (500 to 1000 mg per day.[1–4] The average amount of cholesterol in the American diet has remained relatively constant at about 500 mg per person per day since 1909.

The various facets of cholesterol metabolism, absorption, synthesis, transport, conversion to bile acids (about 33% of the daily production of cholesterol), and excretion are each regulated separately, so that measurement of plasma cholesterol, which involves equilibrium with less than 20% of the body pool, is not a precise indicator of cholesterol metabolism.[5,6]

Absorption

The sources and daily amount of cholesterol available for absorption in the duodenum and jejunum are:

food	500 to 750 mg
bile	750 to 1250 mg
intestinal mucosal secretion	small (large in rats)
intestinal synthesis	unknown

Cholesterol esters are hydrolized by pancreatic cholesterol esterase in the intestines to free cholesterol. The cholesterol from this and the other sources form micelles, containing bile acids, fatty acids (from hydrolysis of triglycerides), and other sterols. Absorption of cholesterol takes place only from these micelles, so that absorption is increased by the presence of dietary fat (the source of the fatty acids) and decreased by the presence of competing sterols (such as plant sitosterols). Cholesterol absorption is highly variable from person to person and from day to day, but on the average, about 50% of the dietary cholesterol is absorbed.[1,7]

Synthesis

Cholesterol absorbed from the intestine inhibits synthesis of cholesterol by the liver by its effect on the enzyme HMG-CoA reductase, which affects the rate-limiting step in cholesterol synthesis. Although about 90% of the cholesterol synthesized in humans is by the liver and intestine (note that intestinal synthesis is not inhibited by exogenous cholesterol), nearly all body cells except mature erythrocytes can synthesize cholesterol. The major source of the carbon atoms is acetate produced from the metabolism of protein, carbohydrate, and fat. The synthesis starts with condensation of the acetate with the enzyme acetyl CoA and involves about 20 steps and more than 25 enzymes before final conversion to cholesterol. Synthesis of cholesterol in the liver is increased by increased caloric intake and decreased by caloric restriction. Total body synthesis of cholesterol is decreased by bile acids, probably because of decreased synthesis by the intestine.

Degradation and Excretion

Quantitatively, the major pathway for removal of cholesterol (200 to 300 mg per day) from the body is by liver conversion to bile acids, cholic and chenodeoxycholic acids, which are conjugated with glycine or taurine to form bile salts. These are excreted in the bile along with free cholesterol, which passes through the biliary duct into the duodenum. About 98% of the bile acids are reabsorbed and returned to the liver through the portal circulation. In the liver, the bile acids are extracted and resecreted in the bile. This pool of 2000 to 3000 mg of bile acids then is recycled. The unabsorbed bile acids are degraded in the large intestine and excreted in the feces. The formation of bile acids is inhibited by their return to the liver and increased by food ingestion. Effects of specific food types on bile acid synthesis are unclear.

Quantitatively, a minor pathway for removal of cholesterol (40 mg per day) is the synthesis of steroid hormones. A small amount (1 mg per day) is excreted in urine and some (up to 50 mg per day) is excreted as sweat and sebaceous secretion or lost as hair or desquamated skin.

Transport

Cholesterol, insoluble in aqueous solutions, is transported in the plasma lipoproteins, which consist of a polar, membrane-like coating of phospholipid (lecithin), specific apoproteins, and free cholesterol, and a nonpolar core of lipids, including cholesterol esters and triglycerides. Ultracentrifugation and electrophoresis have fractionated plasma lipoprotein into chylomicrons, very low density lipoprotein

(VLDL), intermediate density lipoprotein (IDL), low density lipoprotein (LDL), and high density lipoprotein (HDL), arranged in increasing density and concentration of protein and phospholipid and decreasing concentration of triglycerides.

Chylomicrons and the VLDL formed in the intestinal mucosa are transported in the lymph and secreted through the thoracic duct into the blood. The liver also synthesizes some VLDL. Body tissues remove triglycerides from VLDL by the action of the enzyme lipoprotein lipase, leaving a particle that accumulates cholesterol in its core either by transfer of cholesterol esters from HDL or by esterification of free cholesterol on its surface by the action of the enzyme lecithin-cholesterol-transferase (LCAT). This particle can either be removed by the liver or transformed by unknown mechanisms to IDL and then to LDL.[8]

In man, about 15% (0.4 mg/ml) of plasma cholesterol is in the form of VLDL and about 65% (1.5 mg/ml) is LDL. About 75% of the cholesterol in LDL is esterified with long-chain fatty acids.[3] Tissue cells bind LDL from the plasma at specific receptor sites. The number of receptor sites on each type of tissue cell seems to be related to the cell's need for cholesterol. The daily uptake is estimated at 1500 mg. The esterified cholesterol is then hydrolyzed and the free cholesterol is utilized within the cell or incorporated in the cell membrane, and the excess is excreted. The excreted cholesterol is either recycled to the liver or taken up by HDL and transferred to VLDL. Cholesterol metabolism is diagrammed in Figure 5-1.

About 20% (0.45 mg/ml) of the plasma cholesterol is carried by HDL. Cholesterol accumulation in cells may be prevented by blockage by HDL of cell receptor sites for LDL. Although, in contrast to LDL, the concentration of HDL is relatively insensitive to diet, it is increased by physical activity, moderate alcohol ingestion, and estrogen (HDL concentrations are higher in women after puberty than in men).[9]

The optimal level of cholesterol in blood is in dispute. Some people believe that the lower the level, the less the risk of premature coronary heart disease, while others focus on the relative concentration of VLDL, LDL, and HDL.[10] Blood cholesterol is about 27% in the free form and 73% esterified. Blood cholesterol determinations generally report total cholesterol. No sharp definition of "normal" and "hyper" cholesterol levels is possible because of the many factors affecting blood cholesterol levels. These include the quantity of cholesterol absorbed, cholesterol biosynthesis, production of carrier lipoprotein, uptake of cholesterol by the liver and excretion as bile acids, uptake by cells, and individual variations in response to environmental conditions such as diet, weight gain or loss, exercise, and stress. In very severe hypercholesterolemia, genetics is much more important than environment.[11]

Despite the fact that in one study of men, all of whom were eating exactly the same "normal American diet," blood levels ranged from 190 to 282 mg/dl[12] and that the U.S. vital statistics[13] showed that for males between 45 and 54 years old, 49% had values above 240 mg/dl and 14% above 280 mg/dl, "normal" ranges of 160 to 250 mg/dl or 120 to 220 mg/dl are often cited.

Cholesterol levels change with age, being lowest at birth, rising during early childhood to peak values at between 10 and 12 years of age, falling during adolescence, then rising to at least age 69, with perhaps a slight decrease after that. Females have higher levels than males at birth, during the early years, and at ages between 60 and 80, and lower levels between 30 and 50. Levels are essentially the same in both sexes during late childhood, adolescence, early adulthood, and between 50 and 60 years of age.

The effect of dietary cholesterol (Table 5-3) on plasma cholesterol levels has been extensively examined. It is known that the effect on man is smaller and more variable than in animals fed high-cholesterol diets.

Some of the reports of the effects of di-

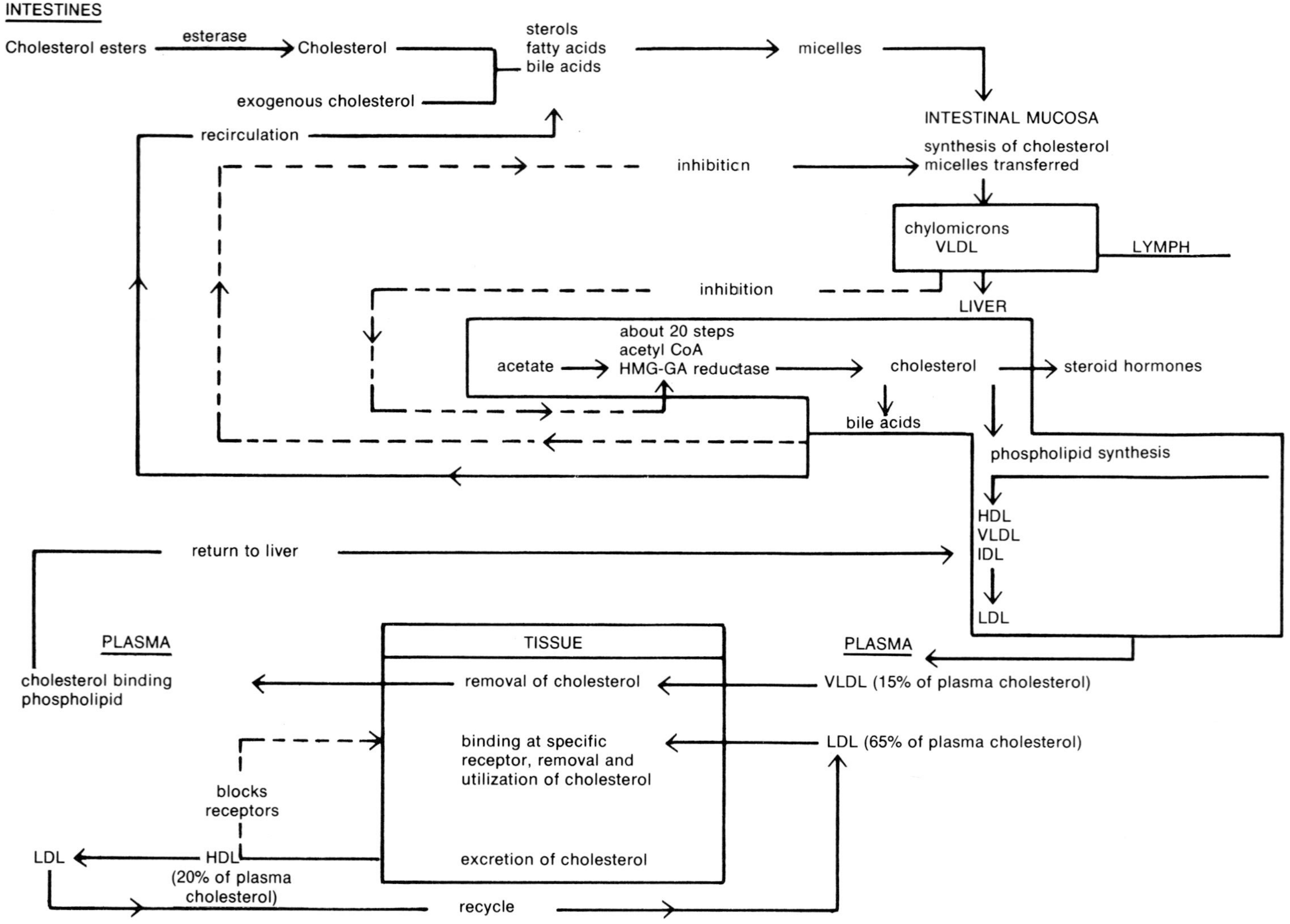

Figure 5-1. Cholesterol Metabolism

TABLE 5-3. Dietary Sources of Cholesterol (mg/100 g of edible portion)

Cholesterol is found in all animal tissues.

Beef	95	Kidney, raw	375
Brains, raw	>2000	Lamb	100
Butter	250	Lard, animal fats	95
Caviar or fish roe	>300	Liver	435
Cheese, cheddar or American	100	Lobster	200
Cheese, cottage, creamed	15	Margarine, all vegetable	0
Cheese, cream	120	Milk, whole	11
Cheese spread	65	Milk, skim	2.2
Chicken	87	Mutton	95
Crab	125	Oysters	>200
Egg white	0	Pork	70
Egg yolk*	1500	Shrimp	125
Fish	50-70	Sweetbreads (thymus)	250
Heart, raw	150	Veal	90
Ice cream	45	Yogurt, 2% fat	7.5

* One large egg contains about 250 mg of cholesterol.
Human milk contains 3 to 6.5 mg/oz.
Plant tissues contain only traces of cholesterol, but contain other sterols.

etary cholesterol are as follows:

1. *Absorbed* cholesterol in the range of 0 to 570 mg per day in vegetarians and nonvegetarians had no effect.
2. Dietary *intakes* in the range of 500 to 700 mg per day raised plasma levels by 5 to 15%.
3. One to two eggs a day (250 to 500 mg cholesterol) did not raise levels in healthy people on customary diets.
4. Plant sterols in normal amounts (250 to 300 mg per day) had neglible effect.
5. Plant sterols (10,000 to 15,000 mg per day) lowered plasma cholesterol 10 to 20%.

For carbohydrates, isocaloric exchange of sucrose for starch at a level of 23% of calories produced no effect. Results of protein studies are conflicting, with most studies reporting no effect, but with one study showing reduction when animal protein was replaced with soy protein. Wheat and bran fiber have no effect, but pectin showed highly variable effects with lowering of levels from 0 to 18%. Whole milk, skim milk, and yogurt have been reported to lower blood levels of cholesterol. Caloric restriction in the obese with hypercholesterolemia lowers blood levels, particularly of VLDL.[11]

A review[14] of the effects of vitamins and minerals on plasma cholesterol concentration reports:

Vitamin C has no effect on plasma cholesterol;

Vitamin D, in large doses, increases the levels;

Vitamin E is not effective in normal persons or in those with hyperlipidemia;

Niacin reduced VLDL but not HDL at very high doses (222 times RDA);

Biotin produced hypercholesterolemia in deficiency, but had no effect in large doses;

Calcium lowers plasma cholesterol at 2 g per day, chiefly affects LDL;

Iron anemia increases cholesterol;

Vanadium—no confirmation of earlier reports of lowering;

Silicon—early reports of lowering in rats not confirmed in man;

Zinc: Copper ratio showed no effect in the only study in man;

Fiber showed a lowering of cholesterol by pectin, but not by wheat fiber. One report of lowering by oatmeal;

Protein had no effect in normal persons, but lowered cholesterol in those with kwashiorkor;

Carbohydrate—no effect in replacement of sugar with starches at 23% of caloric intake (higher than most human diets).

The composition of dietary fat in terms of *cis*-polyunsaturated and long-chain saturated fatty acids is the predominant dietary factor affecting plasma cholesterol levels. If saturated fatty acids are entirely replaced by *cis*-polyunsaturated fatty acids (not the *trans* forms produced when polyunsaturated oils are partially hydrogenated), a 25 to 30% lowering in plasma cholesterol and LDL can be expected. If saturates are only partially replaced by polyunsaturates, cholesterol will be lowered to a lesser degree. The degree of lowering depends on the degree of replacement. This should not be misinterpreted as "polyunsaturated fats lower blood cholesterol." The lowering is only seen when total fat intake represents less than 40 to 45% of total caloric intake, and when polyunsaturates replace long-chain saturates (not the short-chain saturates in butter and dairy products or the monounsaturates of olive oil). The change is brought about in normolipidemic and hypercholesterolemic people by movement of cholesterol into muscle, connective tissue, and adipose tissue. In hyperlipidemic people, there is a marked excretion of fecal steroids.

In general, the studies show little relationship between cholesterol in the diet and serum levels. In addition, people with low serum cholesterol have been found with as severe atherosclerosis as people with high levels. It seems obvious that much more investigation is necessary to clarify the relationship between dietary intake, mechanism of lipid transport, and disease of heart and blood vessels.

REFERENCES—Cholesterol

1. Sabine, J.R.: Cholesterol. New York, Marcel Dekker, 1977.
2. Grundy, S.M.: West. J. Med., *128:*13, 1978.
3. Brown, M.S., and Goldstein, J.L.: Science, *191:*150, 1976.
4. Kaunitz, H.J.: J. Am. Oil Chem. Soc., *52:*293, 1975; Chemistry and Industry, *17:*761, 1977.
5. Kritchevsky, D.: Postgrad. Med., *63:*133, 1978.
6. Dietschy, J.M., and Wilson, J.D.: N. Engl. J. Med., *282:*1128, 1970.
7. Quintão, E., Grundy, S.M., and Ahrens, E.H., Jr.: J. Lipid Res., *12:*221, 1971.
8. Glomset, J.A., and Verdery, R.B.: Expos. Annu. Biochim. Med., *33:*137, 1977 (in English).
9. Thomson, P., and Bortz, W.M., II: J. Am. Geriatr. Soc., *26:*440, 1978.
10. Ahrens, E.H., Jr., and Conner, W.E., co-chmn.: Am. J. Clin. Nutr., *32:*2619, 1979. Special Supplement Report of the Task Force on "The Evidence Relating Six Dietary Factors to the Nation's Health."
11. Grundy, S.M.: Am. J. Clin. Nutr., *30:*985, 1977.
12. Hegsted, D.M.: Food Tech., *32:*44, 1978.
13. Vital and Health Statistics, Total Serum Cholesterol Levels of Adults 18-74 years, 1971-1974. (DHEW Publication No. (PHS) 78-1652, Series 11, No. 205) National Center for Health Statistics, 1978.
14. Truswell, A.S.: Am. J. Clin. Nutr., *31:*977, 1978.

Chapter 6
Protein and Nitrogen

Food proteins provide amino acids for the synthesis of body protein characteristic of each species and supply nitrogen for the synthesis of other tissue constituents. Protein amino acids are necessary for protein synthesis, but the rest of the nitrogen requirement can be met from other nonprotein sources.[1]

Note that the body is in dynamic nitrogen balance, with protein and other nitrogen-containing compounds being degraded and resynthesized continuously. Actually, nitrogen turnover is higher than nitrogen intake requirements since some of the nitrogen is used in resynthesis. The rest of the nitrogenous metabolic products of amino acids are excreted in the urine as urea, creatinine, uric acid, and other nitrogen compounds.

Nitrogen is also lost in feces, sweat and other body secretions, and in sloughed epidermal cells of skin, hair, and nails. Amino acid intake in excess of nitrogen needs is rapidly degraded, with nitrogen excreted as urea and the organic acid that is produced oxidized directly as a source of energy or converted to carbohydrate or fat.

Nitrogen-containing substances in the body include proteins, purines, pyrimidines, creatine, and choline. The renewal rate for protein is not known, but varies with the tissue.

The distribution of protein in the body in terms of actual weight and as a percentage of total body weight is shown in Table 6-1.

Ingested protein is split into amino acids, which are then resynthesized into protein or are degraded and used for energy content. Inorganic sources of nitrogen such as ammonium salts can also be used in protein syn-

TABLE 6-1. Large Protein Stores in Male; Height, 168.5 cm; Weight, 53.8 kg

	Actual Weight kg	Percent of Total Body Weight
Total protein (N × 6.25)	10.006	18.6
Striated muscle	4.680	8.7
Skeleton	1.864	3.5
Skin	0.924	1.7
Adipose tissue	0.361	0.7
Hemoglobin (estimated)	0.750	1.4
Albumin (estimated)	0.250	0.5

thesis of several amino acids. Some amino acids cannot be synthesized by humans. These are

threonine	valine
leucine	isoleucine
lysine	methionine
phenylalanine	tryptophan

These are called "essential" amino acids and must be included in the diet. For children histidine is also essential, and it may be essential for adults. In some cases, arginine may be a limiting factor in growth and development in humans. Other species have other groups of amino acids that are "essential."[2,3]

Some of the essential amino acids are used for the synthesis of some of the "nonessential" amino acids, or specifically, for other nutritional factors. Thus, a portion of the tryptophan is converted to niacin; methionine can be converted to cystine, if insufficient cystine is obtained from the diet; and phenylalanine can be used for the synthesis of other aromatic amino acids if these are deficient in the diet. Because of this interconversion, it is difficult to ascertain the requirements for the individual essential amino acids in the diet, since this depends on the intake of nonessential amino acids.

In feeding studies, various proteins and mixtures of amino acids have been used as standards of comparison. One such recommended pattern and the pattern of dietary intake are shown in Table 6-2.

A number of different patterns of dietary intake have been suggested, such as that in eggs, or milk, or a synthetic mixture (Food and Agriculture Organization of the World Health Organization). The diets are usually expressed as the proportion of each amino acid to tryptophan. Since the results of feeding studies depend not only upon the ratio of the essential amino acids, but also upon the proportion of nonessential amino acids (obviously, the need for an essential amino acid is reduced if the nonessential amino acid into which it is converted is already present), the results are impossible to interpret. No studies have been done by varying one amino acid while holding the others in the diet at the minimum level, because a truly minimal level, independent of all the other amino acids, is not known for any of the amino acids, nor can it be readily determined.

In healthy humans, there is no measur-

TABLE 6-2. Comparison of Tentative Minimum Requirements of Amino Acids with Amino Acid Content of American Diets

Amino Acid	Minimum Requirements (g/day) Women[a]	Men[b]	Amino Acid Content of Food Intakes (g/day) Reynolds[c]	Futrell[d]	Mertz[e]	Wharton[f]
Isoleucine	0.45	0.70	4.2	2.49-5.73	0.7-4.5	2.8-3.1
Leucine	0.62	1.10	6.5	3.28-7.35	1.3-7.8	4.4-4.9
Lysine	0.50	0.80	4.0	1.7-8.6	1.3-5.6	3.5-4.0
Methionine						
+ Cystine	0.55	1.10	3.0	0.90-2.54	0.7-2.7	0.9-1.0
Phenylalanine	0.22	1.10	4.1	1.98-4.88	0.9-3.77	2.5-2.7
Tyrosine	0.90					
Threonine	0.31	0.50	2.8	1.68-3.44	0.9-3.8	1.6-2.9
Tryptophan	0.16	0.25	0.9	0.5-1.28	-	0.4-0.5
Valine	0.65	0.80	4.2	2.85-5.39	0.8-4.9	3.1-3.4

[a] Leverton, R.M.: *In* Protein and Amino Acid Nutrition, A.A. Albanese, ed. New York, Academic Press, 1959, pp. 477-506.
[b] Rose, W.C.: Fed. Proc., *8*:546, 1949.
[c] Reynolds, M.S., Futrell, M.F., and Baumann, C.A.: J. Am. Diet. Assoc., *29*:359, 1953.
[d] Futrell, M.F., Lutz, R.N., Reynolds, M.S., and Baumann, C.A.: J. Nutr., *46*:299, 1952.
[e] Mertz, E.T., et al.: J. Nutr., *46*:313, 1952.
[f] Wharton, M.A., Tyrrell, D., and Patton, M.B.: J. Am. Diet. Assoc., *29*:573, 1953.

able nutritional benefit from intakes that exceed requirements.[4] There is also no evidence that intakes of up to triple the requirements are harmful (humans self-select diets with 9 to 15% of total calories provided by protein). Very small premature infants showed serious toxicity on diets in which protein provided 16% or more of total calories.[5] In addition, large intakes of protein may interfere with calcium utilization.[6] The factors considered in setting amino acid requirements are as follows:

1. An assumption that measurement of the minimum nitrogen intake that prevents nitrogen loss provides a direct estimate of the requirements for maintenance, to which must be added nitrogen for growth in pregnant women and children and nitrogen for milk during lactation. This assumption does not take into account the efficiency of utilization of protein at various protein intakes[7–10]; nor does it take into account the improved nitrogen conservation adaptation in low-protein or protein-free diets or the exponential form of the nitrogen loss curve, with time.[11,12]
2. The standard deviation of individual variability is about 15%. Thus, 30% was added to the average value.[13]
3. The requirements for growth in infants are based on the quantity of protein in the milk needed to assure a satisfactory growth rate.[13]
4. The requirements in children and young adults are based on growth.[14–16]
5. The requirements in pregnancy are based on fetal growth.[17–19]
6. The requirements in lactation are based on milk production.[20]

In addition to the above factors, other conditions that affect protein requirements and protein utilization are as follows:

1. Since the conversion of food to metabolic energy has the first priority in nutrient utilization, protein, no matter how inadequate the diet, will be used as an energy source unless energy can be obtained from an adequate intake of carbohydrate and fat. Thus, when the diet is restricted calorically (by starvation diets or weight-loss diets), lean body mass is lost. In addition, efficiency of protein utilization decreases when energy intake is low. This factor is not allowed for in setting the RDA. Intake of protein, therefore, should be at or above the RDA, with the recognition that protein utilization in low-calorie diets cannot be improved without raising the caloric content of the diet.[21,22]

2. No convincing evidence exists that increase in muscle use affects the need for protein, except the small amounts that are added to the muscle mass during muscle conditioning. There is an initial increase in nitrogen excretion in sweat during heavy work, sports activity, or work in a warm environment. The body soon becomes acclimated, however, and the nitrogen loss drops. No addition was made to the RDA, because the effect is small and temporary.[10,12,23]

3. Extreme environmental and physiologic stresses increase nitrogen loss. Infection, fever, and surgery increase urinary nitrogen loss and also increase energy expenditure. No special allowance is made in the RDA for normal stresses of living, on the assumption that the human subjects used for estimating the nitrogen requirements were exposed to stresses of the same order as the general population. Severe infections and surgery are abnormal conditions requiring special dietary treatment. Special attention should be given to the need for additional protein and energy during convalescence to replace depleted stores and rebuild wasted muscle.

Another problem in setting the RDA is that proteins differ in nutritive value because they differ in digestibility and amino acid composition.[24] The biologic value of a protein is species specific. It is defined as the percent of absorbed nitrogen retained by the body, as determined from nitrogen intake and loss measurements made under standard conditions. In addition, a coefficient of digestibility is determined from measurement of fecal nitrogen loss with and without dietary protein. The product of these two factors gives the net protein utilization.[25]

In practice, the nutritional value of a protein may be evaluated by comparing the amino acid composition to that of a reference material which is assigned a value of 100. Although a common reference protein is that of whole egg, the Food and Nutrition Board has chosen casein as the reference. The percentage by which each essential amino acid in the dietary protein differs from that of the reference casein is calculated. The amino acid showing the greatest deficit is considered the limiting amino acid (usually tryptophan in foods of animal origin or lysine in foods of vegetable origin). The amount of this amino acid in the protein, expressed as a percent of the amount in the reference, gives the chemical score, which corresponds closely to the biologic value if the protein is completely digested.

The story of protein quality does not stop here. Determining chemical score or biologic value, while useful for single products such as infant formulas, does not give correct information about the protein quality of a complex diet. The protein quality of a diet must be based on the total amino acid pattern present in a given meal. Thus, the protein quality of a food low in a particular amino acid may be improved by simultaneous ingestion of a protein high in that particular amino acid. Protein quality of diet, as compared with protein quality of a single food, may be enhanced by eating correct combinations of complementary proteins. Many civilizations have discovered the complementary combination of a grain plus a legume, such as the Italian pasta e fagioli, the Mexican tortilla and refritos, the Spanish Christianos e Moros (white rice and black beans), and the oriental rice and bean curd.

Another complicating factor is that the efficiency of protein utilization decreases as protein intake approaches adequacy.[26] Studies in humans on mixed diets containing high-score protein in amounts approaching adequacy showed 60 to 75% utilization efficiency.

The RDA was modified on the assumption that some people whose source of dietary protein was not of such high quality and not as digestible as that on the test diet might have protein utilization efficiencies of only about 50%.[27,28]

Since plant protein is generally less well digested than animal protein, an additional allowance to the RDA should be made when the diet is composed largely of cereal grains and rootcrops or when plants are an important source of amino acids, such as in a strictly vegetarian diet.

The RDA for maintenance (adult) is set on the basis of 0.45 g of protein per kg per day, determined by nitrogen balance studies, increasing this by 30% to 0.6 g/kg per day to take individual variation into account, then correcting for 75% utilization by increasing it to 0.8 g/kg per day.

In pregnancy, an additional 30 g per day from the second month of pregnancy to birth was deemed adequate. This is based on a nitrogen retention value of 16 mg/kg per day and an assumption of 50% utilization of ingested protein. This translates to 1.3 g/kg per day for pregnant mature women, but 1.5 g/kg for 15 to 18 year olds and 1.7 g/kg for those younger than 15, in order to provide for both the fetus and the maturation needs of the mother.[29–33]

In lactation, 20 g per day above the maintenance level was deemed adequate, based on an assumption of 70% utilization and an average protein concentration in human milk of 1.29 g/dl and an average daily production of 850 ml.

For infants, the RDA is based on the amount of milk protein known to assure a satisfactory growth rate. This is estimated at 2 to 2.4 g/kg per day for the first month, gradually falling to 1.5 g/kg per day in the sixth month.[13]

For infants over 6 months, the requirement of 1.5 g/kg per day has been adjusted to allow for 75% utilization efficiency of protein in a mixed diet.

TABLE 6-3. Protein Supplements for Oral Use

Product Name	Manufacturer	Dosage Form	Dose	Calories	Protein g	Carbohydrates g	Fats g
Casec	Mead Johnson	Powder	tbsp	17	4.0	Trace	0.1
Gevral Protein	Lederle	Powder	26 g	97.8	15.6	6.6	0.52
Nutri-100	Syntex	Liquid	300 ml	313	10.1	3.3	16
Prototabs	North American	Tablet	1	—	0.25*	—	—

* Contains amino acids in proper proportions for a utilization factor of 1.00.
Note that gelatin is not considered a protein supplement. Its chemical score is 0 because it lacks tryptophan. This is destroyed in the production process, which utilizes acid or alkaline hydrolysis.

For the 1 to 18 year old group, an amount of protein, adjusted for an assumed protein utilization efficiency as found for maintenance in adults, is added to the maintenance allowance. The allowances decrease from 2.0 g/kg at 1 year to 0.8 g/kg at 18 years.[14–16]

The RDA for protein is set specifically for people in the United States. Values suggested by the Food and Agriculture Organization of the World Health Organization (FAO/WHO) and values developed for Canada and India are similar. Considerably higher values have been recommended in Australia, Japan, the German Democratic Republic, the United Kingdom, the Netherlands, and Finland.[34]

The need for protein in persons over 50 years old has been investigated with conflicting results.[35,36] Generally, recommended caloric intake/kg decreases with increasing age, but the amount of protein/kg required for nitrogen balance does not decrease. Prudently, therefore, the proportion of calories supplied by protein should increase with advancing age to a minimum value of 12%.

Protein Deficiency

In man, deficiency has many different symptoms, depending on overall deficiencies and deficiencies of specific amino acids. Protein supplements for oral use are listed in Table 6-3; amino acid products, in Table 6-4.

TABLE 6-4. Amino Acid Products

I. L-Lysine—improves utilization of vegetable protein
Dose: 334-1000 mg/day

A. Enisyl (Person & Covey)—334 mg/tablet
B. L-Lysine (Nature's Bounty)—500 mg/tablet

II. Amino Acid Combinations

A. Lycolan Elixir (Lannett)—glycine, lysine
B. Prostade Capsules (Pharmacare)—glycine, alanine, glutamic acid
C. DEQUAsine Tablets (Miller)—lysine, cysteine, methionine, vitamin C, Fe, minerals, yeast, amino acids
D. L-Glutavite Capsules (Berlex)—monosodium glutamate, Fe, B_1, B_2, B_6, B_{12}
E. Lysmins Tablets (Miller)—lysine, methionine, Fe, Cu, I, K, Mg, Mn, Zn
F. Aminoprel Tablets (Pasadena)—lysine, methionine, protein hydrolysate, Fe, Cu, I, K, Mg, Mn, Zn

III. Protein Hydrolysates—utilization factor is *0* for *chemical* hydrolysates, unless tryptophan is added

A. A/G-Pro (Miller)—with lysine, methionine, Fe, Cu, I, K, Mg, Mn, Zn
B. P.D.P. Liquid Protein (Wesley)—enzymatic hydrolysate
C. Protinex (Brunswick)—vitamins, minerals

IV. Protein

A. Pro-Mix (Brunswick)—whey protein
B. Powdered Skim Milk

1. Early symptoms
   a. loss of weight
   b. retarded growth
   c. fatigue and lack of energy
   d. irritability
   e. personality change
   f. retarded wound healing
   g. long convalescence
   h. lowered resistance to many stresses
2. Serious effects
   a. liver insufficiency
   b. hypoproteinemia (due to disturbance of homeostasis rather than deficiency of protein)
   c. nutritional edema due to disturbance of water balance
   d. impaired antibody formation?
   e. damage to endocrine system
   f. in protracted malnutrition, impairment of metabolism so that body does not return to normal when the diet again becomes adequate

Excessive Protein Intake

1. Dietary protein in excess of requirements is utilized for energy.
2. Adaptation to a high-protein diet takes place gradually; normal dietary level is 9 to 15% of total calories.
3. Sudden dietary increase in protein may produce
   a. decreased utilization efficiency (conversion of protein to muscle)
   b. fluid imbalance
      Note: metabolic needs for water
      100 calories of protein requires 350 g of water
      100 calories of carbohydrate—50 g
      100 calories of fat—50 g
   c. increase in nitrogenous compounds in blood
4. Effects of excessive protein intake that are *not* true
   a. produces or aggravates hypertension
   b. causes complications in pregnancy
   c. raises metabolic rate and thus increases stress in fevers
   d. damages kidneys (except when there is danger of accumulation of metabolic products)
   e. damages liver (except when ability to use amino acids is impaired)

Genetic Disorders

Disorders of protein metabolism due to abnormal metabolism of specific amino acids have been identified. They are usually treated by dietary restriction of the offending amino acid to the amounts actually needed for protein synthesis, thus allowing growth without toxicity. These disorders are as follow:

1. Phenylketonuria
2. Maple syrup urine (caused by

TABLE 6-5. Products for Aminoacidurias

Product	Source
Phenylketonuria	
Lofenalac	Mead Johnson
Phenyl-Free	Mead Johnson
Maple Syrup Urine	
GIBCO amino acid mixture	Grand Island Biological Co. Grand Island, NY
MSUD Diet Powder	Mead Johnson
Homocystinuria	
Low-methionine Isomil	Ross
Product 3200 K	Mead Johnson
Tyrosinemia	
Product 3200 AB	Mead Johnson

Notes: 1. As a vitamin-mineral-calorie supplement to amino acid mixtures, Product 80056 is available from Mead Johnson.
2. Amino acid mixtures are also available from Milner Scientific and Medical Research Co., Liverpool, England.

branched-chain amino acids, leucine, isoleucine, and valine)
3. Tyrosinemia
4. Homocystinuria (caused by deficiency of cystathionine synthase)
   a. one form responds to pyridoxine
   b. another form requires the restriction of methionine and a supply of cysteine
5. Histidinemia
6. Alkaptonuria (homogentisic acid from abnormal metabolism of phenylalanine and tyrosine is excreted)
7. Gout

Products for aminoacidurias are listed in Table 6-5.

REFERENCES—Protein

1. Waterlow, J.C., and Stephen, J.M.L., eds.: Human Protein Requirements and Their Fulfillment in Practice. Food and Agriculture Organization of the United Nations, Rome, 1957, FAO Nutrition Meetings Rept. Ser. No. 12.
2. Holt, L.E., Jr., and Synderman, S.E.: Nutr. Abstr. Rev., *35:*1, 1965.
3. Heird, W.C., et al.: J. Pediatr., *81:*162, 1972.
4. Holt, L.E., Jr., Halac, E., Jr., and Kajdi, C.N.: JAMA, *181:*699, 1962.
5. Goldman, H.I., et al.: J. Pediatr., *85:*764, 1974.
6. Anand, C.R., and Linkswiler, H.M.: J. Nutr., *104:*695, 1974.
7. Sumner, E.E., and Murlin, J.R.: J. Nutr., *16:*141, 1938.
8. Bricker, M., Mitchell, H.H., and Kinsman, G.M.: J. Nutr., *30:*269, 1945.
9. Hegsted, D.M., et al.: J. Lab. Clin. Med., *31:*261, 1946.
10. Calloway, D.H., and Margen, S.: J. Nutr., *101:*205, 1971.
11. Waterlow, J.C.: Lancet, *2:*1091, 1968.
12. Holmes, E.G.: World Rev. Nutr. Diet., *5:*237, 1965.
13. Food and Agriculture Organization/World Health Organization, Ad Hoc Expert Committee, WHO Tech. Rept. Ser. No. 522, FAO Nutrition Meetings Rept. Ser. 52. Geneva, WHO, 1973, 118 pp.
14. Widdowson, E.M., and Dickerson, J.W.T.: Chemical Composition of the Body, *In* Mineral Metabolism. Vol. II, Part A. C.L. Comar and F. Bronner, eds. New York, Academic Press, 1963.
15. Foman, S.J.: Infant Nutrition, 2nd Ed. Philadelphia, W.B. Saunders, 1974.
16. Hathaway, M.L.: Heights and Weights of Children in the United States. Home Econ. Res. Rept. No. 2, Institute of Home Economics, Agricultural Research Service, U.S. Dept. of Agriculture, Washington, DC, U.S. Government Printing Office, 1957.
17. Naismith, D.J.: Proc. Nutr. Soc., *28:*25, 1969.
18. Hytten, F.E., and Leitch, I.: Physiology of Human Pregnancy, 2nd Ed. Oxford, Blackwell Scientific Publications, 1971.
19. National Research Council, Committee on Maternal Nutrition: Maternal Nutrition and the Course of Pregnancy: Summary Report. Washington, DC, National Academy of Sciences, 1970.
20. Report of Expert Committee, World Health Organization: Nutrition in Pregnancy and Lactation. Tech. Rept. Ser. No. 302. Geneva, WHO, 1965.
21. Munro, H.N.: Physiol. Rev., *31:*449, 1951.
22. Calloway, D.H., and Spector, H.: Am. J. Clin. Nutr., *2:*405, 1954.
23. Darke, S.J.: Br. J. Nutr., *14:*115, 1960.
24. Block, R.J., and Mitchell, H.H.: Nutr. Abstr. Rev., *16:*249, 1946.
25. Allison, J.B.: Physiol. Rev., *35:*664, 1955.
26. Mitchell, H.H.: J. Biol. Chem., *58:*905, 1924.
27. Inoue, G., Fujita, Y., and Niiyama, Y.: J. Nutr., *103:*1673, 1973.
28. Scrimshaw, N.S.: N. Engl. J. Med., *294:*136, 1976.
29. Committee on Maternal Nutrition, National Research Council: Nutritional Supplementation and the Outcome of Pregnancy. Washington, DC, National Academy of Sciences, 1973, ex Recommended Dietary Allowances, 9th Ed. Washington, DC, National Academy of Sciences, 1980, p. 53.
30. King, J.C., Calloway, D.H., and Margen, S.: J. Nutr., *103:*772, 1973.
31. King, J.C.: Clin. Perinatol., *2:*243, 1975.
32. Appel, J., and King, J.C.: Fed. Proc., *38:*388, 1979, Abstr. 848.
33. Beaton, G.H., and Swiss, L.D.: Am. J. Clin. Nutr., *27:*485, 1974.
34. Cheng, A.H.R., et al.: Am. J. Clin. Nutr., *31:*12, 1978.
35. Uauy, R., Scrimshaw, N.S., and Young, V.R.: Am. J. Clin. Nutr., *31:*779, 1978.
36. Zanni, E., Calloway, D.H., and Zezulka, A.Y.: J. Nutr., *109:*513, 1979.

Chapter 7
The Fat-Soluble Vitamins

VITAMIN A

Different degrees of Vitamin A activity are shown by various stereoisomers of all-*trans* retinol. In addition, various carotenes may be absorbed through the intestinal wall and converted in various degrees to *trans*-retinol.

Formerly, vitamin A activity in food was expressed as international units (IU). One IU is equivalent to 0.3 μg of retinol, 0.344 μg of retinyl acetate, 0.535 μg of retinyl palmitate or 0.6 μg of beta-carotene.[1] These relationships were derived from studies in rats and may not hold for humans. Because the five chemicals are available, the international unit is no longer recognized by the Food and Drug Administration and a proposal is currently (1981) before the World Health Organization (WHO) to abandon the international unit reference standard. The USP unit is identical with the IU.

Because carotenoids are slowly and variably converted to vitamin A by the human body, they are not desirable for use in therapy. Vitamin A, then, in practice, refers to synthetic retinol, retinyl acetate, and retinyl palmitate. These are predominantly in the all-*trans* form, but with a small but variable percentage of the 13-*cis* form (neoretinol), which has about 75% of the biologic activity of the all-*trans* form[2] (Figure 7-1).

The evaluation of vitamin A available from foods is difficult and confusing. The various retinol isomers have various but always lower activity than the all-*trans* forms. The various provitamins (carotenes and cryptoxanthine) have variable activity and variable absorption. Thus, diet has to be specified in terms of both retinol and provitamin. Based on recommendations of the Food and Agriculture Organization (FAO) of WHO and practices adopted in the United Kingdom, the Food and Nutrition Board has recommended that in the United States, vitamin A in foods be expressed as "retinol equivalents" calculated as follows:[3]

μg retinol + μg β-carotene/6 + μg other carotenoids/12

This formula assumes that all retinol is in the *trans* form, although it is known that there are *cis* forms in cooked vegetables[4] and that the retinol from them is completely absorbed; that overall utilization of beta-carotene is 1/6 that of retinol, and that overall utilization of non-beta-carotenes and cryptoxanthine is 1/12 that of retinol.

As yet, food tables do not separate retinol and its esters, beta-carotene, and other provitamin A (Table 7-1). In chemical assay, beta-carotene and retinol are equivalent; thus, the vitamin A content of foods with a high carotene content is overstated.

Vitamin A: Retinol (all-*trans*)

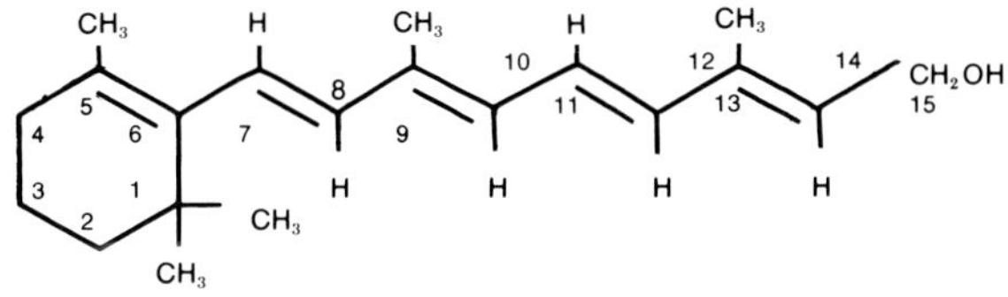

Retinal

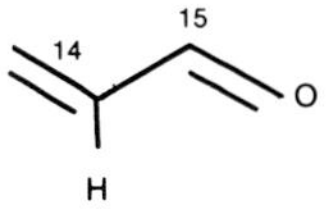

Neovitamin A: 13-*cis* retinol

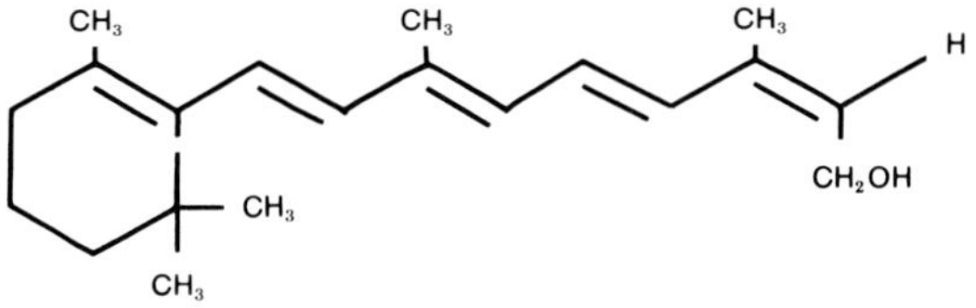

Provitamin A: beta-carotene

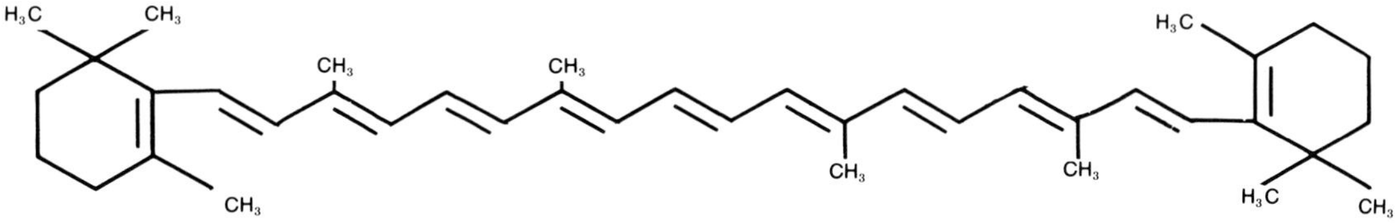

Figure 7-1. Structures of Retinols and Carotenes

Recommended Dietary Allowances

A summary of various studies on vitamin A needs in humans[5] indicates a minimum requirement of 500 to 600 μg of retinol for adults to prevent all deficiency symptoms and maintain an adequate blood level. Intake above this level is thought to be necessary in order to produce storage in the liver.

A study in the United States[6] indicated that foods available to the consumer had about half the vitamin A activity available as retinol, the other half as provitamin A carotenoids. Thus, the old (1974) RDA of 5000 IU translates by the formula above into 1000 (μg) retinol equivalents. This is the level recommended for adult males. For adult females, because of smaller body size, the level is set at 80% of the male level, or 800 retinol equivalents. This is increased to 1000 retinol equivalents during pregnancy to allow for fetal storage, and to 1200 retinol equivalents during lactation to allow for excretion in the milk. According to the study, actual adult intakes ranged from 1150 to 1500 retinol equivalents.

Recommendations for vitamin A intake for infants are based on the levels in human milk (about 0.49 μg/ml); so that for 850 ml of daily milk production, about 420 μg are excreted. For infants 6 months to 1 year old, the recommendation of 400 retinol equivalents is based on milk plus solid food, so that 300 equivalents are retinol and 100 equivalents are provitamin A.

For children and adolescents, the RDA is interpolated from infant and male adult rec-

TABLE 7-1 Chief Dietary Sources of Vitamin A

Based on food tables in International Units, assuming that values given are based on beta-carotene in plants and retinol in fish and meat.

Food	Retinol Equiv per 100 g	Food	Retinol Equiv. per 100 g
Apricots	270	Mango	480
apricot nectar	168	Papaya	1,750
Bok choy	310	Peaches	133
Broccoli	250	Pumpkin	160
Carrots	1,050	Squash, winter	1,700*
Cantalope	340	Sweet potato	870**
Greens, cooked			
beet	510	Butter	3,300
chard	280	Cheese (hard)	1,200
collard	700	Crabmeat	21,700
dandelion	1,170	Liver	
kale	890	beef	44,000
mustard	580	calf	22,500
turnip	760	chicken	12,100
Greens, raw		pork	10,900
endive	330	lamb	50,500
escarole	330	turkey	17,500
romaine	190	liverwurst	6,530
watercress	490	swordfish	2,050
		whitefish	12,000

* Summer squash contains little.
** In contrast, yams have only a trace.

ommendations. They are based on body weight plus an amount estimated to be needed for growth. There is no fixed ratio between the recommendations and body size.

Chemistry

Retinol and carotenoids are insoluble in water, soluble in fats, and easily oxidized by air. In the absence of oxygen, they are stable to heat and the presence of acids and alkalis.

Absorption

In oral doses not greatly exceeding the physiologic requirement, retinol and its esters are completely absorbed if fat is present and fat absorption is normal.

In large doses, fat malabsorption, low protein intake, liver or pancreatic disease absorption is incomplete.

Water-miscible preparations of retinol and its esters are absorbed more rapidly from the gastrointestinal (GI) tract than are oil preparations, and at high doses produce somewhat greater liver storage.[7] Retinol esters are hyrolyzed to retinol in the intestines by pancreatic enzymes. The retinol is then absorbed.

Normal Distribution

After absorption, retinol is esterified, mostly to retinyl palmitate. This enters the circulation by transport in the chylomicrons in lymph. Peak plasma levels occur 3 to 4 hours after ingestion of water-miscible preparations and 4 to 5 hours after ingestion of oily preparations. Peak levels are higher for water-miscible preparations than for the same amount administered in oil.

LIVER

About 90 to 95% of the vitamin A in the body is stored as retinyl palmitate (with small amounts of retinol and retinal) in the liver. Small amounts of the ester are stored in kidneys, lungs, adrenals, retinas, and interperitoneal fat. Carotenes are stored mainly in fatty tissues. Retinol concentration in the liver can reach 300 μg/g, which represents enough to meet body needs for more than 1 year.[8,9]

PLACENTAL BARRIER

Vitamin A does not readily cross the placenta. Levels in umbilical cord blood are about 50% of that in the maternal circulation.

SERUM

Retinol is released from the liver bound to a specific alpha$_1$-globulin, retinol-binding protein (RBP). Retinol release from the liver is conditional on several factors, including zinc and protein. RBP circulates complexed with a pre-albumin; thus, RBP levels are reduced in protein malnutrition.

Normal serum levels of vitamin A are 0.3 to 0.7 μg/ml in adults, 0.2 to 0.5 μg/ml in infants. In adults, the vitamin A consists of 0.2 to 0.5 μg/ml of retinol and 0.2 to 2.0 μg/ml of carotenes. Maternal serum levels slowly drop during pregnancy to about 75% of the normal level at term. Normal levels also decrease with age, being noticeably lower for men over 70. About 10% of the retinol is present as esters, and at a somewhat higher proportion shortly after retinol intake. Serum levels are not necessarily a good indicator of vitamin A nutritional status, since they depend on RBP concentration and do not reflect liver storage until that storage is very low.

During therapy in deficiency states, the retinal deficiency is satisfied first, followed by liver accumulation. Serum levels are normal until the liver is saturated.

Abnormal Distribution

At large intakes, the binding capacity of RBP may be exceeded. Unbound retinol is carried into the circulation by lipoprotein. This unbound retinol is responsible for most of the toxic effects on cell membranes.

In glomerulonephritis, lipoid nephrosis, or chronic renal disease with uremia, serum levels of vitamin A increase because of RBP storage abnormalities.[10]

Serum levels are depressed in patients with defective fat absorption such as is associated with celiac disease, cystic fibrosis, sprue, and obstructive jaundice.

Blood levels of vitamin A decrease in chronic febrile conditions such as rheumatic fever and infectious hepatitis.

Cirrhosis of the liver results in very low or completely absent liver storage, thus lowering serum levels.

Cancer, tuberculosis, chronic infections such as pneumonia, chronic nephrosis, urinary tract infections, and prostate disease may be associated with increased excretion, thus requiring larger intakes.[8] In lobar pneumonia, serum levels may drop to zero.

Metabolism

Retinol is conjugated with glucuronic acid. The beta-glucuronide in the enterohepatic circulation is oxidized to retinal and retinoic acid. The retinoic acid is decarboxylated, conjugated with glucuronic acid, secreted into the bile, and excreted in the feces. Retinoic acid, retinal and water-soluble metabolites are also excreted in urine. Normally, no retinol is excreted (except in milk); but in the diseases previously listed, retinol from dietary sources may be excreted.

Vitamin A is also converted to retinal in the eye, and is used as a component of the visual pigments.

Vitamin A metabolism may be outlined as shown in Figure 7-2.

Pharmacology

Vitamin A is essential to vision. The various transformations are shown in Figure 7-3. Retinol is necessary for the maintenance of epithelial cells by its effect on factors that promote mucous secretion. It stimulates cell growth (epithelial cells, odontoblasts, and bone), and is necessary for the stability of the lipoprotein membrane of all cells and the subcellular particles.[12] Retinol or retinoic acid are necessary for maintenance of growth; retinol, but not retinoic acid, is necessary to both sexes for reproduction.

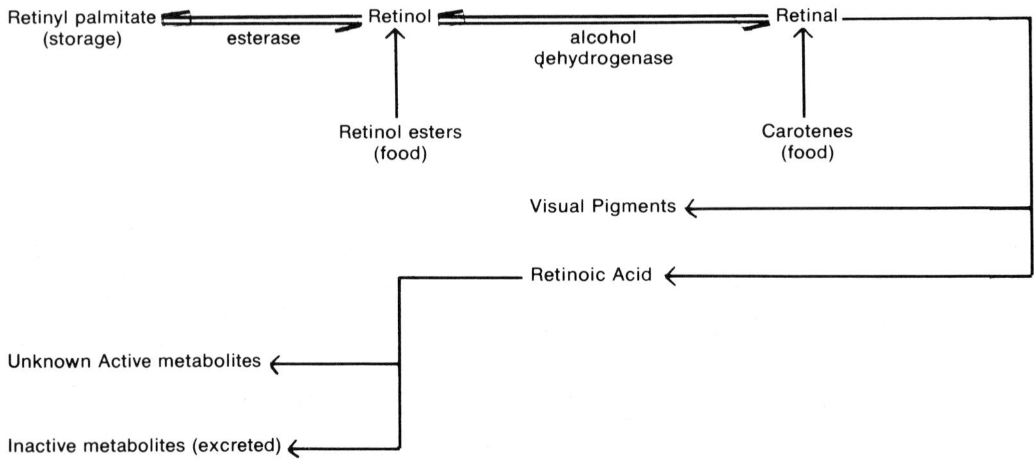

Figure 7-2. Vitamin A Metabolism

Deficiency

Measurement of dark adaptation is the most sensitive test for vitamin A deficiency. Levels of retinal in the cornea fall before there is a drop in serum retinol.[13]

SYMPTOMS[14]

1. Loss of resistance to infection because of breakdown of mucous membrane.
2. Nyctalopia (night blindness).
3. Xerophthalmia (drying and thickening of the conjunctiva, leading to keratomalacia (edema and ulceration). This is a common cause of blindness in children in Asia, Africa, and South America.[15,16]
4. Bitot's spots (microscopic dry spots on the conjunctival membrane).
5. Epithelial atrophy followed by metaplastic hyperkeratinization (follicular hyperkeratosis).
6. Impairment of epiphyseal bone formation.
7. Delayed or improper tooth formation.
8. Photophobia.
9. Conjunctivitis.
10. Asthenopia (weakness of sight).
11. Multiple malformations of fetus.
12. General debility.

POPULATIONS AT RISK[16]

Although nyctalopia is usually the first symptom of vitamin A deficiency in adults, the following (Table 7-2), listing symptoms and causes of vitamin A deficiency in various populations, may aid diagnosis.

Toxicity (hypervitaminosis A)

EFFECTS ON THE FETUS

Safety of maternal doses larger than 1.8 mg (6000 IU) of retinol per day has not been established. Toxic effects on the fetus of excessive intake include:

1. Birth defects
2. Early epiphyseal closure
3. Retarded growth

ACUTE[13]

Infants: 5.1 mg (17,000 IU) retinol to 9.9 mg (33,000 IU)/kg.
Children: more than 7.5 mg (25,000 IU)/kg.
Adults: 9 mg (30,000 IU) retinol to 22.5 mg (75,000 IU)/kg.

Symptoms in Adults

In 6 to 8 hours:

1. Severe headache centered in forehead and eyes.

TABLE 7-2.

Population at Risk	Cause of Deficiency	Symptoms
Pregnant women	Deficient diet Depletion of repeated pregnancy	Low serum levels Xerophthalmia (rare) Bitot's spots (occasional)
Fetus	Maternal deficiency	Low liver reserve Birth defects Spontaneous abortion(?)
Up to 1 year	Low vitamin A in milk Infection	Xerophthalmia (common) Bitot's spots (rare)
1 to 5 years	Nursed for too long Dietary deficiency Infection	Conjunctival xerosis Xerophthalmia Bitot's spots (occasional)
5 to 18 years	Dietary deficiency (vitamin A, carotene, fat, protein)	Conjunctival xerosis (main symptom) Bitot's spots (main symptom) Nyctalopia Follicular hyperkeratosis (occasional)
Adults	Dietary deficiency Infection Cirrhosis of the liver Pancreatic disease	Nyctalopia (main symptom) Bitot's spots (occasional) Xerophthalmia (rare) Follicular hyperkeratosis (occasional)

2. Dizziness.
3. Drowsiness.
4. Nausea and vomiting.

In 12 to 20 hours:

5. Erythemia and swelling of skin, followed by generalized peeling lasting up to several weeks.

Symptoms in Infants

Within 12 hours:

1. Increased intercranial pressure shown by bulging of fontanelles (openings in skull covered by membrane).
2. Loss of appetite.
3. Hyperirritability.
4. Vomiting.

Within a few days:

5. Flaking-off of skin.

Note: Acute vitamin A intoxication has been reported after eating polar bear liver [6 mg (20,000 IU)/g].[17]

CHRONIC[18]

Premature: Lowest recorded dose to cause toxicity: 1.7 (5700 IU) retinol/kg for 7 days.

Less than 1 year: 3.6 mg (12,000 IU) retinol to 105 mg (350, 000 IU) per day or 5.5 mg (18,500 IU) per day for one to three months

1 to 5 years: 11.25 mg (37,500 IU) retinol to 180 mg (600,000 IU) per day

Adults: 1.2 mg (4000 IU)/kg per day for 6 to 15 months

Symptoms in Adults

1. Anorexia (loss of appetite)
2. Muscle soreness after exercise
3. Hair loss
4. Maculoerythematous eruption (reddish pimples) on shoulders and back
5. General drying and flaking of skin
6. Pruritis
7. Symptoms of hypercalcemia
8. Cracking and bleeding of lips, reddened gums, nosebleed
9. Increased cerebrospinal fluid pressure (pseudotumor cerebri) and papilledema (swelling of optic nerve) seen in about half of patients; causes headache and blurred vision.
10. Anemia

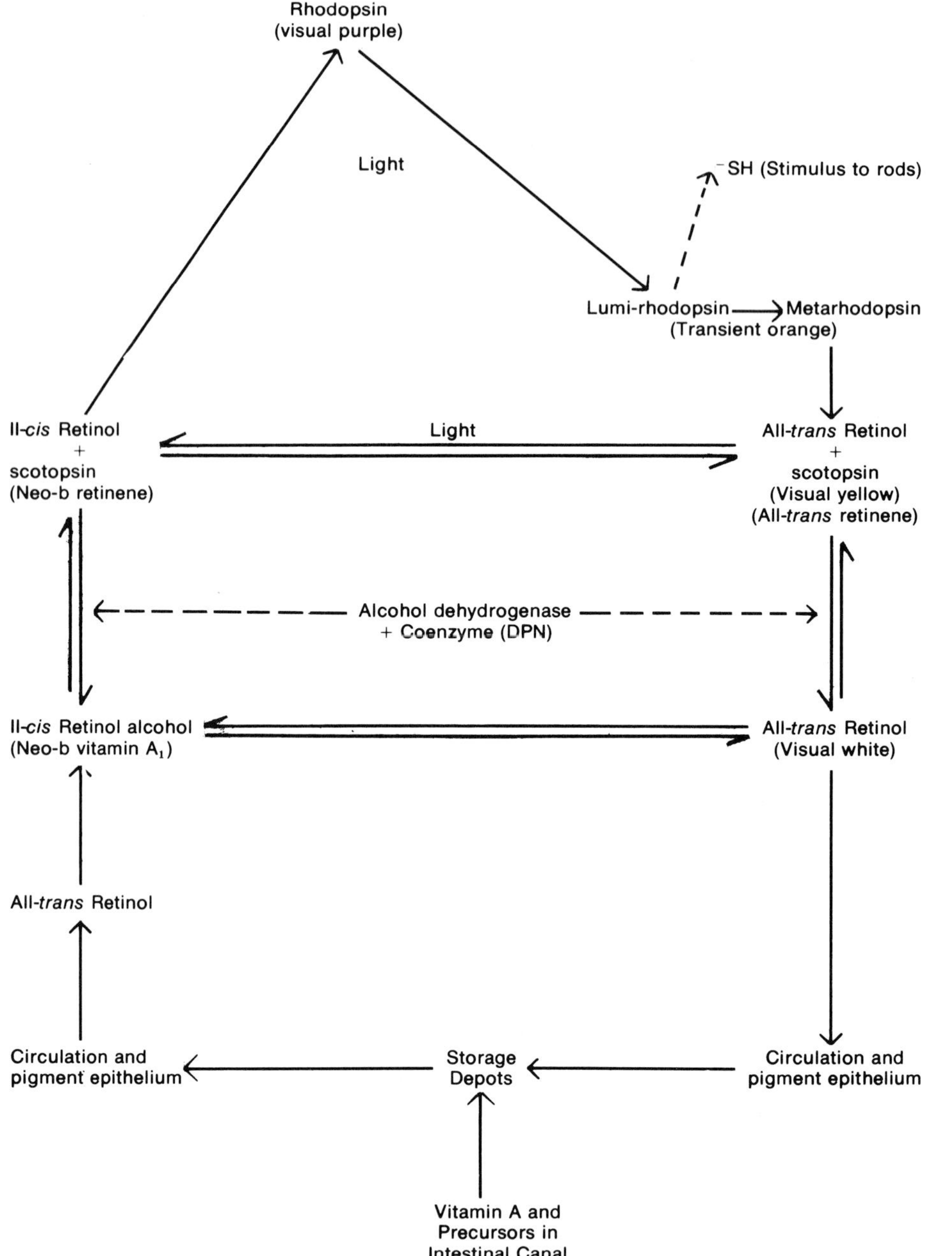

Figure 7-3. Probable Transformations During the Retinol Cycle[11]

11. Painful subcutaneous swellings
12. Painful swelling in area of muscle attachment caused by bone overgrowth
13. Mild fever
14. Excessive sweating

Other Reported Symptoms

1. Brittle nails
2. Erythema
3. Hyperpigmentation
4. Massive desquamation
5. Hypomenorrhea
6. Hepatosplenomegaly
7. Cirrhosis
8. Jaundice
9. Elevated SGOT and SGPT
10. Urinary complaints
11. Leukopenia

12. Leukocytosis
13. Thrombocytopenia

Toxicity is usually accompanied by increased plasma levels of vitamin A. The level does not correlate with the severity of the toxicity.

Sequelae[19]

1. Irreparable liver damage, cirrhosis, and fibrosis.
2. Portal hypertension and ascites (serous fluid in peritoneal cavity).
3. Permanent stunting of bone growth.

TREATMENT

1. Discontinue vitamin A.
2. Institute supportive therapy for symptoms. Symptoms begin to improve within a few days, but recovery may take weeks or months.

Uses in Therapy

DIETARY SUPPLEMENT (Table 7-3)

Infants to 6 months: 0.45 mg (1500 IU) per day

6 months to 3 years: 0.45 mg (1500 IU) to 0.6 mg (2000 IU) per day

4 to 6 years: 0.75 mg (2500 IU) per day

7 to 10 Years: 1.0 mg (3300 IU) to 1.05 mg (3500 IU) per day

Adult: 1.2 mg (4000 IU) to 1.5 mg (5000 IU) per day

The oral route is used for all ages.

MALABSORPTION SYNDROME

Adults: 3 mg (10,000 IU) to 15 mg (50,000 IU) per day, orally, with periodic monitoring of serum levels.

DEFICIENCY SYNDROME

Prophylaxis

Children: 30 mg (100,000 IU) to 120 mg (400,000 IU) in oil once every 3 to 6 months, orally. This routine is sometimes used by health teams in underdeveloped countries to prevent keratomalacia and blindness.

Treatment

1. Adults with corneal changes:
   Orally: 15 mg (50,000 IU) to 30 mg (100,000 IU) per day for 1 to 7 days.
   Intramuscular: 15 mg (50,000 IU) to 30 mg (100,000 IU) per day for 3

TABLE 7-3. Vitamin A Products

Oral Solutions	Retinol Equivalents	International Units
Aquasol A Drops (USV)	15,000	50,000
Injection (Water miscible)		
Aquasol A (USV)*	15,000	50,000
Capsules (Water miscible)		
Various labels	3,000	10,000
	7,500	25,000
	15,000	50,000
	30,000	100,000
Aquasol A (USV)*	7,500	25,000
	15,000	50,000
Capsules		
Various labels	1,500	5,000
Alphalin (Lilly)	3,000	10,000
A-Caps (Drug Industries)*	15,000	50,000
Acon (Endo)*	15,000	50,000
Alphalin Gelseals (Lilly)*	15,000	50,000
Tablets		
Various labels	3,000	10,000
	7,500	25,000
Sust-A (Miller)	1,500	5,000

Note: In order to guarantee the labeled potency for 18 to 24 months, manufacturers use overages up to 40% of label claim. In order to prevent unexpected toxicity, overages should be limited to 25%.

* Prescription required.

days, followed by 15 mg (50,000 IU) per day for 14 days.

Advanced xerophthalmia responds slowly.

2. Adults without corneal changes:
   Orally: 3 mg (10,000 IU) to 7.5 mg (25,000 IU) until clinical improvement (usually 7 to 14 days).
3. Children with xerophthalmia
   Intramuscular: 1.5 mg (5000 IU) to 4.5 mg (15,000 IU) per day for 10 days.
   Orally: 1.5 mg (5000 IU)/kg per day for 5 days or until recovery.

Interferences With Laboratory Tests

1. Vitamin A may give high values for cholesterol determined by the Zlatkis-Zak reaction.
2. It may give high values for bilirubin determined by Ehrlich's reagent.

Drug Interactions

1. Warfarin-produced hypoprothrombinemia is potentiated by large doses of vitamin A.
2. Cholestyramine decreases vitamin A absorption, probably by decreasing bile acids and decreasing micelle formation.
3. Neomycin may decrease vitamin A absorption.

REFERENCES—Vitamin A

1. WHO Expert Committee on Biological Standardization, 18th Report, World Health Organization Tech. Rept. Ser. No. 329. Geneva, World Health Organization, 1966.
2. Bauernfeind, J.C.: Vitamin A Technology, *In* Vitamin A Xeropthalmia and Blindness. Vol. III. Office of Nutrition, Technical Assistance Bureau, Agency for International Development, U.S. Dept. of State, 1973, ex Federal Register: *44:* 16164, March 16, 1979.
3. Committee on Dietary Allowances, Food and Nutrition Board, National Research Council: Recommended Dietary Allowances, 9th Ed. Washington, DC, National Academy of Sciences, 1980.
4. Sweeney, J.P., and Marsh, A.C.: J. Am. Diet. Assoc., *59:*238, 1971.
5. Food and Nutrition Board, National Research Council, Recommended Dietary Allowances, 8th Ed. Washington, DC, National Academy of Sciences, 1974.
6. Consumer and Food Economics Research Division, Agricultural Research Service, U.S. Dept. of Agriculture: Dietary Levels of Households in the U.S., Spring 1965. Preliminary Report ARS 62-17, U.S. Dept. of Agriculture, Washington, 1968, ex Recommended Dietary Allowances, 9th Ed. Washington, DC, National Academy of Sciences, 1980.
7. Ellingson, R.C., et al.: Pediatrics *8:*107, 1951.
8. Lui, N.S.T., and Roels, O.A.: Vitamin A and Carotene, *In* Modern Nutrition in Health and Disease, 6th Ed. R.S. Goodhart and M.E. Shils, eds., Philadelphia, Lea & Febiger, 1980.
9. Yagishita, K., Sundaresan, P.R., and Wolf, G.: Nature, *203:*410, 1964.
10. Smith, F.R., and Goodman, D.S.: J. Clin. Invest., *50:*2426, 1971.
11. Wald, G.: Retinal Chemistry and the Physiology of Vision, Symposium No. 8, Vol. 1 of Visual Problems of Color. London, Her Majesty's Stationery Office, 1958.
12. Lucy, J.A., and Dingle, J.T.: Nature, *204:*156, 1964.
13. Frame, B., et al.: Ann. Inter. Med., *80:*44, 1974.
14. Moore, T.: Vitam. Horm., *18:*499, 1960.
15. McLaren, D.S.: Nutr. Rev., *22:*289, 1964.
16. McLaren, D.S., and Halasa, A.: Postgrad. Med. J., *40:*711, 1964.
17. Notes, Nutr. Rev., *19:*318, 1961.
18. McLaren, D.S.: Trans. R. Soc. Trop. Med. Hyg., *60:*436, 1966.
19. Russell, R.M., et al.: N. Engl. J. Med., *281:*435, 1974.

VITAMIN D

Vitamin D occurs as ergocalciferol (D_2) and cholecalciferol (D_3) which in man, seem to have the same biologic activity.[1] Ergocalciferol is produced in plants by ultraviolet irradiation of ergosterol. Cholecalciferol is produced in animals by ultraviolet irradiation of 7-dehydrocholesterol (7-DHC) in the skin. About 3 to 4% of skin weight is 7-DHC. The amount formed depends on the length and intensity of exposure and the amount and density of skin pigments. The induction of pigmentation by ultraviolet exposure serves as a partial regulatory mechanism. Since the 7-dehydrocholesterol is found in the deeper layers of the skin, heavy pigmentation can absorb up to 95% of the incident radiation.[2] Atmospheric pollution can considerably attenuate ultraviolet radiation. The rate of cholecalciferol production in man is unknown.

One international unit (IU) of vitamin D is defined as the activity of 0.025 μg of cholecalciferol. In the United States, it is recommended that intakes of vitamin D be expressed as cholecalciferol rather than as IU. The original IU was the activity of 1 mg of irradiated ergosterol.

Recommended Dietary Allowances

During the period of human growth (infants, children, adolescents), a daily intake of 2.5 μg (100 IU) of cholecalciferol per day prevents all clinical symptoms of deficiency and produces satisfactory rates of growth and bone mineralization. At intakes of 10 μg per day (400 IU), there seems to be an increase in calcium absorption and some increase in growth. This is the recommended level of intake. Because the level of vitamin D in human milk is inadequate for needs and exposure to sunlight of infants is often inadequate,[3] it is recommended that the full amount (10 μg) be added as a supplement to the diet beginning in the first 2 weeks of life. This is in excess of the actual need. Products containing oleovitamin D, ergocalciferol, or cholecalciferol are listed in Table 7-4.

When skeletal growth stops, calcium needs drop and therefore the need for vitamin D decreases. The RDA for the 19 to 22 age group is reduced to 7.5 μg (300 IU) and further reduced for older people to 5 μg (200 IU). The adult requirement can be met by adequate exposure to sunlight.

During gestation, an increase in maternal calcium intake is needed to provide for fetal needs, thus increasing the need for vitamin D. The RDA is set by adding 5 μg (200 IU) to the maternal recommendation.

During lactation, there is also an increased need for calcium intake. In addition, in nursing women, an increase in the serum level of 1, 25-dihydroxycholecalciferol, an active metabolite of vitamin D, has been observed.[4] The RDA is set by adding 5 μg (200 IU) to the maternal recommendation.

Vitamin D is potentially toxic. Because there is no evidence of any health benefits for intakes above the RDA, it is recommended that the RDA not be exceeded either for infants or for adults.

Chemistry

Vitamin D is stable in foods, being unaffected by storage, processing, or ordinary cooking.

Availability

Vitamin D occurs in sufficient quantities naturally in fatty fish, egg yolk, liver and butter. In the United States, most fresh milk, all evaporated milk, and some powdered milk is fortified to a level of 10 μg/quart of product. Margarine, milk flavorings, breakfast cereals, bread, and chocolate bars have varying amounts of

TABLE 7-4. Products* Containing Oleovitamin D, Ergocalciferol, or Cholecalciferol**

Brand	Manufacturer	Content of Unit
Capsules		
Deltalin Gelseals	Lilly	50,000 IU oleovitamin D
Drisdol	Winthrop	1.25 mg (50,000 IU) ergocalciferol
Tablets		
Calciferol	Kremers-Urban	1.25 mg (50,000 IU) ergocalciferol
Oral Liquid		
Drisdol	Winthrop	200 μg (8000 IU)/ml ergocalciferol
Injection		
Vitamin D_2	CMC	12.5 mg (500,000 IU)/ml ergocalciferol

* All of the products listed here require a prescription.

** Oleovitamin D is a solution of vitamin D in fish liver oil or edible vegetable oil. The vitamin is present as ergocalciferol or cholecalciferol obtained by the activation of ergosterol or of 7-dehydrocholesterol from natural sources.

added vitamin D. Chief dietary sources of vitamin D are shown in Table 7-5.

Human skin exposed to sunlight contains about 0.025 μg (1 IU) per square centimeter, with skin on the back reaching levels of 0.375 μg (15 IU) per square centimeter. About 50 to 75% of the activity is found deep in the epidermis, the rest in the corium adjacent to the epidermis. Biosynthesis of vitamin D is diagrammed in Figure 7-4.

Absorption

After synthesis in the skin, cholecalciferol is absorbed in the subepidermal microcirculation and mixes with circulating cholecalciferol and ergocalciferol from dietary sources.

Ingested vitamin D (cholecalciferol and ergocalciferol) is mostly absorbed in the duodenum and jejunum into lymphatic channels, but only in the presence of lipids and bile salts.[5] In healthy humans, vitamin D is almost completely absorbed from food, oily preparations, and aqueous suspensions.[6]

Distribution

Vitamin D enters the blood as chylomicrons of lymph and associates primarily with a specific alpha-globulin vitamin D-binding protein. The vitamin D is sequestered by the liver for biotransformation or stored in depots in adipose tissue and muscle.[7,8]

Metabolism

In the liver, ergocalciferol and cholecalciferol are converted to the 25-hydroxy derivatives (25-OHD_2 and 25-OHD_3) by the enzyme vitamin D 25-hydroxylase. This enzyme system is controlled by feedback inhibition, which does not function efficiently if large doses of vitamin D are ingested.[9–11] Dihydrotachysterol, a biologically inactive sterol, is activated to 25-hydroxydihydrotachysterol. The structures of analogs and metabolites of vitamin D are shown in Figure 7-5.

In the kidneys, 25-OHD is converted by vitamin D 1-hydroxylase, in the presence of molecular oxygen, malate, and magnesium ion, into calcitriol [1, 25-dihydroxycholecalciferol; 1, 25 $(OH)_2D_3$] and 1, 25-dihydroxyergocalciferol [1, 25 $(OH)_2D_2$]. These are the most biologically active metabolites. This system is regulated by circulating levels of the products, by parathyroid hormone, and by serum concentration of calcium and phosphate ions. The metabolism of vitamin D is influenced by cortisol, estrogens, prolactin, and growth hormone.[9,11,12] Some of the 1, 25 $(OH)_2D$ is stored in adipose tissue and muscle, which act as an almost limitless reservoir for vitamin D and its active metabolites.[13]

When circulating levels of the 1, 25-dihydroxy compounds are adequate, they are further hydroxylated in the kidney at position 24, which produces a marked decrease in biologic activity. It is supposed that further degradation is produced by liver microsomal enzymes, although the metabolic products have not been identified.

Excretion

Metabolites are excreted principally in bile and feces. No active metabolites are excreted in urine. After large doses of ergocalciferol, 25-OHD_2 may be excreted in milk. It is not known if calcitriol is excreted in milk.

TABLE 7-5. Chief Dietary Sources of Vitamin D

Food	IU/100 g	Food	IU/100 g	Food	IU/100 g
Butter	8-60	Liver		Mackerel	300-400
Egg	200	calf	10	Salmon, canned	200-800
Herring	1800	pork	40	Tuna, canned	400-1500

Note: With the exception of oily fishes, there are no food sources rich in vitamin D.

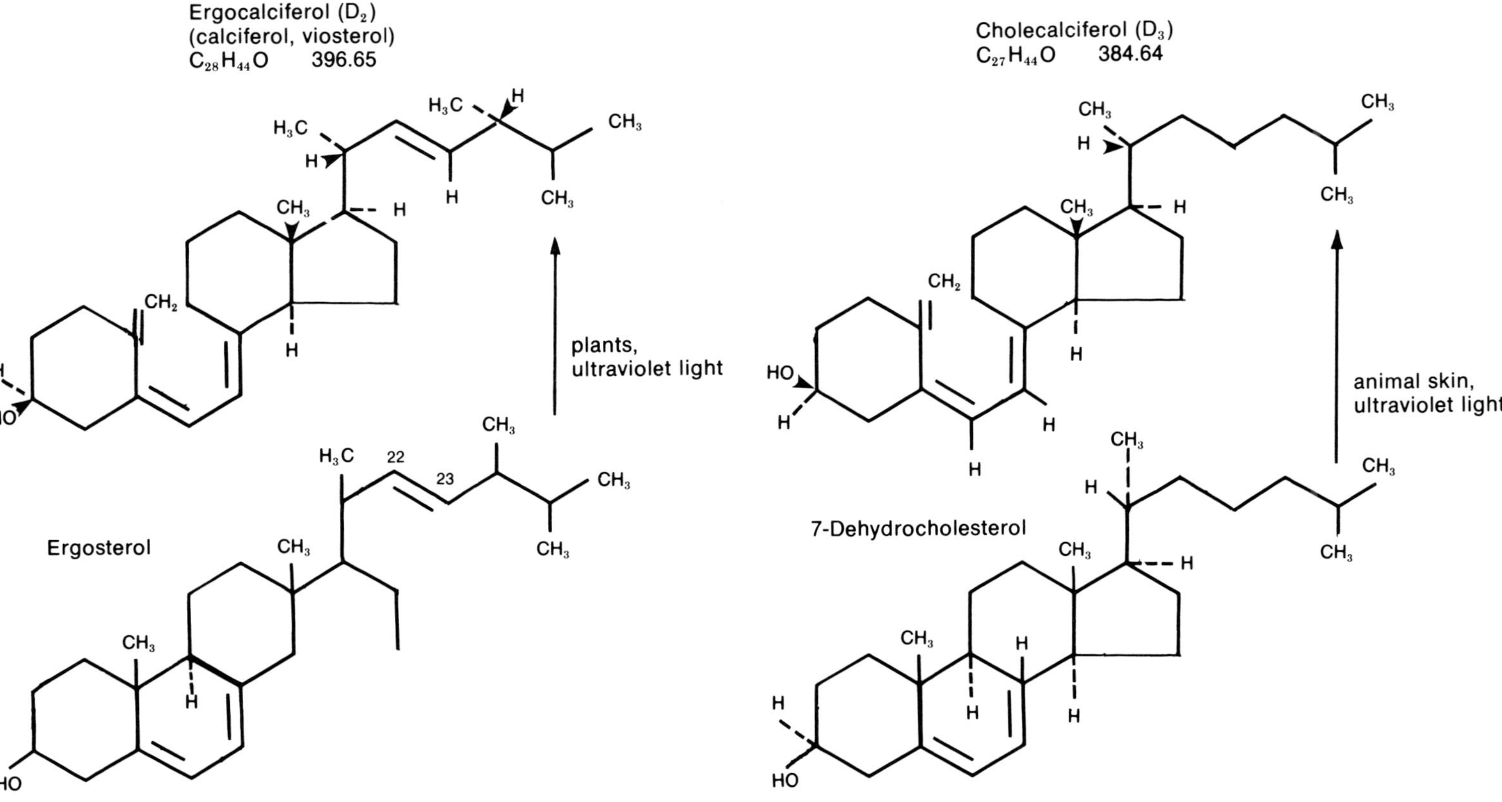

Figure 7-4. Biosynthesis of Vitamin D

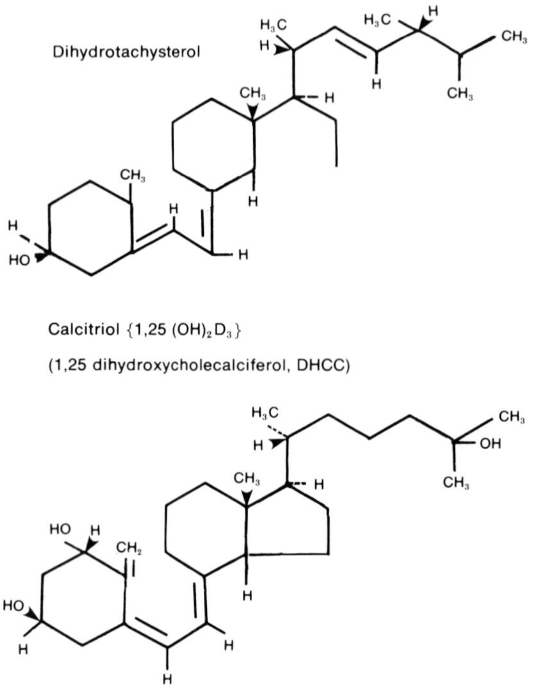

Dihydrotachysterol

Calcitriol {1,25 $(OH)_2D_3$}

(1,25 dihydroxycholecalciferol, DHCC)

Figure 7-5. Analogs and Metabolites of Vitamin D

Normal Laboratory Values

Serum

1. 25-OHD—17 to 23 ng/ml[14]
2. 1, 25 $(OH)_2D$—29 ± 2 pg/ml, adults; 49 to 66 pg/ml, 9 to 18 year olds[15]
3. Vitamin D (colorimetrically with antimony trichloride)
   Children—21 to 52.5 ng/ml
   Adults—17.5 to 77.5 ng/ml

Deficiency

The chief effect of vitamin D deficiency is progressive demineralization of bone and failure of mineralization of new bone, producing weakening of the skeleton. This produces rickets in children and osteomalacia in adults. Vitamin D deficiency may be produced by:

1. Lack of sunlight and vitamin D-deficient diet.
2. Skin hyperpigmentation and vitamin D-deficient diet.
3. Impairment of vitamin D absorption (celiac disease, idiopathic steatorrhea).

In addition to these failures of ingestion and absorption which may be corrected by supplying adequate quantities of the vitamin, there are conditions that resist treatment with vitamin D. These are as follows:

1. Renotubular acidosis.
2. Renal insufficiency.
3. Primary vitamin D resistance (failure to form 1, 25 $(OH)_2D$).
4. Fanconi's syndrome
   a. hypophosphatemia
   b. hypophosphaturia
   c. renal glucosuria
   d. aminoaciduria

RICKETS

1. Characterized chiefly by lack of mineralization at the epiphysis and other rapidly growing bones.
2. Symptoms
   a. delayed closure of fontanelles
   b. craniotabes (softening of skull)
   c. protuberance of forehead
   d. widening of epiphysis (ends of long bones), with disorganization of the epiphyseal disc and formation of a cupped structure instead of the normal straight boundary. Cartilage cells do not degenerate; capillaries cannot penetrate into area
   e. bending of long bones (genu valgum)
   f. thickening of the syncochondroses of the ribs; enlargement of the costochondral junction, forming knobs: "rachitic rosary"
   g. projection of sternum: "pigeon breast"
   h. narrowing of pelvis
   i. kyphosis (spinal curvature)
   j. enlargement of joints (wrist, ankle, knees: "knock knees")
   k. poor muscle development
      (1) delayed walking
      (2) protruding abdomen: "pot belly"
   l. restlessness and nervous irritability
   m. delayed tooth eruption and tooth

malformation with high incidence of cavities

n. occasionally, tetany due to slight lowering of the serum calcium and marked lowering of serum phosphate. There is a rise in serum alkaline phosphatase.

OSTEOMALACIA

1. Frequently associated with fat malabsorption.
2. Symptoms
   a. softening of skeleton, deformity of legs, spine, thorax and pelvis
   b. pain in legs and lower back; may be misdiagnosed as rheumatism
   c. general weakness, particularly in walking; difficulty in climbing stairs and characteristic waddle
   d. spontaneous multiple fracture

POPULATIONS AT RISK

There are few data on recent vitamin D intake in the United States. A report on adults in St. Louis on random diets showed a weekly average of 42.75 μg (1710 IU) or about 6 μg per day, which was in good agreement with serum levels.[10] Various surveys of infants and children show wide variations, with only a minority ingesting approximately at the RDA level, but with most ingesting less than or considerably more than the RDA.[16,17] This wide variation was also seen in Canadian and British surveys. A survey of vitamin D availability (sunlight, food, supplements) to the population of the United States is needed. Definitive evidence of rickets beyond infancy is rare except in heavily pigmented populations and those of low socio-economic levels.

Deficiency symptoms may appear in adults ingesting less than 1.75 μg (75 IU) per day if there is no exposure to sunlight. This may occur in shut-in or immobilized adults, usually women. Premature infants, migratory immigrants, and people on fat-free diets may also be at risk.

DRUG-INDUCED DEFICITS

1. Epileptics treated with phenobarbital and or phenytoin had lowered serum calcium and vitamin D-active metabolite levels and increased incidence of symptoms of vitamin D deficiency.[16–20]
2. Binding of bile acids by cholestyramine resin may interface with vitamin D absorption.[5] Colestipol resin may prevent vitamin D absorption.
3. Large overdoses of mineral oil may prevent vitamin D absorption.
4. Corticosteroids may inhibit conversion to active metabolites.

Toxicity (hypervitaminosis D)

1. Hypercalcemia and accompanying electrolyte abnormalities
   a. Common first symptoms
      (1) weakness
      (2) fatigue
      (3) malaise
      (4) dry mouth
      (5) vague muscle and bone pains
      (6) headache
      (7) metallic or bad taste
   b. gastrointestinal response to hypercalcemia
      (1) nausea
      (2) vomiting
      (3) anorexia
      (4) diarrhea
      (5) weight loss
   c. other responses to hypercalcemia
      (1) thirst
      (2) polyuria
      (3) nocturia
      (4) burning sensation in eyes
      (5) conjunctivitis
      (6) photophobia
      (7) generalized pruritis
      (8) diminished libido
      (9) pancreatitis
      (10) kidney stones
      (11) diminished hearing acuity
      (12) rhinorrhea
      (13) hypertension
      (14) hyperthermia (in children)

(15) hemiplegia (paralysis of one side of the body)
(16) mental retardation
(17) cardiac rhythm abnormalities

2. Indirect effects due to calcification of organs
   a. kidney (nephrocalcinosis)
      (1) renal insufficiency, proteinuria
      (2) azotemia (reversible)
   b. heart
   c. blood vessels (generalized vascular calcification)
3. Osteoporosis (due to mobilization of calcium from bone when calcium intake is inadequate).

Note: Deaths from cardiovascular or renal failure have been reported.

TOXIC INTAKES

1. Patients with clinical disorders, particularly sarcoidosis may be unusually sensitive to small doses.[21] Sarcoidosis is the presence of granulomas in lymph nodes, skin, lungs, and long bones. The cause is unknown.
2. Self-medication with vitamin supplements may produce kidney stones in adults at levels as low as 27.5 μg (1100 IU) per day.[22]
3. Excessive calcium intakes (more than 1 g per day) may give same symptoms as vitamin D toxicity.[23]
4. Wide range of individual susceptibility to toxicity.

Acute

1. At 2500 μg (100,000 IU) per day about 20% of persons develop hypercalcemia.[24]
2. Data indicating high levels of ingestion before production of toxic symptoms have generally been obtained from patients treated with vitamin D or its active metabolites for clinical disorders such as hypoparathyroidism, primary vitamin D resistance, renal disease, and chronic liver disease, all of which reduce absorption or utilization of vitamin D. These reported levels are many times higher than those for normal, healthy people.

Chronic

1. Above 50 μg (2000 IU) per day for long periods
   a. hypercalcemia in infants
   b. nephrocalcinosis in infants and adults
2. 45 to 158 μg (1800 to 6300 IU) per day in children may inhibit linear growth.[25]
3. It appears that for adults, chronic ingestion of vitamin D of greater than 25 μg (1000 IU) per day may be toxic and contribute to the formation of kidney stones and myocardial infarction.

PREGNANCY

In pregnancy, the safety of doses above 10 μg (400 IU) per day has not been established. Animal studies have shown fetal abnormalities associated with hypervitaminosis D for several species.

DRUG-INDUCED

Concurrent administration of thiazide diuretics with therapeutic doses of vitamin D or analogs may produce hypercalcemia and hypoparathyroidism.

TREATMENT

1. Withdrawal of vitamin D.
2. Low calcium diet.
3. Large fluid intake.
4. Acidification of urine.

In acute hypercalcemic crisis (dehydration, stupor, coma, azotemia), the following are indicated:

1. Hydration with intravenous saline may increase calcium excretion.
2. Diuretics acting on the renal loop (furosemide, ethacrinic acid) increase calcium excretion.
3. Citrates, sulfates, phosphates, corticosteroids, edetate (EDTA), and mithramycin increase calcium excretion.
4. Hemodialysis.

Because of storage of vitamin D and its active metabolites, hypercalcemia following chronic administration can persist for more than 2 weeks. After the hypercalcemia is corrected, dosage at a lower level should be started.

Uses in Therapy

Note that the range between a therapeutic dose and a toxic dose of vitamin D is very narrow. Adequate dietary calcium is necessary for response to therapy.

1. Vitamin D-resistant rickets:
   300 to 2500 μg (12,000 to 1,000,000 IU) per day. Readjust downward as soon as there is clinical improvement. Individualize dose, follow with frequent determination of serum and urine calcium, potassium, and urea.
2. Hypoparathyroidism:
   1250 to 5000 μg (50,000 to 200,000 IU) plus 4 g of calcium lactate 6 times a day. Parathyroid hormone and/or dihydrotachysterol may be required. Individualize dose by keeping blood calcium concentration between 9 and 10 mg/dl. Determine serum calcium, phosphrous, and urea at least every 2 weeks. Long bones should be radiographed monthly until condition is stable.

To prevent metastic calcification, patients with hyperphosphatemia should have serum phosphate levels normalized by dietary restriction of phosphate intake and/or administration of aluminum hydroxide gels to bind intestinal phosphate.

3. Some patients with hypocalcemia who are on chronic renal dialysis have shown reduction of elevated parathyroid hormone levels when treated with calcitriol (available as Rocaltrol, Roche, in capsules containing 0.25 μg and 0.5 μg).

   Since calcitriol is the most potent of the vitamin D metabolites, vitamin D from other sources should be eliminated and the patient carefully monitored (at least twice weekly initially, then weekly for 12 weeks, then monthly, if stabilized) to maintain serum calcium levels between 9 and 10 mg/dl and the calcium times phosphate product below 70. Dosage is usually once a day, with some patients requiring 0.25 μg only every other day. The usual dose is 0.5 to 1 μg per day.

   The drug has been used investigationally as follows:
   a. children undergoing hemodialysis: 0.25 to 2 μg per day
   b. children with renal failure not undergoing hemodialysis: 14 to 41 ng/kg per day
   c. hypoparathyroidism and pseudohypoparathyroidism:
      adults—0.25 to 2.7 μg per day
      children—40 to 80 ng/kg per day
   d. vitamin D-dependent rickets:
      children and a few adults—1μg per day
      adults resistant to therapy—12 to 17 μg per day
   e. familial hypophosphatemia (vitamin D-resistant rickets): 2.1 μg per day plus oral phosphate
   f. hypocalcemia in premature infants: 1 μg per day for 5 days. For hypocalcemic tetany, 50 ng/kg per day intravenously for 5 to 12 days.
4. Dihydrotachysterol, a vitamin D analog, is used in the treatment of hypocalcemia associated with hypoparathyroidism and familial hypophosphatemia. It is available as Hytakerol, Winthrop, in capsules containing 125 μg/ml and as an oral solution in sesame oil containing 250 μg/ml. Tablets are available containing 125 μg, 200 μg and 400 μg. These should be stored in light-resistant containers below 8°C. Capsules, tablets, and solutions are also available as generics.

   Dihydrotachysterol has weak antirachitic properties, but after bioactivation, it may be more effective than vitamin D in mobilizing calcium from bone and increasing serum calcium levels. Thus, 1 mg of dihydrotachysterol is equivalent to 3 mg (120,000 IU) of ergocalciferol.

It is used in treatment of hypoparathyroidism or pseudohypoparathyroidism at the following dosages:

Adults—0.75 to 2.5 mg per day for several days *or* a loading dose of 4 times the selected maintenance dose for 2 days, followed by twice the selected maintenance dose for an additional 2 days. (This loading increases chances of toxicity.)

Maintenance dose is usually 0.2 to 1.0 mg per day, with some patients requiring up to 1.5 mg per day.

Children—Initial loading with 1 to 15 mg for 4 days. The maintenance dose is 0.5 to 1.5 mg day.

As usual, treatment should be supplemented with oral calcium and/or parathyroid hormone intramuscularly or intravenously.

Investigationally, dihydrotachysterol has been used as follows:

1. Familial hypophosphatemia (vitamin D-resistant rickets):
   Adults and children—0.5 to 2.0 mg per day until healing of bones is demonstrated, then maintenance at 0.2 to 1.5 mg per day accompanied by oral administration of phosphates.
2. Prophylaxis of hypocalcemic tetany after thyroid surgery: 0.25 mg per day plus calcium supplements until danger of tetany has passed.
3. Renal osteodystrophy and hyperparathyroidism associated with kidney failure:
   Children and adolescents—0.1 to 0.6 mg per day.
4. Osteoporosis: 0.6 mg per day with calcium and fluoride supplements.

In 1980, calcifediol (25-hydroxycholecalciferol) was marketed as Calderol, by Upjohn. It is recommended for treatment of metabolic bone disease associated with renal dialysis in chronic renal failure. It has a longer duration of action and lower potency than calcitriol, as might be expected from the metabolic conversion of cholecalciferol to calcifediol which, in turn, is converted to calcitriol. The lower potency may allow better control of plasma calcium levels than is possible with calcitriol. The dose is usually 50 to 100 μg per day or 100 to 200 μg on alternate days, with some patients responsive to as little as 20 μg every other day. Cautions and side effects are similar to those for calcitriol. Calderol is available in 20 or 50 μg capsules.

Interference with Laboratory Tests

Vitamin D may give a false increase in serum cholesterol determined by the Zlatkis-Zak reaction.

REFERENCES—Vitamin D

1. Cousins, R.J., and DeLuca, H.F.: Vitamin D and Bone, *In* Biochemistry and Physiology of Bone, 2nd Ed. Vol. II. G.H. Bourne, ed. New York, Academic Press, 1972.
2. Loomis, W.F.: Science, *157;*501, 1967.
3. Lapatsanis, P., Deliyanni, V., and Doxiadis, S.: J. Pediatr., *73:*195, 1968.
4. Kumar, R., et al.: J. Clin. Invest., *63:*342, 1979.
5. Thompson, G.R., Ockner, R.K., and Isselbacher, K.J.: J. Clin. Invest., *48:*87, 1969.
6. Committee on Nutrition: Pediatrics, *31:*512, 1963.
7. Rosenstreich, S.J., Rich, C., and Volwiler, W.: J. Clin. Invest., *50:*679, 1971.
8. Mawer E.B., and Schaefer, K.: Biochem. J., *114:*74P, 1969.
9. Avioli, L.V., and Haddad, J.G.: Metabolism, *22:*507, 1973.
10. Haddad, J.G., and Stamp, T.C.B.: Am. J. Med., *57:*57, 1974.
11. Gray, R., Boyle, I., and DeLuca, H.F.: Science, *172:*1232, 1971.
12. DeLuca, H.F.: N. Engl. J. Med., *287:*250, 1972.
13. Haddad, J.G., Jr., and Birge, S.J.: Biochem. Biophys. Res. Commun., *45:*829, 1971.
14. Haddad, J.G., and Chyu, K.J.: J. Clin. Endocrinol. Metab., *33:*992, 1971.
15. Eisman, J.A., et al.: Science, *193:*1021, 1976.
16. Hahn, T.J., et al.: N. Engl. J. Med., *287:*900, 1972.
17. Hahn, T.J., et al.: N. Engl. J. Med., *292:*550, 1975.
18. Dent, C.E., et al.: Br. Med. J., *4:*69, 1970.
19. Richens, A., and Rowe, D.J.F.: Br. Med J., *4:*73, 1970.
20. Sotaniemi, E.A., et al.: Ann. Intern. Med., *77:*389, 1972. Science, *193:*1021, 1976.
21. Harrell, G.T., and Fisher, S.: J. Clin. Invest., *18:*687, 1939.
22. Taylor, W.H.: Clin. Sci., *42:*515, 1972.
23. Bauer, W., Marble, A., and Claflin, D.: J. Clin Invest., *11:*47, 1932.
24. Hess, A.F., and Lewis, J.M.: JAMA, *91:*783, 1928.
25. Jeans, P.C., and Stearns, G.: J. Pediatr., *13:*730, 1938.

VITAMIN E

The original international standard for Vitamin E, dl-alpha-tocopheryl acetate (1 asymmetric carbon atom at 2) is no longer available. The international unit (IU) was the activity of 1 mg of that compound. The commercially available dl-alpha-tocopheryl acetate (all-racemic) has three asymmetric carbon atoms (at 2, 4 and 8) and is assumed to have the same biologic activity as the original international standard. Synthetic dl-alpha-tocopherol has a potency of 1.1 IU/mg. The naturally occurring d-alpha-tocopherol (RRR-alpha-tocopherol) has a potency of 1.49 IU/mg.

For labeling, the USP unit is numerically equivalent to the IU. Only alpha-tocopherols are recognized as sources of vitamin E for vitamin E supplements for humans. The equivalents are as follows:

1 mg dl-alpha-tocopheryl acetate = 1 USP unit

1 mg dl-alpha-tocopheryl acid succinate = 0.89 USP unit

1 mg dl-alpha-tocopherol = 1.1 USP unit

1 mg dl-alpha-tocopheryl acetate = 1.36 USP unit

1 mg d-alpha-tocopherol = 1.49 USP units.

1 mg d-alpha-tocopheryl acid succinate = 1.21 USP units

The USP states that the d and dl forms of alpha tocopherol and its esters shall not be present in the same preparation except as a consequence of the dilution of a dl form with a suitable vehicle which may contain some d form.

For mixed diets in the United States, the d-alpha-tocopherol equivalents are calculated by the formula: mg d-alpha tocopherol + 0.5 (mg beta-tocopherol) + 0.1 (mg gamma-tocopherol) + 0.3 (mg alpha-tocotrienol).

If only the alpha-tocopherol content of a food is reported, the value should be multiplied by 1.2 to obtain the total alpha-tocopherol equivalents to account for the biologic activity of the other isomers that are present. The structures and activities of vitamin E are shown in Figure 7-6.

Recommended Dietary Allowances

Since there is no clinical or biochemical evidence that normal people eating balanced diets in the United States have suboptimum levels of the vitamin, the dietary level is considered adequate.[1,2] Note, however, that the requirement of vitamin E by body tissue is related to the polyunsaturated fatty acid (PUFA) content of the cells. Thus, the requirements for vitamin E may be higher if the diet contains much more PUFA than usual. Fortunately, in the United States, foods high in PUFA are also high in vitamin E. Diets in the United States have a ratio of mg-d-alpha-tocopherol equivalents: g PUFA of 0.4[1,3] and this ratio has been found satisfactory in infant diets.[4] The chief dietary sources of vitamin E are shown on Table 7-6.

Adults: The dietary intake should be enough to maintain blood concentration of total tocopherols above 0.5 mg/dl. The dietary range that supplies this amount is 7 to 13 mg (10 to 20 IU) of d-alpha-tocopherol equivalents in diets supplying 1800 to 3000 kcal. Some high-fat diets contain more.

Recommended: 10 mg equivalents (15 IU) of d-alpha-tocopherol.

Pregnancy and Lactation: About 2 to 3 mg equivalents extra are needed to supply fetal needs and to compensate for vitamin E secreted in milk. This is normally provided by the increased calorie intake.

Recommended: In pregnancy, an additional 2 mg equivalents (3 IU); during lactation, an additional 3 mg equivalents (4.5 IU).

Infants: Breast-fed infants of normal weight show a steady rise in tocopherol blood levels from birth, reaching the adult level in about 2 weeks. The 1.3 to 3.3 mg/L of d-alpha-tocopherol equivalents in human milk is considered adequate. Intakes in that range should be provided to infants on other diets until they weigh about 9 kg (about 1 year old).

Low-birth-weight infants are a spe-

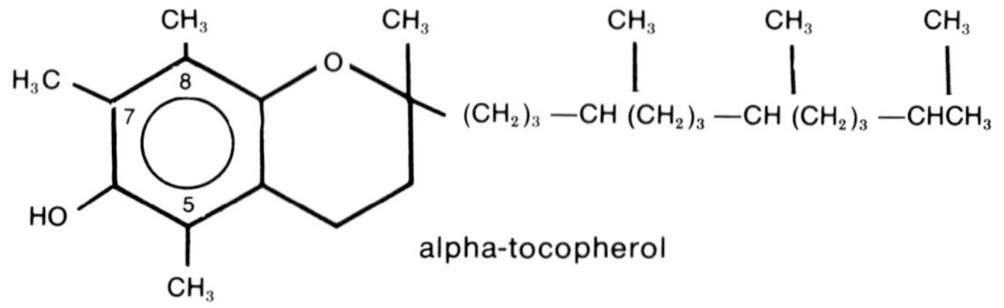

beta = 5,8 diMe, 7 H
gamma = 7,8 diMe, 5 H
delta = 8 Me, 5,7 diH

alpha-tocopherol

	Relative Activity*
alpha	100
beta	33
gamma	10
delta	1

* Antisterility in female mice; only alpha form seems active in humans.

Figure 7-6. Vitamin E Structures and Activities

cial problem. Because of reduced fat absorption, tocopherol absorption is impaired. To provide adequate intakes, the Committee on Nutrition of the American Academy of Pediatrics recommends that formulas for these infants provide 0.7 IU/100 kcal and at least 1.0 IU/g of linoleic acid, plus an oral supplement of 5 IU of water-solubilized alpha-tocopherol per day.[5]

Recommended: Birth to 6 months, 3 mg equivalents (4.5 IU); 6 months to 1 year, 4 mg equivalents (6 IU).

Children: It is assumed that requirements increase with body weight until maturity. Thus, the recommendation is from 3.3 mg equivalents (5 IU) at 1 year (9kg) to 8 mg equivalents (12 IU) at 14 years (40 kg). This is deemed satisfactory for a diet containing linoleic acid as 4 to 7% of calories.

Absorption

Tocopherols are readily destroyed in the digestive tract. The esters, as used in commercial preparations, are stable. The esters are hydrolyzed in the intestinal wall and the free alcohol is absorbed.

Absorption in the gastrointestinal tract depends on the presence of bile and fat. As the dose of vitamin E increases, the fraction absorbed decreases, so that only 20 to 60% of the dietary intake is absorbed. For a dose of 1 mg, absorption varied between 55 and

TABLE 7-6. Chief Dietary Sources of Vitamin E*

Food	IU. alpha-tocopherol/100 g
Oil	
coconut	3.6
cottonseed	56
peanut	11
soybean	10
Margarine	28
Oatmeal	2
Sweet potato	4
Brown rice	1.2
Turnip greens	2.25

* Vitamin E is not present in appreciable amounts in foods of animal origin. The vitamin is widespread in vegetables, with its chief source in nuts, dark green leafy vegetables, and beans. Other sources include: apples, bacon, bananas, beef, carrots, celery, cornmeal, eggs, grapefruit, haddock, lamb, onions, oranges, pork, tomatoes.

78%.[6] In patients with obstructive jaundice and steatorrhea, absorption was between 6 and 16%. In chronic pancreatic insufficiency with malabsorption, values were 32 to 39%. In adults with celiac disease, absorption was 23 to 58%, with significant correlation between absorption and steatorrhea. In two cases of intestinal lymphangiectasis (dilation of lymphatic vessels), absorption was 29%, even though absorption of fat was over 85%.

For absorption of supplements, better results were obtained in premature infants with d-alpha-tocopheryl polyethylene glycol 1000 succinate (TPEGS) than with alpha-tocopheryl acetate.[7] Addition of bile salts or emulsification with Tween 80 did not affect absorption in a patient with xanthomatous biliary cirrhosis.[8] In children and adults with cystic fibrosis, best absorption was obtained with alpha-tocopheryl-polyethylene glycol 1000 succinate in combination with pancreatic enzymes.[9]

After splitting of the esters by pancreatic enzymes, vitamin E reaches the circulation in lymph chylomicrons and then is transported in association with beta-lipoproteins.

Distribution

Vitamin E is distributed to all tissues and stored in adipose tissue. Total body stores are estimated at 3 to 8 g in the adult, representing a supply of more than 4 years' needs.

Placental transfer of vitamin E is poor. Newborns have levels of 20 to 30% of the maternal values. Plasma levels of vitamin E correlate poorly with vitamin E nutritional status or body stores. Vitamin E deficiency is defined as levels below 5 μg/ml of plasma or 800 μg/g of plasma lipids.

After ingestion of a large dose, serum levels of vitamin E peak in 5 to 9 hours, then fall exponentially with a half-life of 53 hours.[10] Several investigators using varying doses have found peak levels 4 hours after administration in healthy adults, others confirm 6 to 9 hours.[11,12] In general, the fraction of the dose absorbed decreased with increasing dose. In patients with severe deficiency, plasma levels were unaffected even when a substantial percentage of the dose was absorbed.[13]

Metabolism

Vitamin E is metabolized in the liver to tocopheronic acid glucuronide.

Excretion

Vitamin E metabolites are excreted primarily in bile. Small amounts are excreted in the urine. Human milk contains 2 to 5 IU/L.

Pharmacology

The exact biologic function of vitamin E in humans is not known. It is thought to be an antioxidant which protects polyunsaturated fatty acids in the cell membranes and other oxygen-sensitive substance (vitamin A, vitamin C) from oxidation. This is supported by the finding that symptoms of vitamin E deficiency in animals are prevented by ubiquinone, selenium, chemical antioxidants, and some sulfhydryl amino acids.

Deficiency

Signs of vitamin E deficiency are not very marked in humans. the following conditions are associated with severe deficiency.[14]

1. Widespread deposition of oxidized lipids (ceroid pigments).
2. Creatinuria.
3. Intolerance of the erythrocyte lipid membrane to oxidants (increased hemolysis rate in vivo).

SYMPTOMS

Deficiencies of vitamin E in animals cause a bewildering array of symptoms, depending on species, age, and nutritional state. These include the following:

1. Impaired reproduction and resorption of the fetus (rats, mice, guinea pigs).
2. Muscular dystrophy, usually with creatinuria (monkeys, mice, others).
3. Formation of ceroid pigments (monkeys, mice, pigs).

4. Increased in vitro red cell hemolysis (rats, chickens).
5. Liver necrosis (rats).

The reproductive symptoms in rats are used in the advertising of vitamin E for humans.

POPULATIONS AT RISK

Plasma concentrations in the normal newborn are about one third those of adults. In low-birth-weight (LBW) infants the plasma level is less than one third of the adult level, due either to the lowered plasma lipid level in LBW infants or the inefficient transfer of vitamin E to the placenta. Within a few days following birth, plasma lipid and vitamin E levels rise. The rise is more rapid in breast-fed infants (2 weeks to adult levels) than in those who are formula fed (4 weeks to adult levels).

In some studies, low-birth-weight infants fed commercial formula made with polyunsaturated fat and low vitamin E content have shown edema and anemia attributed to vitamin E deficiency. New FDA regulations (January, 1981) prevent marketing of incorrectly formulated products.[15,16]

One study showed that mothers with low plasma vitamin E levels (below 0.7 mg/dl) had infants with very low plasma vitamin E. Supplementation for these mothers in the last trimester of pregnancy was recommended.[17]

There is a risk of deficiency in people who have conditions that interfere with fat absorption and, hence, absorption of fat-soluble vitamins, such as in chronic obstructive jaundice, prolonged steatorrhea, cirrhosis of the liver and a-beta-lipoproteinemia.[14]

Toxicity

Vitamin E has very low toxicity. Unpublished data by R.M. Salkeld in the FDA OTC, Volume 150121, showed that doses of 3000 IU/day for 11 years and doses of 55,000 IU/day for a few months had no detrimental clinical or biochemical effects. There were complaints of gastrointestinal symptoms in about 8% of those at the higher dosage. There have been rare reports of other toxic symptoms. These include the following:

1. Creatinuria (at 2 to 4 g per day for several months)[18]
2. Nausea, diarrhea, cramps
3. Fatigue, weakness
4. Headache, blurred vision
5. Rash
6. Contact dermatitis (topical application)
7. Gonadal dysfunction
8. Increase in serum levels of creatine kinase, cholesterol, and triglycerides
9. Increase in urinary estrogens and androgens
10. Decreased serum thyroxine and triiodothyronine
11. Thrombophlebitis[19]

On the basis of animal studies,[20] caution in chronic ingestion of large doses is urged because of the possibility of reduction of vitamin A levels.

Megavitamin doses (1800 IU per day for 4 weeks) showed, in healthy college students, no subjective muscular disorders, gastrointestinal disorder, or effects on work performance or sexuality. Objectively, there were no effects on serum cholesterol, prothrombin time, serum creatinine phosphokinase, or total leukocyte count.

Megavitamin doses caused an increase in serum triglycerides in females, especially those taking oral contraceptives, and a reduction in serum thyroxine and triiodothyronine, except in females taking oral contraceptives.[21]

There is one report of 50 persons with thrombophlebitis, most of whom were taking more than 400 IU per day. The symptoms disappeared when vitamin E was discontinued and conventional therapy for thrombophlebitis was instituted.[19]

Uses in Therapy

The only indications for therapy are to raise low plasma levels to normal and to reduce in vitro peroxide erythrocyte hemolysis to normal. Doses must be individualized

TABLE 7-7. Vitamin E Products

	Brand	Manufacturer	Content, IU	Form*
*Injections***	Generic	Various	200/ml	—
	E-Ferol	O'Neal, Jones & Feldman	200/ml	2
Drops	Aquasol E	USV	50/ml	2
Capsules	Generic	Various	100, 200, 400 600, 800, 1000	—
	Aquasol E	USV	30, 100, 400	1
	Eprolin Gelseals	Lilly	50, 100	2
	Viterra E	Pfipharmecs	100, 200, 400, 600	2
	CEN-E	Century	100, 200, 400	1
	Epsilan-M	Adria	100	1
	Tocopher Caps	Columbia	100	1
	Tokols-100	Ulmer	100	1
	EGo	Coastal	200	2
	D'Alpha-E	Alto	200	1
	Pheryl-E	Miller	100	3
	E-Ferol Succinate	O'Neal, Jones & Feldman	200, 400	3
	Dalfatol	Tutag	400	1
	E-Ferol Acetate	O'Neal, Jones & Feldman	400	1
	Tokols-400	Ulmer	400	1
	Vita-Plus E	Scot-Tussin	400	1
	Tocopher M	Columbia	1000	4
Chewable Tablets	Generic	Various	100, 200	—
	Vitamin E	Squibb	200, 400	2
	Chew-E	North American	200	2
Tablets	Pheryl-E	Miller	100, 400	3

* Forms: 1. d-alpha-tocopheryl acetate 2. dl-alpha-tocopheryl acetate 3. dl-alpha-tocopheryl succinate 4. mixed tocopheryls concentrate
** Prescription only.

and are in the range of 10 to more than 400 IU per day. Vitamin E products are listed in Table 7-7.

INADEQUATELY SUBSTANTIATED THERAPIES

Many claims of subjective benefit of vitamin E therapy have been made for a wide variety of conditions. These claims of benefit have been denied by objective evaluation.[22–27] The conditions in which vitamin E has been claimed to have an effect include:

1. Improved human fertility.[28,29]
2. Cardiovascular disease.[30,31]
3. Dupuytren's contracture (marked contraction of the hand marked by flexion of the third and fourth digit on the palm, chiefly afflicting adult males).
4. Peyronie's Disease (induration of the corpus cavernosa and hardening of the erectile tissue around the clitoris or penis).[32,33]
5. Relief of leg cramps.[34]
6. Porphyria.[35]
7. Anemia of protein-calorie malnutrition.[36]
8. Anemia of low-birth-weight infant.[15,37]
9. Increased pulmonary resistance to photochemical smog.[38]
10. Prevention of retrolental fibroplasia in infants being given oxygen.
11. Prevention of bronchopulmonary dysplasia in infants.
12. Treatment of beta-thalassemia.
13. Treatment of sickle cell anemia.
14. Habitual abortion.
15. Peptic ulcer.
16. Burns.
17. Neuritis.
18. Chronic progressive hereditary (Huntington's) chorea.

19. Chronic cystic mastitis.
20. Cancer prevention.
21. Increased physical endurance.
22. Menopausal syndrome.

Because of its low toxicity, vitamin E does no apparent harm except to deny use of more vigorous measures. It is unfortunate, however, that this lack of toxicity allows for exaggerated and unproven claims of benefit.

Nutrient Interactions

1. Dietary requirement for vitamin E increases when the intake of polyunsaturated fats increases.[10]
2. Vitamin E seems to increase the absorption, lymphatic transport, and storage of vitamin A and may also stabilize vitamin A in cell membranes. Thus, it may counter hypervitaminosis A. While small doses enhance carotene utilization (in rats), larger doses reduce conversion and storage of vitamin A from carotene.[20,39,40]
3. Red blood cell fragility to hydrogen peroxide was increased in children with vitamin E sufficiency but with iron deficiency anemia. This sensitivity was increased on treatment with iron dextran. The rise could be prevented by administering vitamin E with iron.[41] Thus, low-birth-weight (LBW) infants treated with iron for iron deficiency anemia may develop hemolytic anemia unless the iron is accompanied by vitamin E, although this has been disputed.[30]

Drug Interactions

1. Vitamin E or its metabolites may have anti-vitamin K effects. Patients receiving anticoagulants may be at risk in hemorrhage following large doses of vitamin E. (Note that large doses of vitamin E do not affect blood clotting in normal people). The effect was due to a decline of vitamin K-dependent coagulation factors II, VII, IX, and X.[10]

REFERENCES—Vitamin E

1. Bieri, J.G., and Evarts, R.P.: J. Am. Diet. Assoc., *62:*147, 1973.
2. Underwood, B.A., et al.: Am. J. Clin. Nutr., *23:*1314, 1970.
3. Witting, L.A., and Lee, L.: Am. J. Clin. Nutr., *28:*571, 1975.
4. Lewis, J.S., et al.: Am. J. Clin. Nutr., *26:*136, 1973.
5. Committee on Nutrition, American Academy of Pediatrics: Pediatrics, *60:*519, 1977.
6. MacMahon, M.T., and Neale, G.: Clin. Sci., *38:*197, 1970.
7. Melhorn, D.K., and Gross, S.: Pediatr. Res., *7:* 404, Abstract 176, 1973.
8. Woodruff, C.W.: Am. J. Clin. Nutr., *4:*597, 1956.
9. Melhorn, D.K.: RI Med. J., *57:*100, 1974.
10. Corrigan, J.H., Jr., and Marcus, F.I.: JAMA, *230:*1300, 1974.
11. Goldbloom, R.B.: Pediatrics, *32*,36, 1963.
12. Hashim, S.A., and Schuttringer, G.R.: Am. J. Clin. Nutr., *19:*137, 1966.
13. Kelleher, J., and Losowsky, M.S.: Biochem J., *110:*20P, 1969.
14. Binder, H.J., et al.: N. Engl. J. Med., *273:*1289, 1965.
15. Ritchie, J.H., et al.: N. Engl. J. Med. *279:*1185, 1968.
16. Panos, T.C., et al.: Am. J. Clin. Nutr., *21:*15, 1968.
17. Tancredi, P., et al.: Pediatria (Napoli), *76:*571, 1968 (in Italian).
18. Briggs, M.H.: Lancet, *1:*220, 1974.
19. Roberts, H.J.: Angiology, *30:*169, 1979.
20. Bieri, J.G.: Am. J. Clin. Nutr., *26:*382, 1973.
21. Tsai, A.C., et al.: Am. J. Clin. Nutr., *31:*831, 1978.
22. Committee on Nutritional Misinformation: Supplementation of Human Diets With Vitamin E. Washington, DC, National Academy of Sciences, 1973.
23. Olson, R.E.: Circulation, *48:*179, 1973.
24. Baker, S.J., Pereira, S.M., and Begum, A.: Blood, *32:*717, 1968.
25. Lovric, V.A., et al.: J. Pediatr., *72:*431, 1968.
26. Watson, C.J., Bossenmaier, I., Cardinal, R.: Arch. Intern Med., *131:*698, 1973.
27. Byström, J., et al.: J. Plast. Reconstr. Surg., *7:*137, 1973.
28. Swyer, G.I.M.: Br. J. Nutr., *3:*100, 1949.
29. Williams, H.T.G., Fenna, D., and Macbeth, R.A.: Surg. Gynecol. Obstet., *132:*662, 1971.
30. Asfour, R.Y., and Firzli, S.: Am. J. Clin Nutr., *17:*158, 1965.
31. Hodges, R.E.: Drug Therapy, *3:*101, 1973.
32. Horton, C.E., and Devine, C.J, Jr.: Plast. Reconstr. Surg., *52:*503, 1973.
33. Devine, C.J., and Horton, C.E.: J. Urology, *111:* 44, 1974.
34. Ayres, S., Jr., and Mihan, R.: Cal. Med., *111:*87, 1969.
35. Nair, P.P., et al.: Arch. Intern. Med., *128:*411, 1971.
36. Darby, W.J.: Vitam. Horm., *26:*685, 1968.
37. Oski, F.A., and Barness, L.A.: Am. J. Clin. Nutr., *21:*45, 1968.
38. Mustafa, M.G.: Nutr. Rpts. Intern, *11:*473, 1975.

39. Weigelt, T.O., and Maehder, K.: Tierärzliche Umschau, *28*:348, 1978.
40. McCuaig, L.W., and Motzok, I.: Poultry Science, *49*:1050, 1970.
41. Melhorn, D.K., and Gross, S.: J. Lab. Clin. Med., *74*:789, 1969.

VITAMIN K

Two classes of substances with vitamin K activity occur naturally. These are phytonadione (K_1, phylloquinone, or 2-methyl-3-phytyl-1,4 naphthoquinone) in green plants and menaquinones (K_2) in bacteria and animals. Menaquinones are designated by the number of isoprene units attached to the carbon atom at position 3 of the naphthoquinone ring. The naturally occurring substances range from menaquinone-6 to menaquinone-13. Another method of designating menaquinones is as K_2 followed by the number of carbon atoms at position 3 in parentheses. Thus menaquinone-6 is also K_2(30).

Naphthoquinone derivatives with vitamin K activity have been synthesized. These are a provitamin K, menadione (K_3 2-methyl-1,4 naphthoquinone), which requires introduction of a side chain at position 3 for activation, and a vitamin K analog, menadiol sodium diphosphate (K_4). Structures associated with vitamin K activity are shown in Figure 7-7.

Safe and Adequate Intake

Vitamin K is synthesized by intestinal flora in normal people and is variably absorbed. Estimated total needs are about 2 μg/kg.[1] Because of the uncertainty of intestinal synthesis and absorption of vitamin K, there is no RDA. An estimate of the range of dietary intakes considered to be adequate is given in Table 1-3. For adults, the lower level of the range is based on an assumption that one half is provided by diet. The upper level assumes that all the requirements will be provided by the diet. For infants, it was assumed that there was no contribution from intestinal flora. The recommendation of 12 μg/day is in the range provided by human milk (15 μg/L).

Chemistry

Vitamin K is stable to heat and reducing agents. It is decomposed by alkali, strong acids, oxidizing agents, and light. Its pharmaceutical preparations should be protected from light.

Absorption

Phytonadione and menaquinones are absorbed from the gastrointestinal tract only in the presence of bile. The substances are transported in the lymph. Absorption is poor and variable, ranging from 10 to 15%.[1] Some of the vitamin K is transformed by intestinal bacteria into menadione, which can be absorbed in the absence of bile salts.

Distribution

Vitamin K is not stored in the tissues. After large doses, accumulations are found in the liver and spleen[2] for a short time.

Vitamin K does cross the placental barrier, but apparently with increasing difficulty as pregnancy advances. There seems to be little transfer to the infant when it is close to term.

Metabolism

All forms of vitamin K are converted into a single form, having 20 isoprenoid carbons at position 3.[3] Little is known about its metabolism or storage, except that tissue concentrations are low and there are no major storage sites.[4]

Excretion

Little is known about vitamin K excretion; but after administration of radioactive vitamin K to rats, radioactivity was found in the urine and bile.[5,6]

Laboratory Values

1. Partial Thromboplastin Time (activated) (Prothrombin Consumption Time):
   Normal Adult—more than 30 seconds (25 to 37 seconds)
   Abnormal—less than 20 seconds
   Hemophilia—14 to 15 seconds

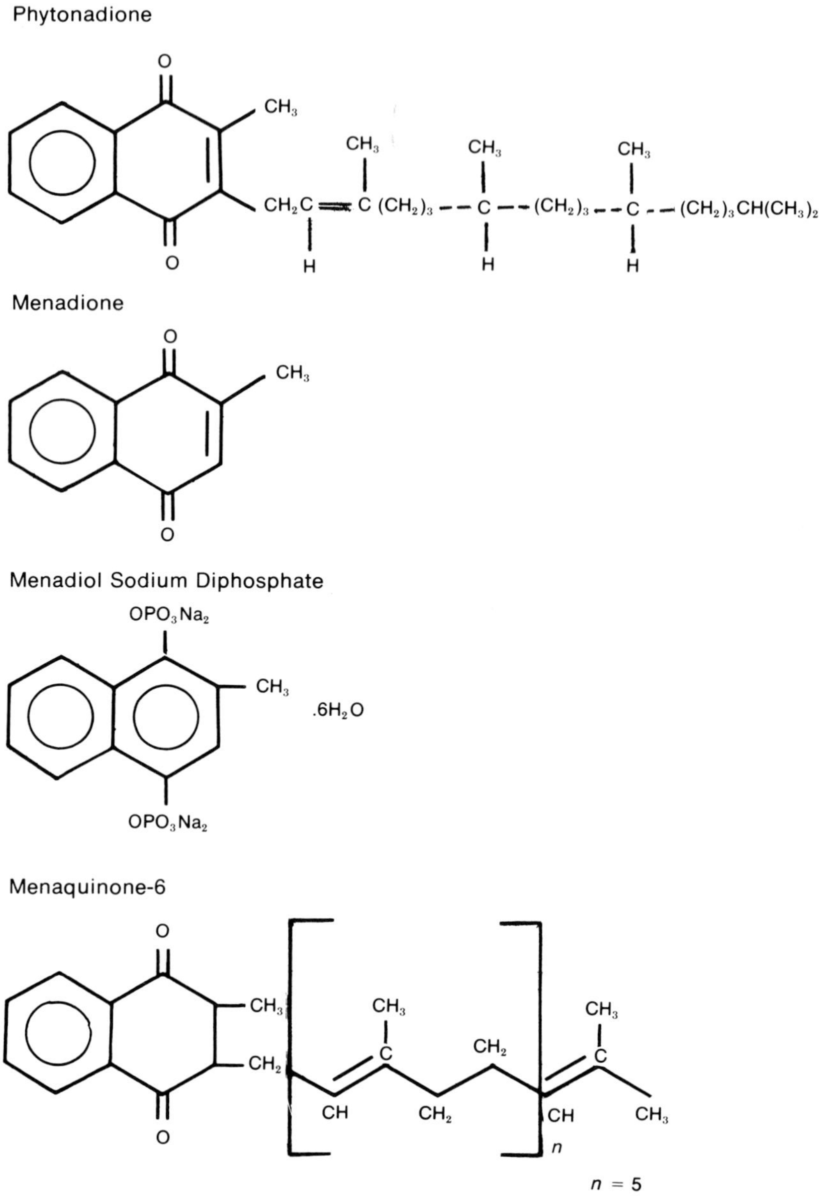

Phytonadione

Menadione

Menadiol Sodium Diphosphate

Menaquinone-6

$n = 5$

Figure 7-7. Structures Associated with Vitamin K Activity

Note that *coagulation time* usually remains normal until the thromboplastin time falls below 20 seconds.

2. Prothrombin:
   Normal Adults—60 to 140 mg/dl

Deficiency

Vitamin K is involved in the clotting mechanism. It is responsible for the maintenance of normal prothrombin time. Prolonged clotting time is caused by lack of one or more of the four coagulation factors produced in the liver; prothrombin (Factor II), proconvertin (Factor VII), thromboplastin (Christmas factor, Factor IX) and Stuart factor (Factor X). Large doses of vitamin K, either orally or parenterally, promote the synthesis of these factors by the liver.

TABLE 7-8. Vitamin K Products
(All are by prescription only)

Brand	Company	Data
Phytonadione (K_1)		
Mephyton	MSD	5 mg tablets
Konakion	Roche	For intramuscular injection, 2 and 10 mg/ml contains polysorbate 80
Aquamephyton	MSD	For parenteral use, 2 and 10 mg/ml Colloidal dispersion Contains polyoxyethylated fatty acid derivative
Menadione (K_3)		
Generic	Burgin-Arden Lilly	For parenteral use, 25 mg/ml 5 mg tablets
Menadiol Sodium Diphosphate (K_4)		
Kappadione	Lilly	For parenteral use, 10 mg/ml
Synkayvite	Roche	5 mg tablets
Synkayvite	Roche	For parenteral use, 10 and 37.5 mg/ml

Note dose relationships; Menadione has about three times the potency of phytonadione; Menadiol Sodium Diphosphate has about one half the potency of Menadione.

Because of the low water solubility of phytonadione and menadione and the uncertain, but always less than 100% absorption of oral doses and the criticality of dissolution of all forms of the drug to obtaining the desired effect, the FDA has proposed bioequivalence requirements for all vitamin K-type coagulants.[13]

Products containing vitamin K are listed in Table 7-8.

SYMPTOMS

The only symptom of vitamin K deficiency is bleeding caused by hypoprothrombinemia.

POPULATIONS AT RISK

There is seldom a lack of available vitamin K for adults. Dietary sources of vitamin K are shown in Table 7-9. Deficiency may be produced by one of the following:

1. Faulty absorption due to lack of bile in the intestine
   a. insufficient secretion of bile salts
   b. biliary obstruction (jaundice)
   c. biliary fistula
   d. surgery on the intestines
   e. therapy with drugs that remove bile acids, such as cholestyramine resin
2. Greasy diarrhea which sweeps vitamin K and other fat-soluble vitamins out of the body
   a. mineral oil in excessive doses
   b. sprue
   c. celiac disease
   d. cystic fibrosis
   e. ulcerative colitis
   f. regional ileitis
   g. pellagra
3. Limitation of vitamin K production by intestinal bacteria when dietary intake

TABLE 7-9. Dietary Sources of Vitamin K

Food	mg/100 g
Primary	
Brussel sprouts	0.8 to 3.0
Cabbage	3.2
Cauliflower	3.6
Spinach and other dark green leafy vegetables	0.4 to 3.0
Other Important Sources	
Carrots	0.1
Cereals	0.04 to 0.3
Pork liver	0.04 to 0.8
Green peas	0.3
Tomatoes	0.4

is low due to intestinal chemosterilization by
a. neomycin
b. quinine
c. quinidine

4. The coagulation process does not function fully in all newborn. Usually, the concentrations of vitamin K and Factors II, VII, IX, and X are low, especially during the first few days. There is considerable individual variation, and values above normal have been reported. The number and functional state of the thrombocytes are usually normal. Nevertheless, about 0.1 to 1% of newborn not given vitamin K do experience bleeding. Many of these could be helped by vitamin K treatment.[7–9] The vitamin K levels in normal infants fall for the first 3 days, then approach adult values within a week of birth, apparently due to delay in establishment of the intestinal flora.

   The routine administration of vitamin K (especially parenterally) to newborn infants born to nutritionally adequate mothers is highly questionable.

Toxicity

1. No toxicity appears to be associated with orally ingested naturally occurring vitamin K. There are reports of headache and gastric distress during therapy.
2. Little investigation has been done on chronic toxicity of therapeutic doses of vitamin K. Inadequate information exists to judge whether there is an effect on the fertility of human males or females (no reproduction studies in animals exist) or whether there are adverse effects on the fetus.
3. Menadione powder is irritating to the respiratory tract and skin. Contact with its solution in alcohol causes blisters.
4. Menadiol sodium diphosphate, a water-soluble analog, injected in large amounts (5 to 30 mg per day) has caused hemolytic anemia, hyperbilirubinemia and kernicterus (biliary pigmentation accompanied by degeneration of nerve cells), and death in neonates (particularly prematures) or when given to the mother prior to delivery.[10,11] The toxicity is due to binding of sulfhydryl groups on the unsubstituted 3-position.[12]
5. Menadione and menadiol sodium diphosphate can induce erythrocyte hemolysis in patients who have a genetic deficiency of glucose-6-phosphate in the red blood cells.

Uses in Therapy

A. Prevention and treatment of hypoprothrombinemia.

   Phytonadione is the drug of choice, and the oral route is preferred. Because the oral dose may require 6 to 10 hours to act and even parenteral doses require several hours for action, in cases of severe bleeding, fresh whole blood or plasma is needed.

   If the patient has decreased bile secretion, the oral dose is given with 300 mg of ox bile or 500 mg of dehydrocholic acid. The dose is adjusted or repeated as needed on the basis of laboratory determination of the prothrombin time.

   Subcutaneous or intramuscular administration is contraindicated in hypoprothrombinemia because of the possibility of inducing hemorrhage or hematoma at the injection site. These routes, however, may have to be used if the patient cannot retain an oral dose.

   WARNING: If no other routes are possible, phytonadione as a colloidal water dispersion may be given intravenously at a rate not exceeding 1 mg per minute, usually well diluted with 5% dextrose, 0.9% saline, or 5% dextrose in 0.9% saline. No other diluents should be used. The drug should be administered immediately after dilution. Any unused portion of the dilution and any unused portion of the original ampule should be discarded. The infusion bottle must be protected from light at all times.

Even with the above precautions, risk of severe reactions is high. The reactions resemble hypersensitivity or anaphylaxis and include shock, cardiac and/or respiratory arrest, and death.

The action of the vitamin is usually detectable within 1 hour, and hemorrhage is usually controlled in 3 to 6 hours. Normal prothrombin levels are obtained in 12 to 14 hours.

B. Treatment of anticoagulant-induced prothrombin deficiency.

The structure of vitamin K is similar to the anticoagulant coumarin derivatives (dicumarol, phenprocoumon, warfarin) and the indanone derivatives (anisindione, phenindione) but is dissimilar to heparin. The anticoagulant effect of heparin is not antagonized by vitamin K therapy.

When bleeding is *not* present or immediately threatened, 2.5 to 10 mg phytonadione can be given orally, intramuscularly, or subcutaneously. Note that dosage should be carefully adjusted to prevent lowering of the anticoagulant drug activity below desired levels. If response is not satisfactory, repeat the oral dose in 12 to 48 hours or the parenteral dose in 6 to 8 hours.

When bleeding is present, 10 to 50 mg of phytonadione may be given by *slow* intravenous injections (see WARNING under A). If needed, repeat every 4 hours.

Vitamin K does not directly antagonize the effect of the anticoagulants. Action is by competition, with vitamin K promoting the synthesis of clotting factors by the liver.

C. Prophylaxis of hemorrhagic disease of the newborn whose mothers have received anticonvulsive therapy during pregnancy is accomplished by intramuscular or subcutaneous administration of 0.5 to 1 mg of phytonadione (in water-dispersible form) to the newborn immediately after delivery and repeated, if necessay, 6 to 8 hours later. Larger doses may be necessary.

D. Hypoprothrombinemia due to malabsorption, drug therapy that inhibits vitamin K synthesis by bacterial flora, and the effect of salicylates:
   Adults—Orally or parenterally, 2 to 25 mg repeated as necessary
   Children—5 to 10 mg
   Infants—2 mg

E. Patients on prolonged hyperalimentation or total parenteral nutrition that is vitamin K deficient (this should not occur):
   Adults—5 to 10 mg phytonadione, once a week, intramuscularly
   Children—2 to 5 mg phytonadione, once a week, intramuscularly

F. When diet contains less than 100 μg vitamin K/L:
   Infants—1 mg phytonadione, once a month, intramuscularly

INADEQUATELY SUBSTANTIATED THERAPIES

A. Hereditary hypoprothrombinemia.
B. Hypoprothrombinemia due to severe liver disease. (High doses of phytonadione may aggravate the disease.)

Note: Failure to respond to usual doses of vitamin K indicates a condition that is not vitamin K-dependent (Koller Test). Large or repeated doses of vitamin K are contraindicated.

REFERENCES—Vitamin K

1. Olson, R.E.: Vitamin K, *In* Modern Nutrition in Health and Disease, 6th Ed. R.S. Goodhart and M.E. Shils, eds. Philadelphia, Lea & Febiger, 1980.
2. Dam, H., Prange, I., and Søndergaard, E.: Acta Pharmacol. Toxicol. (Kbh), *10:*58, 1954 and *11:*90, 1955.
3. Martius, C.: Schweiz. Med. Wochschr., *93:*1264, 1963 (in German).

4. Hollander, D., and Rim, E.: Gut, *17:*450, 1976.
5. Jaques, L.B., Millar, G.J., and Spinks, J.W.T.: Schweiz. Med. Wochschr., *84:*792, 1945 (in English).
6. Taylor, J.D., et al.: Can. J. Biochem. Physiol., *34:*1143, 1956.
7. Committee on Nutrition, American Academy of Pediatrics: Pediatrics, *28:*501, 1961.
8. Vietti, T.J., et al.: J. Pediatr., *56:*343, 1955.
9. Wefring, K.W.: J. Pediatr., *61:*686, 1962.
10. Warner, E.D.: Vitamin K Malnutrition, *In* Clinical Nutrition, 2nd Ed. N. Jolliffe, ed. New York, Harper Brothers, 1962.
11. Hayes, K.C., and Hegsted, D.M.: Toxicity of the Vitamins, *In* Toxicants Occurring Naturally in Foods, 2nd Ed. Washington, DC, National Academy of Sciences, 1973.
12. Owen, C.A., Jr.: Vitamin K XI. Pharmacology and Toxicology, *In* The Vitamins, 2nd Ed. Vol. 3. W.H. Sebrell, Jr. and R.S. Harris, eds. New York, Academic Press, 1971.
13. Federal Register: *45:*14063-7, March 4, 1980.

Chapter 8

The Water-Soluble Vitamins

BIOTIN

Biotin is a water-soluble substance widely distributed in low concentrations. It is also known as vitamin H, coenzyme R, Factor S, Factor W, and Factor Y.

Safe and Adequate Intake

Average diet in the United States provides 100 to 300 μg of biotin per day. It is synthesized by intestinal microflora in man, so that urinary excretion frequently exceeds dietary intakes and biotin deficiency in humans does not take place on biotin-free diets.[1] Deficiency may be produced in humans by feeding large amounts of avidin (found in raw egg white), which binds biotin, making it nutritionally unavailable.[2]

It is assumed that fecal excretion measures biotin synthesis by intestinal microflora. It is also assumed that urinary excretion measures the amount of biotin absorbed. Assuming 50% absorption of dietary biotin, 100 μg of intake would provide 46μg of urinary excretion, the highest level reported.

Since biotin urinary excretion of infants older than 0.5 years is comparable with that of adults,[3] it is assumed that biotin requirements are proportional to body weight and caloric intake. The recommended amount of intake is 50 μg/1000 kcal.

For intakes in young infants, the biotin content of human milk (10 μg/1000 kcal) and infant formulas (15 μg/1000 kcal) has not been associated with symptoms of deficiency.

No RDA is set, but "safe and adequate" intakes are listed. It is likely that no dietary biotin is needed by healthy humans.

Chemistry

Biotin is a white substance, sparingly soluble in water. It is stable to heat and alkali, and readily oxidized by chemical oxidants but not by air.

Absorption

Biotin is relatively well absorbed[4] following oral administration, as shown by high urinary excretion following large doses. Absorption from the large intestine has been shown by introducing an aqueous biotin solution into the distal colon,[5] producing increases in blood and urine levels. The mechanism of absorption is not known.

Metabolism

Not known.

Excretion

Urinary excretion.

Pharmacology

1. Coenzyme for acetyl coenzyme A carboxylase.
2. Involved in fatty acid synthesis.
3. Involved in carbohydrate metabolism.
4. Necessary for interconversion of amino acids.

Laboratory Values

Normal Blood:
Infants—15 to 55 μg/dl
Adults—12 to 24 μg/dl, slightly lower in pregnancy.

Deficiency[1]

Biotin deficiency in humans has been reported only for those people who ate dozens of raw eggs, and little else, daily for several years. Experimental biotin deficiency in humans produces the following symptoms:

1. Nausea, vomiting, anorexia
2. Glossitis
3. Palor
4. Mental depression
5. Dry, red, scaly dermatitis
6. Neural abnormalities (in severe chronic deficiency)

Dietary sources of biotin are shown in Table 8-1.

Toxicity

Biotin, given parenterally, up to 5 mg per day for 12 days produced no symptoms.[6]

TABLE 8-1. Dietary Sources of Biotin*

Food	μg/100 g
Cauliflower	17
Chocolate	32
Eggs	25
Liver, beef	100
Mushrooms	16
Peanuts, roasted	39

* Biotin is usually present in plants in the range of 2 to 4 μg/100 g and in animals in the range of 5 to 10 μg/100 g. There are wide differences in availability as shown by the fact that biotin from corn and soybean is available to animals but biotin from wheat is nearly unavailable.

Uses in Therapy[3]

1. Leiner's disease (infantile seborrheic dermatitis found in infants nursing from malnourished mothers). Biotin does not always relieve this condition. Furthermore, the symptoms are found in infants fed formulas with high biotin contents. It is now thought that the biotin-responsive symptoms represent an individual abnormality because of the high dose (1 to 5 mg) needed to alleviate the symptoms.

2. Genetic disorders responsive to biotin (very rare, one case each).
   a. beta-methylcrotonyl glycinuria[7]
   b. propionic acidemia[8]

REFERENCES—Biotin

1. Swendseid, M.E., et al.: Am. J. Clin. Nutr., *17:*272, 1965.
2. Sydenstricker, V.P., et al.: JAMA, *118:*1199, 1942.
3. Bonjour, J.P.: Int. J. Vit. Nutr. Res., *47:*107, 1977.
4. Gardner, J., Parsons, H.T., and Peterson, W.H.: Am. J. Med. Sci., *211:*198, 1946.
5. Sorrell, M.F., et al.: Nutr. Rep. Int., *3:*143, 1971.
6. Messaritakis, J., et al.: Arch. Dis. Childhood, *50:*871, 1975.
7. Gompertz, D., et al.: Lancet, *2:*22, 1971.
8. Barnes, N.D., et al.: Lancet, *2:*244, 1970.

CHOLINE

Choline is synthesized in humans by methylation of ethanolamine or de novo. This requires adequate supplies of methionine or vitamin B_{12} and folacin. There is no reliable information about the rate of choline biosynthesis in man or what influences it. It is available commercially as choline bitartrate, choline chloride, and choline citrate.

Generally, choline is not considered as an essential nutrient for humans. The young of animal species may be at risk in deficiency because of either increased needs or less efficient biosynthesis than adults.[1] For this reason, it is recommended that choline be added to infant formulas even in the absence of any demonstration of need.

Intake in the average diet in the United States is 150 to 900 mg per day.

TABLE 8-2. Dietary Sources of Choline*

Food	mg/100 g
Asparagus	130
Beans, green	300
Beef	90
Carrots	95
Cheese, cheddar	50
Egg yolk	1130
Lamb	110
Liver	600
Liverwurst	370
Oats, rolled	150
Peanuts	165
Peanut butter	145
Peas	260
Pork	85
Spinach	240
Wheat germ	400

* Choline is abundant in both plants and animals. Human milk contains about 90 mg/L.

Pharmacology[2]

1. Constituent of phospholipids
   a. sphingomyelin
   b. lecithin
2. Precursor for acetylcholine (neurotransmitter).
3. Source of labile methyl groups for methylation reactions such as synthesis of methionine.

Toxicity[3]

No data for man. Lethal dose in rabbits is 500 μg/kg subcutaneously, in mice 31.3 mg/kg intraperitoneally, in rats and guinea pigs 60 mg/kg. In man, therapy with 3 to 12 g daily for up to 4 months showed no toxicity.

Choline, in therapeutic doses, imparts an odor of dead fish to the body and breath.

Uses in Therapy[2]

In animals, choline deficiency produces fatty infiltration of the liver and hemorrhagic kidney disease. In man, therapy with choline for the fatty liver and cirrhosis associated with alcoholism is no more effective than a balanced diet.

Other lipotropic factors (inositol, betaine) have been used in conjunction with choline.

EXPERIMENTAL

1. Huntington's chorea.
2. Tardive dyskinesia (in combination with lecithin).

Dietary sources of choline are shown in Table 8-2; choline products, in Table 8-3.

REFERENCES—Choline

1. Griffith, W.H., and Dyer, H.M.: Nutr. Rev., *26*:1, 1968.
2. Griffith, W.H., et al.: Choline, *In* The Vitamins. 2nd Ed. Vol. III. W. H. Sebrell and R. S. Harris, eds. New York, Academic Press, 1971.
3. Cornatzer, W.E.: Proc. Soc. Exp. Biol. Med., *85*:642, 1954.

VITAMIN C

Two substances have vitamin C activity in humans: ascorbic acid and dehydroascorbic acid.[1] Dehydroascorbic acid is an oxidation product of ascorbic acid. A consequence of this fact is that even though ascorbic acid is readily destroyed by heating in air to form

TABLE 8-3. Choline Products

	Manufacturer	Strength
Choline		
Powder	Freeda Pharmaceuticals	
Tablets	Generic from various manufacturers	325, 500, 650 mg
Choline Bitartrate		
Tablets	Fibertone	250 mg
Choline Chloride*		
Powder	Generic from various manufacturers	
Choline Dihydrogen Citrate		
Powder	City Chemical	

* By prescription only.

dehydroascorbic acid, which is then further degraded, the substance still may retain considerable vitamin C potency. This has led to some understatement of the vitamin C content of foods, in which vitamin C was determined as ascorbic acid only. Erythorbic acid (isoascorbic acid) salts have reducing properties and are used as food preservatives. They have little or no vitamin C activity, but common analytic procedures do not distinguish between ascorbic and isoascorbic acids.

Recommended Dietary Allowances

The human requirement for vitamin C has been estimated from the amount needed to prevent or cure scurvy, a disease caused by vitamin C deficiency, the amount metabolized daily by the body, and the amount necessary to saturate reserve sites.[2]

A daily intake of 10 mg cures scurvy in humans.[3] Estimates of adequacy have been made, however, by measuring ascorbate concentrations in serum, leukoyctes, erythrocytes, and urine. Maximal plasma concentration is about 1.4 mg/dl. Intakes greater than those required to reach that level produce a sharp rise in urinary excretion.[4] Intakes of over 60 mg per day are required to saturate adult human leukocytes.[5] Use of radioactive ascorbic acid shows body pools in healthy adult males of 1490 to 1560 mg at intakes of 77.5 mg per day[3,6] and 2300 to 2800 mg at intakes of 200 mg per day.[7]

In depletion studies, scurvy was observed when the body pool fell below 300 mg and symptoms disappeared when the body pool was restored to 300 mg. No ascorbic acid was detected in the urine until the body pool approached 1500 mg. A daily intake of 60 mg was necessary to maintain that body pool.[8] The catabolic rate for ascorbic acid ranged from 2.2 to 4.1% of the body pool per day. Thus, for a 1500 mg pool, catabolism accounts for 33 to 61.5 mg per day.[9]

Acute emotional stress and environmental stress such as exposure to elevated temperatures require increased vitamin C intakes of up to 250 mg per day.[10] The effects on plasma levels due to individual variation, age, sex, drugs, smoking, and oral contraceptives have been investigated, but without any conclusions as to the effect on required intakes.

Although little is known about the requirements of the adult female, there seem to be differences in metabolism and retention of vitamin C which may be related to hormonal activity.[5] The requirement is assumed to be the same as for males.

The RDA is set at 60 mg for adults, assuming an average absorption efficiency of 85%,[11] a catabolism rate of $2.9 \pm 0.6\%$,[6] and a desired pool of 1500 mg, which is sufficient to protect the adult male against scurvy for 30 to 45 days. Although a larger pool may be obtained at intakes of 200 mg per day, it is believed that such a pool is unnecessary.

Human milk contains 30 to 55 mg/L of vitamin C, depending on the maternal dietary intake. This provides an average of 35 mg per day to the infant, which is the value adopted for the RDA.

On a weight basis, the vitamin C requirement for children is higher than that for adults. For children up to age 11, the recommendation is 45 mg per day. The full adult recommendation is advised for older children.

Vitamin C levels in plasma fall during pregnancy. The reason is not known. The fetus concentrates vitamin C, so that fetal levels are about 50% higher at term than maternal levels. An extra allowance of 20 mg per day is recommended in pregnancy.

During lactation, an extra allowance of 40 mg per day is recommended to replace the approximately 35 mg per day excreted in milk.

Chemistry

Ascorbic acid is water-soluble. It darkens on exposure to light. Solutions, particularly if they are alkaline, are rapidly oxidized in air. Vitamin C structures are shown in Figure 8-1.

Absorption

Ascorbic acid is readily absorbed by an active process, similar to the process of

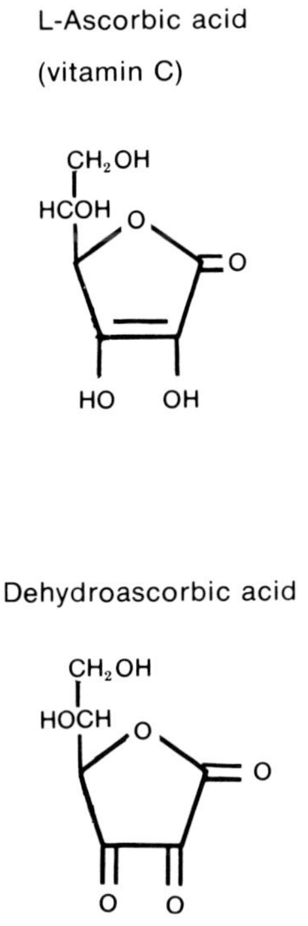

L-Ascorbic acid

(vitamin C)

CH_2OH / HCOH / O / =O / HO OH

Dehydroascorbic acid

CH_2OH / HOCH / O / =O / O O

Figure 8-1. Vitamin C Structures

absorption of glucose and other carbohydrates.[12] Because of this, large doses may not be fully absorbed (50% absorption for 1.5 g dose). It probably passes the membranes as the more lipid-soluble dehydroascorbic acid, which is then reduced to ascorbic acid.[13]

Distribution

About 25% of ascorbic acid in plasma is bound to protein. About 20% of the vitamin C activity is as dehydroascorbic acid.

Metabolism

Ascorbic acid is reversibly oxidized to dehydroascorbic acid. Some ascorbic acid is metabolized to inactive compounds, which include ascorbic acid-2-sulfate and oxalic acid.

Excretion

Very little ascorbic acid is excreted in feces. The inactive metabolites are excreted in urine. Ascorbic acid in excess of that needed to saturate body pools is excreted in the urine. The renal threshold (concentration in plasma above which urinary excretion occurs) is about 1.4 mg/dl.

Ascorbic acid is removed by hemodialysis.

Physiologic Functions

A. Ascorbic acid and dehydroascorbic acid form a reduction-oxidation system with semidehydroascorbic acid as a highly reactive transient intermediate. The symptoms of scurvy are due to failure of ascorbic acid-dependent hydroxylations requiring molecular oxygen. These include:
   1. Proline to hydroxyproline (formation of collagen).[15]
   2. Dopamine to noradrenalin.
   3. Hydroxylations in steroid synthesis.[15]
B. Another function of ascorbic acid is as a reducing agent (electron donor) in the following:
   1. Protection of parahydroxy-phenylpyruvic acid hydroxylase (tyrosine metabolism).[16]
   2. Folic acid to tetrahydrofolate.[17,18]
C. It also is required for the incorporation of iron into ferritin.
D. Dehydroascorbic acid is needed in the conversion of tryptophan to 5-hydroxytryptophan (in presence of copper ion).
E. The presence of 25 to 75 mg of ascorbic acid in meals enhances the absorption of iron.[19]

Laboratory Values (Table 8-4)

The nutritional status of vitamin C may be evaluated by a saturation test. An oral dose of 11 mg of ascorbic acid/kg is given, and urinary ascorbate excretion is measured for 24 hours. Excretion of less than 20% of the dose suggests deficiency. Normal subjects excrete more than 50% of the dose.

Deficiency

Vitamin C deficiency results in scurvy (ascorbutic syndrome).

TABLE 8-4 Ascorbic Acid

	Whole Blood mg/dl		Plasma or Serum mg/dl	
	Mean	95% Range	Mean	95% Range
Men, 20-30	0.507	0.224-0.880	0.476	0.196-0.876
Women, 20-30	0.884	0.517-1.28	0.897	0.624-1.41
Children, 10-13	—	—	0.6	0-1.5
Normal Saturated Adult	—	—	—	1.0-2.0
Scurvy				Below 0.15

SYMPTOMS

The manifestations of vitamin C deficiency include the following:

1. Fatigue
2. Spontaneous hemorrhage
   a. swollen, bleeding gums
   b. swollen joints
   c. muscle aches and pains
   d. extensive hemorrhagic patches under the skin
3. Follicular hyperkeratosis
4. Personality changes
5. Changes in bone structure and growth
   a. characteristic loss of tooth enamel
   b. destruction of bone starting at metaphysis in infants
   c. subperiostial bleeding in infants

Diagnosis is made only by correlation of the physical symptoms with low blood levels of ascorbic acid.

POPULATIONS AT RISK

Average consumption of vitamin C in the daily American diet ranges from 30 to 250 mg per day. The lower amount is sufficient to prevent symptoms of scurvy; the higher amount is sufficient to sustain a maximal body pool. Dietary sources of vitamin C are listed in Table 8-5.

Ascorbic acid needs are increased in the following conditions,[20–22] but not beyond the ability to be met by a carefully selected diet.

1. Achlorhydria
2. Peptic ulcer
3. Chronic diarrhea
4. Burns
5. Surgical wounds
6. Neoplastic disease
7. Hyperthyroidism
8. Pregnancy
9. Lactation

Cigarette smokers have lower plasma/serum/leukocyte levels than nonsmokers, but this varies with vitamin C intake, differences disappearing at intakes of 100 to 500 mg per day.[23]

Oral contraceptives, antibiotics, and salicylates have been reported to decrease plasma levels, but there is no evidence that this requires additional ascorbic acid, or that ascorbic acid supplements would affect the levels.

Toxicity

1. Doses of 4 to 15 g per day may produce nausea and diarrhea due to osmotic effects.[24]
2. Doses greater than 1 g may produce an increase in vitamin C (which acidifies urine), calcium, uric acid, and oxalate excretion, which may enhance formation of crystals (stones) in the kidney and bladder.[25] This would be a particular problem for people with high intakes of foods containing oxalates (spinach, rhubarb, chocolate, tea), those who have higher than normal conversion of ascorbate to oxalate, and those with diseases of the small intestine, particularly those who have had resections (increase in oxalate excretion).
3. Sickle cell crisis has been reported after ingestion of large doses of vitamin C, which increased blood acidity.
4. Patients with glucose-6-phosphate dehydrogenase deficiency showed hemolysis after large oral or intravenous doses.

TABLE 8-5. Dietary Sources of Vitamin C
(As normally served, vegetables cooked and drained)

Food	mg/100 g
Apricots	
raw	10
Asparagus	
fresh or frozen	26
Avocados	14
Beans	
lima	
fresh or frozen	17
canned	6
green	10
yellow	13
Beet greens	15
Broccoli	
fresh	90
frozen	73
Brussel sprouts	87
Cabbage	
raw	47
cooked	24
Cauliflower	
fresh cooked	55
frozen	41
Chard, Swiss	16
Coleslaw	29
Collard greens	46
Endive	
raw	10
Grapefruit	
fresh	38
canned	30
Grapefruit juice	30
Kale	63
Lemon juice	
fresh	46
Lettuce	
romaine	18
Lime juice	
fresh	32
Liver	
beef	27
calf	37
chicken	16
pork	27
Mango	
fresh	35
Melon	
canteloupe	33
honeydew	23
frozen	16
Mustard greens	
fresh	48
frozen	20
Okra	
fresh	20
frozen	12
Oranges	50
Orange juice	
fresh	50
canned	40
reconstituted	45
Papaya	56
Parsnip	10
Peas	
green snow	24
green	
fresh	20
canned	8
blackeyed	
fresh	17
canned	3
Peppers	
sweet green	128
red	204
Persimmon	66
Pineapple	
raw	17
Pineapple juice	10
Potato	
baked	16
mashed	9
reconstituted	3
chips	16
Radishes	26
Raspberries	
fresh	25
frozen	21
canned	9
Rutabaga	26
Sauerkraut	14
Sauerkraut juice	
canned	18
Scallions	
whole	25
Spinach	
fresh	28
canned	14
frozen	19
Squash	
summer	10
winter	
baked	13
boiled	8
Strawberries	
fresh	39
frozen	55
Sweet Potato	
baked in skin	22
boiled in skin	17
candied	10
canned	8
Tangerine	31
Tomato	24
Tomato juice	
canned	16
Turnip	22
Turnip greens	
fresh	47
frozen	19

TABLE 8-6. Vitamin C Products

Brand	Company	Strength
Ascorbic Acid or Sodium Ascorbate		
Capsules, Extended Time Release		
Generic	Various	250 mg, 500 mg
Ascor	Pharmex	250 mg
Ascorbicap	ICN	500 mg
Ascor-B.I.D.	Pharmex	250 mg
Ascorbineed	Hanlon	250 mg
Best-C	Hauck	500 mg
Cetane Timed	O'Neal, Jones & Feldman	500 mg
Cevi-Bid	Geriatric	500 mg
Cevita Kaycaps	Kay	500 mg
C-Long Granucaps	Tutag	500 mg
C-Span	Edwards	500 mg
Dura-C 500 Graduals	Amfre-Grant	500 mg
SpanCap C	North American	500 mg
Tablets		
Generic	Various	25, 50, 250, 500, 1000 mg
Cevalin	Lilly	100, 250, 500 mg
Cevita	Kay	250, 500 mg
Vitacee	CMC	25, 50, 100, 250, 500 mg
Viterra-C	Pfipharmecs	250, 500 mg
Tablets, Chewable		
Generic	Various	100, 250, 500, 1000 mg
Ascorbajen	Jenkins	100 mg
Cevita	Kay	250 mg
Tablets, Timed release		
Generic	Various	1000 mg
Arco-Cee	Arco	750 mg
Cemill	Miller	250, 500 mg
Oral Liquids		
Generic	Various	500 mg/5 ml
Ce-Vi-Sol	Mead Johnson	35 mg/0.6 ml
Cecon	Abbott	100 mg/ml
Liqui-Cee*	American Critical Care	1000 mg/5 ml
Tega C-Syrup-500	Ortega	500 mg/5 ml
Vitamin C	CMC	20 mg/ml
*Injection,** Ascorbic Acid		
Generic	Various	50, 100, 200, 250 mg/ml
Cevalin	Lilly	100, 500, mg/ml
Vitacee	Cencil	50 mg/ml
*Injection,** Sodium Ascorbate		
Generic	Various	250 mg/ml
C-Ject	Lincoln	200 mg/ml
Cevita	Kay	250 mg/ml
Cenolate	Abbott	250 mg/ml
*Injection,** Calcium Ascorbate		
Calscorbate	O'Neal, Jones & Feldman	100 mg/ml

* On prescription only.

5. Prolonged use of large doses may produce accelerated metabolism of ascorbic acid, thus producing scurvy when intake is reduced to normal. Neonatal scurvy is produced in this way, when large doses of the vitamin have been ingested during pregnancy.

Uses in Therapy

The oral route is preferred. When oral administration is not possible or when malabsorption is suspected, intramuscular injection is the preferred parenteral route, although subcutaneous and intravenous administration is possible. Vitamin C products are listed in Table 8-6.

1. Scurvy:
   Adults—100 to 250 mg, once or twice daily for 2 days to 3 weeks. Larger doses are not advantageous.
   Infants and Children—100 to 300 mg per day in divided doses.
2. Chronic hemodialysis:
   Adults—100 to 200 mg per day
3. Urinary acidification:
   4 to 12 g per day. The 0.2 pH unit reduction is usually not clinically significant.[26,27]
4. Reduction of tyrosinemia in premature infants:
   100 mg per day.[28]
5. Specific antidote for symptoms of reaction between disulfuram and alcohol.
6. As an adjunct to iron removal in deferoxamine therapy:
   200 to 2000 mg (unconfirmed efficacy).
7. Colds:
   1000 to 3000 mg per day or more. Studies show that frequency of colds is not significantly affected. Average duration was shortened from 15 to 14.5 days, with fewer working days lost (University of Toronto study 1971 to 1974). Greatest effect was seen when regular supplement was combined with increased ingestion at onset of cold symptoms. No advantage was seen at intakes larger than 250 mg per day.[29] Other clinical trials have given inconsistent or statistically insignificant results.
   Doses of 3000 mg per day failed to protect volunteers from infection by rhinovirus 44.[30]
   Interestingly, one study[31] has shown that ingestion of 2000 mg per day by healthy male volunteers reduced the antibacterial activity of leukocytes.
8. Ascorbic acid in large doses may have pharmacologic effects on the immune system which are not related to its vitamin activity.[32]

INADEQUATELY SUBSTANTIATED THERAPIES

There is no convincing evidence that ascorbic acid has any effect in the following conditions:

1. Atherosclerosis (lowering of blood cholesterol)
2. Allergy or hay fever
3. Mental disease, schizophrenia (megadoses)
4. Corneal ulcers
5. Idiopathic methemoglobinemia (300 to 600 mg per day)
6. Megaloblastic anemia and capillary fragility (unless vitamin C deficiency has been shown by laboratory test)
7. Immobilized patients with pressure sores
8. Adjunct to iron therapy in iron deficiency anemia (at doses of less than 200 mg)
9. Carcinoma
10. Hemorhagic conditions (unless due to scurvy)
    a. hematuria
    b. retinal hemorrhage
    c. anemia
11. Dental problems
    a. caries
    b. pyorrhea
    c. gum infections
12. Acne
13. Infertility
14. Peptic ulcer
15. Tuberculosis
16. Dysentery
17. Leg ulcers

18. Prophylaxis of fatigue
19. Prophylaxis of heat prostration
20. Prophylaxis of vascular thrombosis
21. Fractures
22. Imperfect bone formation
23. Treatment of drug toxicity from
    a. levodopa
    b. succinylcholine
    c. arsenic
24. Mucolysis

Interference with Laboratory Tests

1. False negatives in testing for glucosuria.

   Ingestion of more than 500 mg per day (to produce urinary concentrations of more than 10 mg/dl) gives false negatives with glucose oxidase enzyme test strips.[33]
2. False positives in tests for glucosuria, depending on reduction of cupric ion.
3. False negatives in stool occult blood tests.

   Ingestion of more than 1 g per day (to produce fecal excretion greater than 55 mg per day) gives false negatives with tests using amines (Hemoccult, Derman). If this test is to be done, no vitamin C supplement should be taken in the preceding 3 days.[34]

Interference with Drug Action

1. Blockage of anticoagulant effects of heparin at 200 mg ascorbic acid to 100 units (1 mg) of heparin.[35]
2. Blockage of warfarin anticoagulant action at 16 g ascorbic acid per day.[36]
3. Interferes with effectiveness of disulfuram (large doses).
4. Interferences due to acidification of urine
   a. increases tubule reabsorption of acidic drugs, thus exaggerating their action.
   b. decreases tubal reabsorption of alkaline drugs, thus decreasing their action (amphetamines, tricyclic depressants).
   c. crystal formation with sulfonamides.

REFERENCES—Vitamin C

1. Sabry, J.H., Fisher, K.H., and Dodds, M.L.: J. Nutr., *64:*457, 1958.
2. Irwin, M.I., and Hutchins, B.K.: J. Nutr., *106:*823, 1976.
3. Hodges, R.E., et al.: Am. J. Clin. Nutr., *24:*432, 1971.
4. Friedman G.J., Sherry, S., and Ralli, E.P.: J. Clin. Invest., *19:*685, 1940.
5. Sauberlich, H.E.: Ann. NY Acad. Sci., *258:*438, 1975.
6. Baker, E.M., et al.: Am. J. Clin. Nutr., *24:*444, 1971.
7. Baker, E.M., Saari, J.C., and Tolbert, B.M.: Am. J. Clin. Nutr.,*19:*371, 1966.
8. Kallner, A., Hartmann, D., and Hornig, D.: Am. J. Clin. Nutr., *32:*530, 1979.
9. Baker, E.M., et al.: Am. J. Clin. Nutr., *22:*549, 1969.
10. Visagie, M.E., et al.: S. Afr. Med. J., *48:*2502, 1974.
11. Kallner, A., Hartmann, D., and Hornig, D.: Int. J. Vit. Nutr. Res., *47:*383, 1977.
12. Woodruff, C.W.: Ascorbic Acid, *In* Nutrition. Vol. II. G.H. Beaton and E.W. McHenry, eds. New York, Academic Press, 1964.
13. Martin, G.R.: Ann. NY Acad. Sci., *92:*141, 1961.
14. Barnes, M.J.: Ann. NY Acad. Sci., *258:*264, 1975.
15. Stone, K.J., and Townsley, B.H.: Biochem. J., *131:*611, 1973.
16. La Du, B.N., and Zannoni, V.G.: Ann. NY Acad. Sci., *92:*175, 1961.
17. Stokes, P.L., et al.: Am. J. Clin. Nutr., *28:*126, 1975.
18. Thien, K.R., et al.: J. Clin. Pathol., *30:*438, 1977.
19. Monson, E.R., et al.: Am. J. Clin. Nutr., *31:*134, 1978.
20. Vilter, R.W.: Ascorbic Acid XIII. Pharmacology, *In* The Vitamins, 2nd Ed. Vol. 1. W.H. Sebrell, Jr. and R.S. Harris, eds. New York, Academic Press, 1967.
21. Goldsmith, G.A.: Ann. NY Acad. Sci., *92:*230, 1961.
22. Crandon, J.H., et al.: Ann. NY Acad. Sci., *92:*246, 1961.
23. Yeung, D.L.: Am. J. Clin. Nutr., *29:*1216, 1976.
24. Hodges, R.E.: Ascorbic Acid, *In* Modern Nutrition in Health and Disease. 6th Ed. R.S. Goodhart and M.E. Shils, eds. Philadelphia, Lea & Febiger, 1980.
25. Robertson, W.G., and Peacock, M.: Clin. Sci., *43:*499, 1972.
26. Anderson, T.W., Reid, D.B.W., and Beaton, G.H.: Can. Med. Assoc. J., *107:*503, 1972, and *108:*133, 1973.
27. Hetey, S.K., et al.: Am. J. Hosp. Pharm., *37:*235, 1980.
28. Nahata, M.C., Cummins, B.A., and McLeod, D.C.: Am. J. Hosp. Pharm., *38:*33, 1981.
29. Anderson, T.W., Suranyi, G., and Beaton, G.H.: Can. Med. Assoc. J., *111:*31, 1974.

30. Schwartz, A.R., et al.: J. Infect. Dis., *128*:500, 1973.
31. Shilotri, P.G., and Bhat, K.S.: Am. J. Clin. Nutr., *30*:1077, 1977.
32. Prinz, W., et al.: Int. J. Vit. Nutr. Res., *47*:248, 1977.
33. Mayson, J.S., Schumaker, O., and Nakamura, R.M.: Am. J. Clin. Pathol., *58*:297, 1972.
34. Jaffe, R.M., et al.: Ann. Intern. Med., *83*:824, 1975.
35. Owen, C.A., et al.: Mayo Clin. Proc., *45*:140, 1970.
36. Smith, E.C., et al.: JAMA, *221*:1166, 1972.

THIAMIN

Thiamin is also known as vitamin B_1. It is available commercially as thiamine chloride hydrochloride. Thiamine mononitrate is no longer used because of irrational fear of nitrates as carcinogens.

Recommended Dietary Allowances

Because thiamin is essential in energy metabolism, particularly in the metabolism of carbohydrates, its requirement is related to caloric intake.[1] In starvation, tissue stores are depleted rapidly.[2] On this basis, recommended daily intake is 1 mg to maintain body stores for adults on calorically inadequate diets.

The RDA is set on the basis of the following considerations:

1. Clinical signs of thiamin deficiency occur in adults at intakes below 0.12 μg/1000 kcal.[3] Various levels from 0.35 to 0.5 mg/1000 kcal were reported as being consistent with good health.
2. Urinary excretion studies show a minimum requirement of about 0.34 mg/1000 kcal, but more than 0.5 mg/1000 kcal is needed to maintain tissue saturation.[4]
3. Erythrocyte transketolase activity is maximized at 1.1 mg/1000 kcal,[4] but submaximum activity is not accompanied by ill effects and "normal" values were found at intakes around 0.5 mg/1000 kcal.[5]

The RDA is set at 0.5 mg/1000 kcal, or a minimum of 1 mg per day for adults if they consume less than 2000 kcal per day. Dietary sources of thiamin are shown in Table 8-7.

Studies show that thiamin requirements increase early in pregnancy and remain constant during the course of pregnancy.[6] An increase of 0.1 mg/1000 kcal or not less than 0.4 mg per day is recommended.

Thiamin requirements increase during lactation due to increased energy requirements and secretion of thiamin into the milk. An increase of 0.1 mg/1000 kcal or not less than 0.5 mg per day is recommended.

The few studies on thiamin requirement indicate that it is about 0.27 mg/1000 kcal or 0.03 mg/kg of body weight.[7–9] Although the average thiamin content of human milk (0.27 mg/1000 kcal) is sufficient to protect against thiamin deficiency in the infant, the recommendation is 0.5 mg/1000 kcal to provide a safety margin in milk-substitute formulas.

The few studies on thiamin requirements in children and adolescents show that 0.3 mg/1000 kcal was adequate for preadolescents, but inadequate for 16- to 18-year-old girls; that 0.6 mg/1000 kcal was marginal for the latter group; and that 14- to 17-year-old boys require 0.32 to 0.44 mg/1000 kcal.[10–12] For children and adolescents, the recommended amount is 0.5 mg/1000 kcal or not less than 1 mg per day.

Chemistry (Figure 8-2)

Thiamin is soluble in water. It is decomposed by oxidizing and reducing agents and moist heat in the presence of alkali. Decomposition is retarded by acid. Thiamin $pk_1 = 4.8$ $pk_2 = 9.0$.

Absorption

Intestinal absorption of thiamin is an active process. In healthy humans, the fraction absorbed decreases with increasing dose.[13,14]

Thiamin absorption is significantly reduced in the presence of ethanol (chronic alcoholism) and in the presence of folate depletion.[15,16]

The total amount absorbed after megadoses is in the range of 4 to 8 mg. When administered with food, the rate of absorp-

TABLE 8-7. Dietary Sources of Thiamin in Foods as Usually Eaten

Food	μg/100 g	Food	μg/100 g
Asparagus		Molasses	
cooked	160	blackstrap	110
Avocado	110	Mussels	160
Bacon		Nuts	
fried	510	chestnuts	220
Bamboo shoots	150	filberts (hazelnuts)	460
Barley		"Indian" nuts	1280
pearled	120	peanuts (roasted)	320
Beans		peanut butter	120
white	140	pistachio	167
red	110	pignola	620
lima	180	walnuts	330
Bean sprouts	100	Oranges	100
Bread		Oysters	120
cracked wheat	110	Peas	
enriched white	250	snow	220
rye	170	green	280
pumpernickel	130	canned	100
whole wheat	250	Pineapple	
Buckwheat		fresh or canned	100
whole grain	600	Pork	500
Chicken		Potatoes	
dark meat	120	french fried	120
giblets	170	baked	100
Clams	100	Potato chips	210
Collards	110	Rice	
Corn		brown	90
cooked kernels	110	white	20
Eggs	110	enriched	110
Fish		Sausages and cold cuts	
abalone canned	120	bologna	160
drum (redfish)	150	liverwurst	170
grouper	170	minced ham	730
mackerel	270	pork sausage	290
salmon		salami	250
fresh cooked	140	scrapple	190
canned	30	Syrup	
shad		cane	130
baked	130	Soybeans	
whitefish	110	cooked	310
Heart	200-250	Soybean sprouts	160
Kidney	510	Wheat germ	2010
Lamb	140	toasted	1650
Liver		Yeast	
beef	260	brewer's	4280
chicken	170		
pork	340		

Note that products made with enriched flours: macaroni, spaghetti, and other pasta; cakes and muffins from mixes; breakfast cereals, etc., generally contain about 140 μg/100 g of product as it is usually eaten.

Do not be led astray by tables showing thiamin content of various flours or raw food. Thiamin is not stable to moist heat and much is lost in cooking and processing. Many substances which can be sources of thiamin when freshly cooked lose most of their thiamin during sterilization, if they are canned.

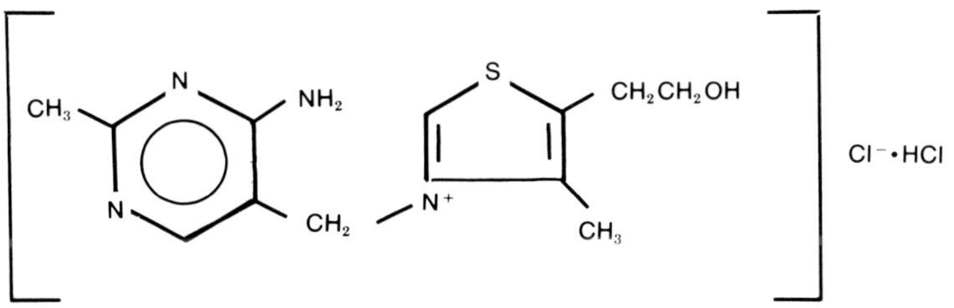

Figure 8-2. Structure of Thiamine Hydrochloride

tion is slowed but the amount absorbed is not affected. Absorption is rapid and complete from intramuscular injection. Thiamin products are listed in Table 8-8.

TABLE 8-8. Thiamin Products

Brand	Manufacturer	Strength
*Injections**		
Generic	Various	100, 200 mg/ml
Betalin S	Lilly	100 mg/ml
Elixirs		
Betalin S	Lilly	2.25 mg/5 ml
Bewon	Wyeth	0.25 mg/5 ml
Tablets		
Generic	Various	5, 10, 25, 50, 100, 250, 500 mg
Betalin S	Lilly	10, 25, 50, 100 mg
Pan-B-1	Panray	50, 100, mg

* By prescription only.

Distribution

Thiamin is widely distributed in tissues. The body pool is estimated to be 30 mg. Thus, with a 1 mg per day turnover, symptoms of thiamin deficiency in a normal adult are not seen for 2 to 3 weeks after complete withdrawal.

Metabolism

Thiamin appears to be metabolized in the liver.

Excretion

At intakes above 0.5 to 0.6 mg per day, urinary excretion rises in proportion to intake and may reach 0.1 mg per day in some diets.[17] Metabolites are also found in the urine. Excretion in human milk is dependent on maternal intake.

Pharmacology

Thiamine functions as a coenzyme in carbohydrate metabolism (2-keto sugars and alpha-keto acids). It combines with adenosine triphosphate (ATP) in the liver, kidneys, and leukocytes to form the active coenzyme thiamine diphosphate (pyrophosphate), also known as cocarboxylase. This acts as a coenzyme in the decarboxylation of pyruvic acid and acetyl coenzyme A (Embden-Meyerhof glycolytic pathway), in the decarboxylation of alpha-ketoglutaric acid to succinyl coenzyme A (citric acid cycle), and in the formation of sedoheptulose phosphate and fructose-6-phosphate (hexose monophosphate shunt). It also aids in transketolation reactions.

Laboratory Tests

TRANSKETOLASE IN PLASMA

Normal adult: 0.017 to 0.060 U/dl (mean: 0.029). A unit is the amount that will catalyze the conversion of 1 micromole of the substrate per minute under standardized conditions.

THIAMIN IN BLOOD

Normal adult: total 1.0 to 7.5 μg/dl (mean 2.8).

URINARY EXCRETION

Measures absorbability or bioavailability of dosage. Urinary level is measured in fasting state and after administration of a 5 mg dose.[18]

Deficiency

Thiamin deficiency produces the following biochemical alterations.[19,20]

1. Increase in blood pyruvic acid and lactic acid
2. Reduction in red blood cell transketolase
3. Neurologic lesions
4. Cardiac lesions

SYMPTOMS

A. Clinical symptoms
   1. Gastrointestinal symptoms
      a. dysphagia (loss of appetite)
      b. achlorhydria (reduction in gastric secretion)
      c. spastic colon
   2. Beriberi
      a. peripheral neuritis ("dry beriberi")[21]
         (1) ascending, symmetrical, bilateral neuritis
         (2) hyperesthesia, anesthesia
         (3) degeneration of peripheral nerve fibers
      b. Cardiovascular symptoms ("wet beriberi")[22]
         (1) general edema (aggravated by low protein intake)
         (2) dyspnea (loss of breath on exertion)
         (3) diminished vital capacity
         (4) enlarged heart
         (5) palpitations (gallop rhythm)
         (6) elevated blood pressure
         (7) myocardial lesions
         (8) abnormal electrocardiogram (EKG shows reversal of T-wave and prolonged QT-interval)
   3. Wernicke's Encephalopathy[23]
      a. usually found in chronic alcoholics
      b. acute hemmorhagic polyencephalitis (brain lesions, convulsions); Korsakoff's syndrome

B. Low erythrocyte transketolase activity, low blood thiamine, reduced urinary excretion, without clinical symptoms.

POPULATIONS AT RISK

1. Alcoholics[24]
2. Patients on chronic renal dialysis[25]
3. Patients with chronic febrile infections[26]
4. Patients with intravenous hyperalimentation deficient in thiamin (should not occur)
5. Those receiving high carbohydrate diets and intravenous administration of dextrose (increased thiamin need)

In Subclinical Deficiency

1. Pregnant women,[27] 35% of those tested
2. Alcoholics[28]
3. Sick and injured,[29] 31% of routine hospital admissions
4. School children[30] in New York, 68% of Blacks, 52% of Caucasians, 6% of Chinese
5. Old people[31]
6. 12% of people tested[32]

Thiaminases occur in raw fish, some vegetables, and tea.[33–35] These are not usually responsible for thiamin deficiency unless intake is abnormally high. A deficiency state can be produced by the administration of the thiamine antagonist, pyrithiamine.[36]

Toxicity

Thiamine is considered to be nontoxic even in very large doses (100 to 500 mg parenterally). There are, however, a considerable number of reports of idiosyncratic reactions to ingestion of extraordinarily large doses or to intravenous administration of therapeutic doses. These include the following:

1. Headache
2. Irritability and restlessness
3. Insomnia
4. Feelings of warmth or tingling
5. Pruritis
6. Weakness
7. Sweating
8. Nausea
9. Gastrointestinal bleeding
10. Angioedema
11. Pulmonary edema
12. Respiratory distress

13. Cyanosis
14. Transient vasodilation and hypotension
15. Vascular collapse
16. Death

Note: Administration is contraindicated in patients with a known sensitivity to thiamin or any other ingredient in the thiamin preparation. Symptoms in sensitive people have been provoked by 5 mg oral doses.[37] An intradermal test dose is recommended if sensitivity is suspected.

Uses in Therapy

Whenever possible, thiamin is administered orally.

1. Wernicke's syndrome:
   Treat as medical emergency with 10 to 20 mg of thiamine hydrochloride intramuscularly or by slow intravenous administration three times a day for 2 weeks. Note that doses over 30 mg three times a day may not be utilized.
   Note: Administration of intravenous glucose may exacerbate the condition. Administer thiamin before the glucose.
2. High-output heart failure ("wet" beriberi):
   Dose as above, preferably intravenously.
3. Deficiency due to malabsorption (critically ill):
   Adults—as above
   Children—10 to 25 mg parenterally
4. Deficiency due to malabsorption (condition not critical):
   5 mg per day to 10 mg three times a day, orally, for 1 month.
5. Genetic enzyme deficiency responsive to thiamin therapy, 10 to 20 mg per day as a single oral dose, up to 4 g per day in divided doses.
6. Dietary supplement (in deficient diet or hyperalimentation):
   Adults—1 to 2 mg per day
   Children—0.5 to 1 mg per day
   Infants—0.3 to 0.5 mg per day

INADEQUATELY SUBSTANTIATED THERAPIES

There is no adequate evidence of benefit in the following conditions

1. dermatoses
2. multiple sclerosis
3. infection
4. drug toxicity
5. cancer
6. edema in infants
7. impotence
8. ulcerative colitis
9. chronic diarrhea
10. as an insect repellant

or, if thiamin intake is adequate, in

1. stimulation of mental responsiveness or improvement of thinking
2. dysphagia and anorexia
3. tiredness
4. neurologic disorders

Interference with Laboratory Tests

1. Uric acid determination by phosphotungstate—false high.
2. Urobilinogen spot test with Ehrlich's reagent—false positive.
3. Serum theophylline by spectrophotometry (Schack and Waxler)—false results.

Interference with Drug Action

Thiamin may enhance the effects of neuromuscular blocking agents. This observation is of unknown therapeutic significance.

REFERENCES—Thiamin

1. Sauberlich, H.E., Herman, Y.F., and Stevens, C.O.: Am. J. Clin. Nutr., *23:*671, 1970.
2. Consolazio, C.F., et al.: Am. J. Clin. Nutr., *24:*1060, 1971.
3. Horwitt, M.K., et al.: Investigations of Human Requirements for B-Complex Vitamins. Bulletin of the National Research Council No. 116, Washington, DC, National Academy of Sciences, 1948.
4. Reuter, H., Gasmann, B., and Böhm, M.: Int. J. Vit. Nutr. Res., *37:*315, 1967.
5. Bamji, M.S.: Am. J. Clin. Nutr., *23:*52, 1970.
6. Heller, S., Salkeld, R.M., and Körner, W.F.: Am. J. Clin. Nutr., *27:*1221, 1974.
7. Holt, L.E., Jr., et al.: J. Nutr., *37:*53, 1949.
8. Knott, E.M., Kleiger, S.C., and Schlutz, F.W.: J. Pediatr., *22:*43, 1943.

9. Knott, E.M., Kleiger, S.C., and Torres-Bracamonte, F.: J. Nutr., *25:*49, 1943.
10. Hart, M., and Reynolds, M.S.: J. Home Econ., *49:*35, 1957.
11. Dick, E.C., et al.: J. Nutr., *66:*173, 1958.
12. Boyden, R.E., and Erikson, S.E.: Am. J. Clin. Nutr., *19:*398, 1966.
13. Morrison, A.B., and Campbell, J.A.: J. Nutr., *72:*435, 1960.
14. Thomson, A.D., and Leevy, C.M.: Clin. Sci., *43:*153, 1972.
15. Thomson, A.D., Baker, H., and Leevy, C.M.: J. Lab. Clin. Med., *76:*34, 1970.
16. Howard, L., Wagner, C., and Schenker, S.: J. Nutr., *104:*1024, 1974.
17. Pearson, W.N.: Am. J. Clin. Nutr., *20:*514, 1967.
18. Sauberlich, H.E., Dowdy, R.D., and Skalen, J.A.: CRC Critical Reviews in Clinical Laboratory Sciences, *4:*236, 1973.
19. Sauberlich, H.E.: Am. J. Clin. Nutr., *20:*528, 1967.
20. McCandless, D.W., and Schenker, S.: J. Clin. Invest., *47:*2268, 1968.
21. Fennelly, J., et al.: Br. Med. J. *2:*1290, 1964.
22. Gelfand, D., and Bellet, S.: Med. Clin. N. Am., *33:*1643, 1949.
23. Philip, G.B., et al.: J. Clin. Invest., *31:*859, 1952.
24. Leevy, C.M., and Baker, H.: Am. J. Clin. Nutr., *21:*1325, 1968.
25. Raskin, N.H., and Fishman, R.A.: N. Engl. J. Med., *294:*204, 1976.
26. Gilbert, V.E., Susser, M.C., and Nolte, A.: Metabolism, *18:*789, 1969.
27. Baker, H., et al.: Am. J. Clin. Nutr., *28:*59, 1975.
28. Leevy, C.M., et al.: Am. J. Clin. Nutr., *16:*339, 1965.
29. Leevy, C.M., et al.: Am. J. Clin. Nutr., *17:*259, 1965.
30. Baker, H., et al.: Am. J. Clin. Nutr., *20:*850, 1967.
31. Brin, M., et al.: Am. J. Clin. Nutr., *17:*240, 1965.
32. U.S. Dept. of Health, Education and Welfare: Ten State Nutrition Survey 1968-70. Vol. IV. Biochemical. DHEW Pub. No. (HSM) 72-8132, 1972, p. IV-219.
33. Krampitz, L.O., and Woolley, D.W.: J. Biol. Chem., *152:*9, 1944.
34. Nakornchai, S., et al.: J. Med. Assoc. Thai., *58:*81, 1975.
35. Vimokesant, S.L., et al.: Nutr. Rep. Int., *9:*317, 1974.
36. Koedam, J.C.: Biochim. Biophys. Acta, *29:*333, 1958.
37. Mills, C.A.: JAMA, *116:*2101, 1941.

RIBOFLAVIN

Riboflavin is also known as vitamin B_2.

Recommended Dietary Allowances

The RDA is based on consideration of the following:

1. Protein needs (0.6 mg/1000 kcal)[1]
2. Energy intake—no relationship to riboflavin need[2]
3. Metabolic body size—not less than 1.2 mg per day
4. Urinary excretion[3,4]
5. Levels producing clinical symptoms of deficiency
6. Erythrocyte glutathione reductase (EGR) activity[5] and its stimulation by flavin adenine dinucleotide (FAD)[6]

   This measure is based on the fact that the availability of FAD in the body depends on the riboflavin stores; thus, if the diet is riboflavin deficient, ERG activity in vitro is increased when FAD is added.

For practical purposes, however, the RDA was computed as 0.6 mg/1000 kcal for all ages, but with a minimum recommended intake of 1.2 mg per day.

Needs for riboflavin increase during pregnancy[7,8]; an extra 0.3 mg per day of riboflavin is recommended.

In lactation, the recommended increase of 0.5 mg per day is based on the riboflavin content of human milk (0.4 mg/L)[9] and an assumed 70% conversion for milk production.[2]

Some data seem to indicate an increased need for riboflavin by women taking oral contraceptives. They are insufficient, however, for making a recommendation for an addition to the recommended intake, because no instances of riboflavin deficiency have been reported for this population.

Some riboflavin is synthesized by intestinal bacteria, particularly when the diet contains large amounts of difficultly digestible carbohydrate.[10] Some of this may be absorbed. Dietary sources of riboflavin are shown in Table 8-9.

Chemistry (Figure 8-3)

Riboflavin is yellow to yellow orange. It is slightly soluble in water and alcohol; oxidized by air; and not stable to alkali or light. Preparations are incompatible with tetracycline, erythromycin, and streptomycin. Riboflavin $pk_a = 10.2$.

Absorption

Absorption of riboflavin occurs primarily in the proximal portion of the intestine. The

TABLE 8-9. Dietary Sources of Riboflavin

Food	μg/100 g	Food	μg/100 g
Almonds	920	Molasses	
Asparagus	180	blackstrap	190
Avocados	200	Mushrooms	
Bacon		fresh or canned	300
fried	340	Mussels	
Canadian		canned	130
fried	170	Okra	180
Beans		Oysters	180
lima		Peanuts	130
fresh, cooked	100	Peanut butter	120
canned, solids	50	Peas	
frozen, cooked	50	blackeyed	110
Beef		snow	110
cooked	200	Pork	200
canned	230	Roe (fish)	
corned	180	raw	720
Beet greens	150	Salmon	
Brazil nuts	120	canned	140
Bread		Sausage and luncheon meat	220
cracked wheat	90	liverwurst	1440
rye	70	Shad	
pumpernickel	80	baked	260
whole wheat	120	Soybean sprouts	
Buckwheat flour	150	raw	200
Dandelion greens	160	Soybeans	
Eggs	300	cooked	130
Goose	240	Spinach	140
Heart		Squash	
beef	1220	cooked	80
Herring		frozen, cooked	40
canned	180	Tuna	
kippered	280	canned	120
Ice cream, ice milk	210	Turkey	
"Indian" nuts	230	roasted	140
Kale	180	Turnip	
Kidney		cooked	50
braised, beef	4800	Turnip greens	
Lamb	250	cooked	240
Liver		Veal	240
beef	4190	Wheat germ	680
chicken	2690	Whitefish	
pork	4360	baked	110
Mackerel		Yeast	
broiled	270	brewer's	4280
Milk		Yogurt	160
cow's	170		
goat's	110		

Note: Enriched bakery products contain 200 μg/100 g. Enriched pasta products contain 100 μg/100 g

absorption is regulated by a saturable active transport mechanism. The extent of absorption is also limited by the duration of contact with the specialized segment of the intestine in which absorption occurs. Absorption is decreased by a deficiency in bile salts. Thus absorption increases if riboflavin is given with food and is decreased in patients with

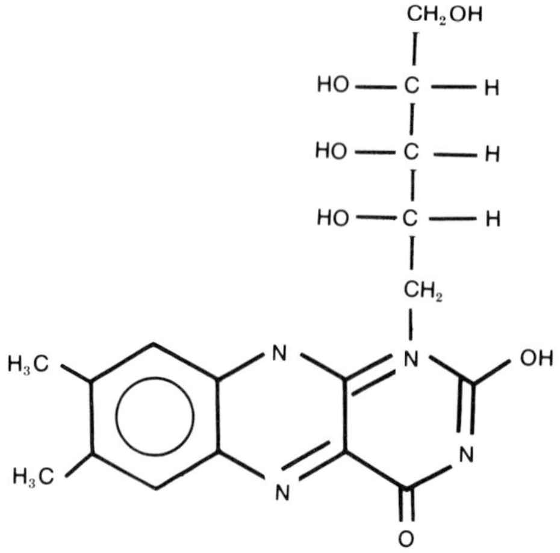

Figure 8-3. Structure of Riboflavin

hepatitis, cirrhosis, and biliary obstruction and in patients taking probenecid. Riboflavin-5-phosphate is converted to free riboflavin rapidly in the intestine before absorption.

Because of the specific intestinal area for absorption, timed release preparations of riboflavin behave erratically.

Distribution

Flavin adenine dinucleotide (FAD) and flavin mononucleotide (FMN) are widely found in the tissues. Free riboflavin is found in the retina. About 60% of FAD and FMN in blood is bound to protein. Riboflavin is stored in limited quantities in liver, spleen, kidney, and heart, mostly as FAD.

Riboflavin crosses the placenta.

Metabolism

In the cells of the gastrointestinal mucosa, riboflavin is phosphorylated to riboflavin-5-phosphate (flavin mononucleotide, FMN). In the liver, FMN is converted to flavin adenine dinucleotide (FAD).

Excretion

Ingestion of riboflavin in the range of the RDA produces excretion of about 9% of the amount unchanged in the urine. The fate of the remainder is unknown. Urinary excretion increases with increased intake. The half-life is 66 to 84 minutes after a single large oral or intramuscular dose.[11]

Pharmacology

A. FMN and FAD are coenzymes which, when combined with apoenzyme, form more than 40 flavoprotein oxidases, including the following:
   1. Aldehyde oxidase
   2. Xanthine oxidase
   3. D-amino acid oxidases
   4. Dehydrogenases, such as
      a. acetyl-coenzyme A dehydrogenase
      b. succinate dehydrogenase
      c. glutathione reductase
   5. L-amino acid oxidase
   6. Cytochrome C reductace
B. Riboflavin is involved in conversion of tryptophan to niacin.[12]

Riboflavin thus is involved in growth and repair of tissues and tissue respiration.

Laboratory Tests

The following are indicative but not diagnostic of riboflavin deficiency.

1. Urinary concentration of less that 27 μg/g of creatine.
2. Daily urinary excretion of less than 50 μg of riboflavin.
3. Riboflavin loading: normal male adults excrete 40% of a 10 mg dose.

Deficiency

Clinical episodes of riboflavin deficiency are rare.

SYMPTOMS

Symptoms of clinical riboflavin deficiency include the following:

1. Atrophy and other epidermal changes, manifested as
   a. angular cheiloses (lesions on lips and mucocutaneous junction at corner of mouth)
   b. glossitis
   c. scaly, greasy, scrotal dermatitis
   d. roughening of skin on nose (shark skin)

2. Eye problems
   a. vascularization of the cornea (early diagnostic sign) with blepharospasm, photophobia, cataract formation, and ulceration
   b. abnormal pigmentation of iris
3. Peripheral neuropathy (in alcoholics, with severe deficiency).
4. Normocytic, normochromic anemia (subjects given riboflavin antagonist).[13]

In Experimental Animals

1. Maternal riboflavin deficiency produces fetal abnormalities.[14]
   a. shortening of long bones
   b. micrognathia (abnormally small jaw, usually the lower)
   c. cleft palate
   d. hydrocephalus
   e. heart malformation
   f. eye lesions.
2. Deficiency enhances tumorigenesis by azo dyes.[15]
3. Degeneration of myelin sheath of nerves.
4. Impaired red blood cell formation, resulting in anemia.

POPULATIONS AT RISK

1. Patients with biliary obstruction:[16]
2. People with large daily intakes of alcohol[17]

In Subclinical Deficiency

1. Pregnancy[18]
2. The sick and injured[19]
3. Schoolchildren[20]
4. Alcoholics, commonly[21]

Toxicity

No toxicity has been reported for oral doses of riboflavin.

Uses in Therapy

1. Biliary obstruction: 2.5 to 5.0 mg per day.
2. Genetic metabolic disease characterized by splenomegaly, microcytic anemia, and deficiency in glutathione reductase.
3. Dietary deficiency: 5 to 10 mg orally, daily, or 50 mg intramuscularly.

Riboflavin products are listed in Table 8-10.

TABLE 8-10. Riboflavin Products

Brand	Manufacturer	Strength
*Injection**		
Generic	Veratex	50 mg/ml
Riobin-50	Pasadena Research	50 mg/ml
Tablets		
Generic	Various	5, 10, 25 mg
	Freeda	50 mg
	Nature's Bounty	100 mg

* By prescription only.

INADEQUATELY SUBSTANTIATED THERAPIES

Riboflavin has not been shown to be effective in well-controlled studies for the following:

1. Acne
2. Migraine headache
3. Congenital methemoglobinemia
4. Muscle cramps
5. "Burning feet"

Interference with Laboratory Tests

1. Large doses of riboflavin produce bright yellow urine.
2. Fluorescent substances in urine and plasma interfere with fluorometric determination of
   a. urobilinogen
   b. catecholamines

Drug Interactions

Delayed but increased absorption with drugs, such as propantheline bromide, decreasing intestinal transit time.

REFERENCES—Riboflavin

1. Horwitt, M.K.: Am. J. Clin. Nutr., *18:*458, 1966.
2. Brö-Rasmussen, F.: Nutr. Abstr. Rev., *28:*1, 369, 1958.
3. Horwitt, M.K., et al.: J. Nutr., *41:*247, 1950.
4. Bessey, O.A., Horwitt, M.K., and Love, R.H.: J. Nutr., *58:*367, 1956.
5. Tillotson, J.A., and Baker E.M.: Am. J. Clin. Nutr., *25:*425, 1972.

6. Pearson, W.N.: Am. J. Clin. Nutr., *20:*514, 1967.
7. Brzezinski A., Bromberg, Y.M., and Braun, K.: J. Lab. Clin. Med., *39:*84, 1952.
8. Heller, S., Salkeld, R.M., and Körner, W.F.: Am. J. Clin. Nutr., *27:*1225, 1974.
9. Roderuck, C., et al.: J. Nutr., *32:*267, 1946.
10. Najjar, V.A., et al.: JAMA, *126:*357, 1944.
11. Windmueller, H.G., Anderson, A.A., and Mickelsen, O.: Am. J. Clin. Nutr., *15:*73, 1964.
12. Lim Sylianco, C.Y., and Berg, C.P.: J. Biol. Chem., *234:*912, 1959.
13. Lane, M., and Alfrey, C.P., Jr.: Blood, *25:*432, 1965.
14. Mackler, B.: Pediatrics, *43:*915, 1969.
15. Rivlin, R.S.: N. Engl. J. Med., *283:*463, 1970.
16. Jusko, W.J., et al.: Am. J. Dis. Childhood, *121:*48, 1971.
17. Rosenthal, W.S., et al.: Am. J. Clin. Nutr., *26:*856, 1973.
18. Baker, H., et al.: Am. J. Clin. Nutr., *28:*59, 1975.
19. Leevy, C.M., et al.: Am. J. Clin. Nutr., *17:*259, 1965.
20. Baker, H., et al.: Am. J. Clin. Nutr., *20:*850, 1967.
21. Leevy, C.M., et al.: Am. J. Clin. Nutr., *16:*339, 1965.

NIACIN

Niacin is also known as vitamin B_3. It consists of two substances, nicotinic acid (niacin) and nicotinamide (niacinamide). The term "niacin" is used generically for both compounds, since the molecular weights differ by less than 1%. It also occurs in tissues in two coenzymatic forms, niacinamide adenine dinucleotide (NAD) and niacinamide adenine dinucleotide phosphate (NADP).

Recommended Dietary Allowances

Practically all the information about human needs for niacin comes from studies on adult humans, spanning a period of more than 20 years, done at two research centers.[1–3] The studies are complicated by the fact that there exists an obligatory split in the pathway for tryptophan metabolism; so that, on the average, ingestion of 60 mg of tryptophan causes the production of 1 mg of niacin. Although variations between individuals are large,[4–6] diets are evaluated by calculating the ingestion of 60 mg of tryptophan as equivalent to 1 mg of niacin. (Niacin content of diet is expressed as "niacin equivalents," with one equivalent representing 1 mg of niacin.) Dietary sources of niacin are listed in Table 8-11.

The studies produced some evidence that niacin needs increase with the amount of energy utilized. Symptoms of deficiency appeared in one subject at an intake of 4.9 niacin equivalents/1000 kcal. In diets containing about 200 mg of tryptophan, urinary excretion of niacin metabolites increased when 8 to 10 mg of niacin were given. This suggests that a daily intake of 11.3 to 13.3 niacin equivalents is adequate to maintain saturation of body stores.

Average diets in the United States contain 500 to 1000 mg of tryptophan or more per day (animal protein contains about 1.47% tryptophan, vegetable protein about 1% tryptophan) and 8 to 17 mg of niacin, thus giving a total of 16 to 34 niacin equivalents. The evaluation of diet, however, is complicated because niacin from grains and other foodstuffs may not be completely available. Note that corn protein has a low tryptophan content (0.6%).[7,8] In addition, abnormally high intakes of leucine may increase the niacin requirement.[8]

On considering all the data, the recommended intake for adults is 6.6 niacin equivalents/1000 kcal, but not less than 13 niacin equivalents per day.

There are no data for niacin requirements for children from infancy through adolescence. Human milk from well nourished mothers contains about 1.7 mg of niacin and 220 mg of tryptophan/L (700 kcal).[9] On this basis, the RDA is set at 8 niacin equivalents/1000 kcal for infants up to 6 months and 6.6 niacin equivalents/1000 kcal, but not less than 8 niacin equivalents daily, for older children and adolescents.

The needs for niacin during pregnancy are not clear. Data can be interpreted as either an increased or a decreased need. The recommendation is an increase of 2 niacin equivalents daily, based on the recommended increase of 300 calories of caloric intake.

During lactation, based on the niacin content of milk and the recommendation of an increase in 500 kcal of energy intake, the recommendation is an additional 5 niacin equivalents per day.

TABLE 8-11. Dietary Sources of Niacin*

Food	mg/100 g	Food	mg/100 g
Almonds	3.5	Liver	
Bacon		beef	16.5
fried	5.2	chicken	11.7
Canadian	5.0	pork	22.3
Barley	3.1	Mackerel	6.0
Beef	5.0	Peanuts	17.1
Bread		Peanut butter	14.0
enriched, white	2.5	Pork	2.7
whole wheat	2.8	Potato chips	4.8
Buckwheat		Salmon	7.3
whole	4.4	Sausages	
Bulgur wheat	2.4	liverwurst	6.5
Chicken	9.0	pork sausage	3.7
Codfish	3.0	salami	4.5
Dates	2.2	Shad	5.4
Finnan haddie	2.1	Shrimp	2.7
Flounder	2.5	Swordfish	11.0
Goose	8.5	Trout	3.0
Haddock	3.2	Tuna	11.5
Halibut	8.3	Turkey	8.0
Ham	4.4	Veal	4.5
Herring	3.5	Wheat germ	4.2
Lamb	4.5	Yeast, brewer's	38.0

* Chief sources are meat, fish, peanuts. Significant quantities may be obtained from enriched products such as breakfast cereals, pasta, rice, cakes, and cookies.

Chemistry (Figure 8-4)

Niacin is incompatible with oxidizing agents. Niacinamide is hydrolyzed by alkali and strong acids. Niacin $pk_a = 4.85$.

Absorption

Niacin and niacinamide are rapidly and completely absorbed from the gastrointestinal tract and from subcutaneous and intramuscular injections.

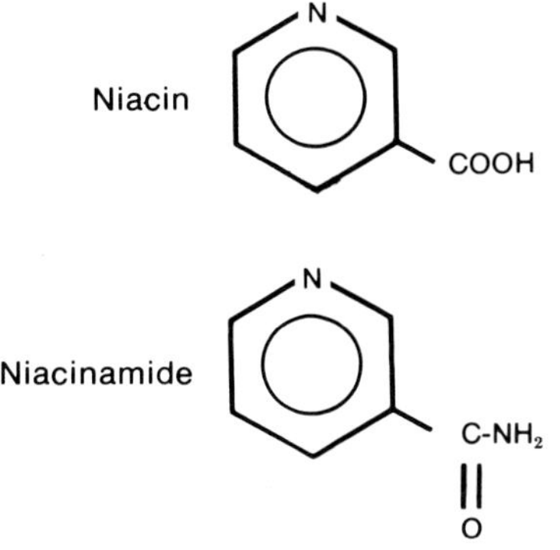

Figure 8-4. Niacin Structures

Metabolism

In usual doses (12 to 18 mg per day), niacin is coverted into niacinamide. (Only a fraction of large doses is converted to niacinamide.) The niacinamide is distributed throughout the body. In the liver, niacinamide is metabolized to N′-methylnicotinamide, N′-methyl-6-pyridone-3-carboxamide, nicotinuric acid (niacin-glycine conjugate), and a variety of N′-methylated derivatives.

Excretion[10]

Niacin and its metabolites are excreted in the urine. On a niacin-deficient diet, urinary excretion drops to a low and constant level before clinical deficiency symptoms appear. The excretory products are influenced by level of niacin intake, body needs for niacin, the availability of methyl donors, the efficiency of the methylating mechanism, and biosynthesis of niacin from tryptophan. After large doses, niacin and/or niacinamide in the urine increases.

Pharmacology

The coenzymes formed from niacinamide, NAD and NADP, are electron transfer agents. They catalyze many biochemical reactions involving carbohydrates, amino acids, and fats, particularly in glycogenolysis, tissue respiration (hydrogen transport as $NADH_2$), and lipid metabolism/liberation of free fatty acids from tissue).[11]

Laboratory Tests

1. Urinary excretion of N′-methylnicotinamide plus N′-methyl-6-pyridone-3-carboxamide less than 2 mg/24 hours indicates deficient intake.
2. Feeding a standard diet of 10 mg niacin + 100 mg tryptophan to patients produces excretion of less than 3 mg per day of products as compared with 7 to 37 mg in adequately nourished people.
3. A normal adult male excretes 50% of a 10 mg test dose.
4. Excretion of less than 0.5 mg N′-methylnicontinamide per g of creatine (best measure) indicates deficiency.

Deficiency

Niacin deficiency produces pellagra (pellis = skin, agra = seizure).

The disease was first diagnosed in Milan, Italy, as an endemic condition characterized by skin covered with tubercules and rough scales and depression, debility, dizziness, and epilepsy. The disease is characteristic of populations who live on diets high in corn. The condition is exacerbated by exposure to sunlight and heavy work.

SYMPTOMS

1. Erythema (dark red color) appearing symmetrically on arms, legs, face, neck, and other regions exposed to air and light. The skin eventually becomes dry, cracked, and brown. The epidermis becomes keratinized and tends to separate from the dermis. The dermis becomes atrophied, and its blood vessels, dilated.
2. Chronic inflammation of the gastrointestinal mucosa
   a. stomatitis
   b. glossitis
   c. gastritis and achlorhydria
   d. diarrhea, frequently bloody
3. Emotional disturbance
   a. delerium
   b. hallucinations
   c. mental confusion

These symptoms are referred to as the "3 D's"—dermatitis, diarrhea, dementia.

The neurologic symptoms usually associated with pellagra—retrobulbar neuritis, chromatolysis of brain ganglion cells, and degeneration of the myelin sheath of motor and sensory nerves—have not been seen in experimental niacin deficiency[12] and may be due to concomitant deficiency of other vitamins.

POPULATIONS AT RISK

1. Alcoholics
2. Food fadists
3. Debilitated patients (loss of appetite? poor absorption?)

Low circulatory levels of niacin were found in the following populations:

1. Children tested in New York[13]: 60% of Puerto Ricans, 54% of Caucasians, 46% of Blacks, 34% of Chinese.
2. Patients in municipal hospitals in New Jersey[14]: 29% of admissions (random sample). Dietary histories showed intakes below the RDA level in one third of these.

Toxicity

NIACIN

Side effects are produced with a single oral dose as low as 50 mg.

1. Flushing of the skin (vasodilation)[15]:

5% of test subjects at 50 mg, 50% at 100 mg, all at 500 mg.

2. At doses larger than 300 mg for various periods[16]
   a. gastrointestinal distress (40%)—dose should be taken with meals
   b. pruritis (25%)
   c. jaundice and hepatic abnormalities (3000 mg)
   d. pigmented hyperkeratosis (3000 mg per day for 24 months)[17]
   e. glucose intolerance (4500 mg per day for 4 weeks); diabetics may need dose adjustment of insulin[18]
   f. cardiac arrhythmia

NIACINAMIDE

No side effects are produced at doses less than 3000 mg. One report of toxicity at a dose of 9000 mg per day for 7 days[19] produced the following symptoms:

1. Nausea and vomiting
2. Liver biopsy showed portal fibrosis and swollen parenchyma. Liver function tests were normal 3 weeks after nicotinamide was stopped.

There are no reports of serious toxicity not reversed by discontinuing administration. Because of the unpleasantness of the flushing syndrome with niacin, niacinamide is the preferred form for therapy of deficiency states. Note, however, that niacinamide is not effective as a vasodilator or as an antilipidemic.

Uses in Therapy

1. Because of the flushing and tingling sensations produced, niacin has a strong placebo effect.
2. Antilipemic (lowering of blood cholesterol): Niacin (usually as aluminum nicotinate to prevent gastritis), but not niacinamide, in large doses (3000 to 7500 mg) lowers blood cholesterol.[20] Note that all patients experience flushing and 26% discontinue therapy because of it. (See toxicity for other side effects.)
3. Pellagra:
   300 to 500 mg per day in divided doses orally. If the oral route is not tolerated, then 50 to 100 mg intramuscularly five or more times daily, or 25 to 100 mg intravenously. The concentration should be not more than 10 mg/ml, and the rate of administration not more than 2 mg per minute, twice a day in 0.9% sodium chloride. Anaphylactic shock has occurred.
4. Hartnup disease (decrease in conversion of tryptophan to niacin).

Niacin products are listed in Table 8-12.

INADEQUATELY SUBSTANTIATED THERAPIES

1. Use of niacin as a vasodilator at 100 to 150 mg, three to five times a day, orally or 300 to 400 mg every 12 hours in an extended release preparation in the treatment of the following:
   a. peripheral vascular disease
   b. vascular spasm
   c. migraine headache
   d. Ménière's syndrome and dizziness
2. Acne
3. Leprosy
4. Motion sickness
5. Livedoid vasculitis (blue-purple mottling of the skin)
6. Alcoholism
7. Central nervous system disorders
   a. schizophrenia
   b. drug-induced hallucination
   c. chronic brain syndrome
   d. hyperkinesis
   e. unipolar depression

Administer with caution in patients with the following disorders:

1. Coronary artery disease
2. Gallbladder disease
3. History of jaundice or liver disease
4. Diabetes mellitus
5. Gout (some reports of mild rise in serum uric acid)
6. Peptic ulcer

TABLE 8-12. Niacin Products

Brand	Manufacturer	Strength
Niacin (Nicotinic Acid)		
Tablets		
Generic	Various	2, 50, 100, 500* mg
SK-Niacin	SKF	50, 100 mg
Nicolar	Armour	500 mg
Tablets—Timed-Release		
Span Niacin	Scrip	150 mg
Capsules		
Wampocap	Wallace	500 mg
Capsules—Timed-Release*		
Generic	Various	125, 250, 400 mg
Diacin	Lemmon	200 mg
Niac	O'Neal, Jones & Feldman	300 mg
Nico-400 Plateau Caps	Marion	400 mg
Nicobid	Armour	125, 250, 500 mg
Nicocap	ICN	400 mg
Nico-Span	Key	400 mg
Nicotym	Everett	400 mg
Tega-Span	Ortega	400 mg
Elixir		
Nicotinex	Fleming	50 mg/5 ml
*Injection**		
Generic	Various	50, 100 mg/ml

Niacinamide (Nicotinamide)

This substance is available under its generic name from many manufacturers. The following forms are available:

Tablets—25, 50, 100, 500 mg
Capsules—500 mg
Injection*—100 mg/ml

Brand	Manufacturer	Strength
Aluminum Nicotinate*		
Tablets		
Nicalex	Merrell	625 mg = 500 mg niacin

Note: As antilipemic: some patients must chew or crush tablets to get adequate absorption of niacin.

Brand	Manufacturer	Strength
Nicotinyl Alcohol*		
Tartrate Salt		
Roniacol	Roche	Tablets: 50 mg Timed-Release Tablets: 150 mg Elixir: 50 mg/5 ml

Classified by FDA as "possibly effective" in conditions associated with deficient circulation.

* By prescription only.

CONTRAINDICATED IN PATIENTS WITH

1. Severe hypotension
2. Arterial hemorrhaging
3. Active peptic ulcer

PREGNANCY

No known effects are associated with doses of niacin as a vitamin supplement in pregnancy. No studies have been done with large doses.

Interference with Laboratory Tests

1. Urine glucose—false positive with tests depending on reduction of cupric ion (Benedict's solution).
2. Urinary catecholamines—falsely high results in fluorometric determinations (niacin may produce fluorescent metabolites).

Drug Interactions

Niacin may potentiate the hypotensive effects of sympathetic ganglionic blocking agents and may produce postural hypotension.

REFERENCES—Niacin

1. Goldsmith, G.A., et al.: J. Clin. Invest., *31:*533, 1952.
2. Goldsmith, G.A., et al.: J. Nutr., *56:*371, 1955.
3. Goldsmith, G.A.: J. Am. Diet. Assoc., *32:*312, 1956.
4. Horwitt, M.K., et al.: J. Nutr., *60*(Suppl. 1):1, 1956.
5. Horwitt, M.K.: J. Am. Diet. Assoc., *34:*914, 1958.
6. Goldsmith, G.A., Miller, O.N., and Unglaub, W.G.: J. Nutr., *73:*172, 1961.
7. Mason, J.B., Gibson, N., and Kodicek, E.: Br. J. Nutr., *30:*297, 1973.
8. Gopalan, C., and Jaya Rao, K.S.: Vit. Horm., *33:*505, 1975.
9. Toverud, K.U., Stearns, G., and Macy, I.G.: Maternal Nutrition and Child Health. Bulletin of the National Research Council No. 123. Washington, DC, Academy of Sciences, Nov. 1950 (Reprinted, 1957).
10. Sauberlich, H.E., Dawdy, R.P., and Skala, J.H.: CRC Critical Reviews in Clinical Laboratory Sciences, *4:*284, 1973.
11. Eaton, R.P., Steinberg, D., and Thompson, R.H.: J. Clin. Invest., *44:*247, 1965.
12. Goldsmith, G.A.: The B Vitamins: Thiamine, Riboflavin, Niacin, *In* Nutrition. Vol. 2. G.H. Beaton and E.W. McHenry, eds. New York, Academic Press, 1964.
13. Baker H., et al.: Am. J. Clin. Nutr., *20:*850, 1967.
14. Leevy, C.M., et al.: Am. J. Clin. Nutr., *17:259,* 1965.
15. Spies, T.D., Bean, W.B., and Stone, R.E.: JAMA, *111:*584, 1938.
16. Belle, M., and Halpern, M.M.: Am. J. Cardiol., *2:*449, 1958.
17. Wittenborn, J.R., Weber, E.S.P., and Brown, M.: Arch. Gen. Psychiatry, *28:*308, 1973.
18. Gaut, Z.N., et al.: Metabolism, *20:*1031, 1971.
19. Winter, S.L., and Boyer, J.L.: N. Engl. J. Med., *289:*1180, 1973.
20. Parsons, W.B., Jr., and Flinn, J.H.: JAMA, *165:* 234, 1957.

PANTOTHENIC ACID

Pantothenic acid is also known as vitamin B_5. Substances with corresponding vitamin activity are D-pantothenic acid, calcium-D-pantothenate (calcium pantothenate), sodium-D-pantothenate, pantothenyl alcohol (dexpanthenol, panthenol), and D-pantothenamide.

Safe and Adequate Intake

The recommended intake of pantothenic acid is based on the 5 to 20 mg per day found in the diet of average healthy American adults (average value about 7 mg per day) and a urinary excretion of 5 to 7 mg per day when the diet contains 10 mg per day.[1] Urinary excretion generally correlates well with intake, but individual variation is high. Synthesis by intestinal microflora is suspected, but amounts and availability are unknown.[2] Clinical evidence of dietary deficiency has not been seen in humans even on intakes of 1.1 mg per day and it is possible that there is no actual requirement for pantothenic acid in the diet.[3]

No RDA is set for pantothenic acid. Daily dietary intakes thought to be "safe and adequate" are in the range of 4 to 7 mg for adults and not less than 2 mg even for infants. Human milk contains about 2 mg/L. Additional amounts may be needed, therefore, during lactation and pregnancy, although there is no recommendation for this. In general, however, recommended allowances are proportional to energy needs. Dietary sources of pantothenic acid are shown in Table 8-13.

Chemistry (Figure 8-5)

Pantothenic acid and pantothenol are water soluble. Their commercial preparations are hygroscopic, viscous oils. Calcium

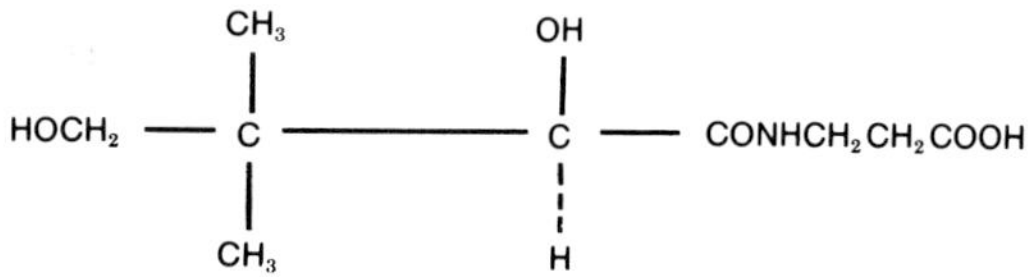

Figure 8-5. Structure of Pantothenic Acid

TABLE 8-13. Dietary Sources of Pantothenic Acid

Best Sources	
Food	mg/100 g
Beef	1.1
Broccoli	1.4
Eggs	2.7
Liver, beef	5.2
Mushrooms	1.7
Oats	1.3
Peas	1.0
Peanuts, roasted	2.5
Soybeans	1.8
Wheat germ	2.0
Other Sources	
Food	μg/100 g
Bread, whole wheat	570
Cauliflower	920
Cheese	600
Chicken	750
Lamb	600
Milk	290
Oranges	340
Oysters	490
Pork	500
Potatoes	500
Sweet potatoes	940
Salmon	900

pantothenate is a white crystalline, water-soluble solid. All are incompatible with strong acids and alkalis. Parenteral dexpanthenol preparations are packed with nitrogen, displacing air.

Absorption

Pantothenic acid and its analogs are well absorbed from oral doses.[4]

Distribution

Most pantothenic acid is found as coenzyme A in erythrocytes, with some free acid in the serum.[5]

Metabolism

All forms are converted to pantothenic acid. Only free pantothenic acid is found in the urine.

Pharmacology[6]

Coenzyme A is involved in acyl transfer reactions, including the following:

1. Synthesis of fatty acids
2. Synthesis of sterols
3. Gluconeogenesis
4. Energy release
5. Normal functioning of epithelium

Deficiency

After many unsuccessful attempts, pantothenic acid deficiency in man has been produced in two people by feeding a pantothenic acid-free diet for 10 weeks.[1] Earlier studies using the pantothenic acid antagonist omega-methylpantothenic acid gave poorly reproducible results, high individual variability of symptoms, and reports of symptoms not alleviated by feeding of pantothenic acid, indicating possible toxic effects of the antagonist. The symptoms included fatigue, insomnia, neurologic disturbances, reduced eosinopenic responses to ACTH, and increased sensitivity to insulin.

Toxicity

1. Pantothenic acid is relatively nontoxic. Daily doses of 10 to 20 g orally produced only occasional diarrhea and water retention.[7]
2. Dexpanthenol administration has resulted in reports of one case of heartburn and a few cases of gastrointestinal cramps.
3. The manufacturer of dexpanthol states that it may prolong bleeding time and should not be given to hemophiliacs.

Uses in Therapy

1. Although some investigators insist that urinary excretion of less than 1 mg per 24 hours shows a deficiency state, no clinical symptoms have been observed. Pantothenic acid concentrations normally range from 14 to 46.4 μg/dl in plasma. Blood levels are higher in infants and adults, lower in pregnant women, and lower in older women. Although administration of supplements increased plasma concentrations, there was no increase of erythrocyte coenzyme A levels.

2. Pantothenic acid deficiency in man has been suspected only in conjunction with deficiency of other B vitamins.
3. Dexpanthenol (Ilopan, Adria) has been suggested for use in the prevention of postoperative abdominal distention.[7] Well controlled trials have failed to substantiate its efficacy. Doses were 250 to 500 mg intramuscularly, repeated in 2 or 4 to 12 hours as needed, or by slow intravenous infusion diluted in 5% dextrose or lactated Ringer's injection.
4. Pantothenic acid has no therapeutic uses as a single entity. Reports of successful use in osteoarthritis and rheumatism at high doses with uncertain results seem to indicate individual metabolic errors rather than ineffective therapy. The original reports (Lancet, 1963) have not been confirmed.

Drug Interactions

On theoretic grounds, the manufacturer suggests waiting 12 hours after neostigmine or other enterokinetic (parasympathomimetic) drugs and 1 hour after succinylcholine chloride (one report of prolongation of muscle relaxant effect, not seen in a controlled trial).

REFERENCES—Pantothenic Acid

1. Fry, P.K., Fox, H.M., and Tuo, H.G.: J. Nutr. Sci. Vitaminol. (Tokyo), *22:*339, 1976.
2. Oldham, H.G., Davis, M.V., and Roberts, L.J.: J. Nutr., *32:*163, 1946.
3. Cohenour, S.H., and Calloway, D.H.: Am. J. Clin. Nutr., *25:*512, 1972.
4. Rubin, S.H., et al.: J. Nutr., *35:*499, 1948.
5. Hatano, M.: J. Vitaminol., *8:*134, 1962.
6. Krehl, W.A.: Borden's Review of Nutrition Research, *15:*53, 1954.
7. Sebrell, W.H., Jr., and Harris, R.S.: The Vitamins. Chemistry, Physiology, Pathology. Vol. II. New York, Academic Press, 1954.

VITAMIN B_6

Vitamin B_6 comprises pyridoxine, found in plants, and pyridoxal and pyridoxamine, found in animals. All three are converted by pyridoxal kinase to pyridoxal phosphate. The physiologically active forms are pyridoxamine phosphate and pyridoxal phosphate (codecarboxylase).

There is no information on the relative biologic activity of the three forms of vitamin B_6 in man, but they are equally active in rats.

The commercially available form is pyridoxine hydrochloride. Structures related to vitamin B_6 are shown in Figure 8-6.

Recommended Dietary Allowances

Estimates of vitamin B_6 nutritional needs are based on information about the following:

1. Level to produce clinical symptoms
2. Level to cure clinical symptoms
3. Plasma levels of pyridoxal phosphate
4. Excretion of tryptophan metabolites after tryptophan loading
5. Activity of serum transaminase
6. Activity of erythrocyte transaminase
7. Urinary excretion of vitamin B_6 or 4-pyridoxic acid[1]

The estimate is complicated by the fact that the requirement increases in high-protein diets.[2] The 1975 Dietary Standard for Canada recommended 0.02 mg of vitamin B_6/g protein. Because of the wide range of protein in the American diet and the lack of knowledge about availability and absorption of vitamin B_6 from dietary sources, the RDA is set at 2.2 mg for adult males and 2.0 mg for adult females, corresponding to ingestion of 110 and 100 g of protein per day, respectively.

The concentration of vitamin B_6 is higher by a factor of 6.6 in umbilical cord blood than in the maternal circulation, thus providing the fetus with a store of the vitamin.[3] Experience with milk-substitute formulas indicates satisfactory results at 0.015 mg/g protein or 0.4 mg/1000 kcal.[4] Supplementation of 0.3 mg per day prevents abnormal tryptophan metabolite excretion.[5] The RDA is set at 0.3 mg for infants and at 0.6 mg for those on mixed diets (0.5 to 1.0 year).

Insufficient data exist to satisfactorily evaluate the needs of children and adolescents. The values are set at intakes of 0.9 mg

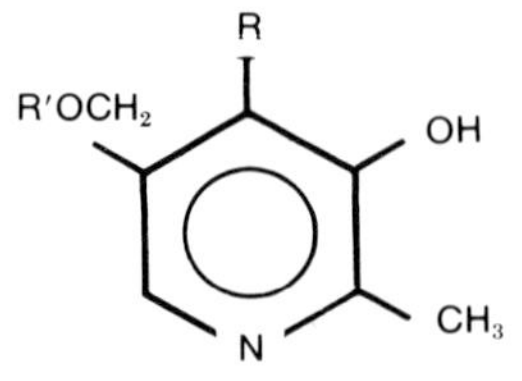

Name	R	R'
pyridoxine	$-CH_2OH$	H
pyridoxal	-CHO	H
pyridoxamine	$-CH_2NH_2$	H
4-pyridoxic acid	-COOH	H
deoxypyridoxine	$-CH_3$	H
pyridoxamine phosphate	$-CH_2NH_2$	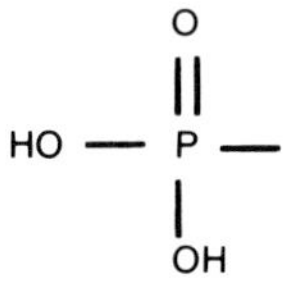 HO — P(=O)(OH) —
pyridoxal phosphate (codecarboxylase)	-CHO	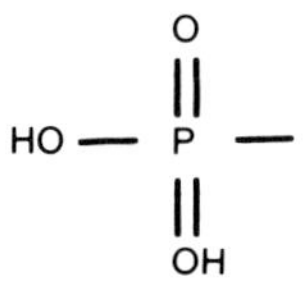 HO — P(=O)(=OH) —

Figure 8-6. Structures Related to Vitamin B_6

for those 1 to 3 years of age, 1.3 mg for 4 to 6 years, 1.6 mg for 7 to 10 years, 1.8 mg for 11 to 14 years, and 2.0 mg for 15 to 18 years.

In pregnancy, theoretically, vitamin B_6 intake should be increased because of the following:

1. Increased protein intake
2. Vitamin B_6 concentration by the fetus
3. Increased tryptophan oxidase activity caused by increase in estrogens

In addition, in pregnancy, biochemical indicators of vitamin B_6 adequacy differ from those in the nonpregnant adult, as follows:

1. In late pregnancy, decreased vitamin B_6 in urine, serum, leukocytes, and erythrocytes
2. Decreased transaminase activity of erythrocytes and leukocytes

The biochemical changes can be prevented by supplementation of 6 to 10 mg per day. Nevertheless, no clinical signs of deficiency occur and routine supplementation during pregnancy does not improve the clinical condition of the mother or fetus, thus casting doubts on the benefits of supplementation.[6] An additional allowance of 0.6 mg per day (total = 2.6 mg per day) is recommended on the basis of protein intake. Higher recommendations would not generally be supplied by diet and would require a recommendation of supplementation. In addition, there is concern that forcing the values of the pregnant female to those of the nonpregnant would produce high levels in the fetus, which might adversely affect synthesis of fetal pyridoxal phosphate enzymes and increase fetal requirements for pyridoxine after birth.[7]

In lactation, vitamin B_6 in milk is related to the nutritional state of the mother. It ranges from 0.01 to 0.02 mg/L during the first days of lactation and gradually increases to 0.10 to 0.25 mg/L.[8] The vitamin B_6:protein ratio was found to be about 13 μg/g at intakes below 2.5 mg per day, rising to 23 μg/g at intakes of 2.5 to 5.0 mg per day. An additional allowance of 0.5 mg per day (total = 2.5 mg per day) is recommended. This provides adequately for the needs of the human-milk-nourished infant.

Use of estrogen-containing oral contraceptives may be accompanied by an increase in urinary tryptophan metabolites and a temporary fall in plasma pyridoxal phosphate concentration. Despite the fact that a reported 10 to 15% of women taking oral contraceptives showed lowered biochemical indices, recent studies using depletion-repletion show that requirements for vitamin B_6 are about the same for users and nonusers of oral contraceptives.[9,10] The effect reported is not considered to be clinically significant.

In the elderly, plasma pyridoxal phosphate decreases, accompanied by a decrease in serum transaminase and a decrease in the conversion of tryptophan. Although transaminase activity can be increased by large doses of pyridoxine, there is no improvement of clinical status.

Chemistry

Pyridoxine hydrochloride is incompatible with alkaline solutions, iron salts, or oxidizing agents. It is slowly decomposed by light.

Absorption

Pyridoxine, pyridoxal, and pyridoxamine are readily absorbed from oral doses.

Distribution

Pyridoxal and pyridoxal phosphate are highly bound to blood protein. Major stores are in the liver, with lesser amounts in muscle and brain. The total body store is estimated at 16 to 27 mg. Pyridoxal crosses the placenta and is concentrated by the fetus.

Metabolism

In the liver, pyridoxine is phosphorylated to pyridoxine phosphate and, in the presence of riboflavin, transaminated to pyridoxal phosphate. Erythrocytes convert pyridoxine and pyridoxamine to the corresponding phosphates. In the liver, pyridoxal is oxidized to 4-pyridoxic acid. The biologic half-life is 15 to 20 days.

Excretion

The metabolic product, 4-pyridoxic acid, is excreted in the urine. This accounts for 20 to 40% of the ingested pyridoxine.

Pharmacology (Figure 8-7)

1. Pyridoxamine phosphate acts in transaminations of amino acids and keto-acids and in the formation of antibodies.
2. Pyridoxal phosphate is a cofactor in more than 60 enzymatic reactions, including the following:[11]
   a. oxidases

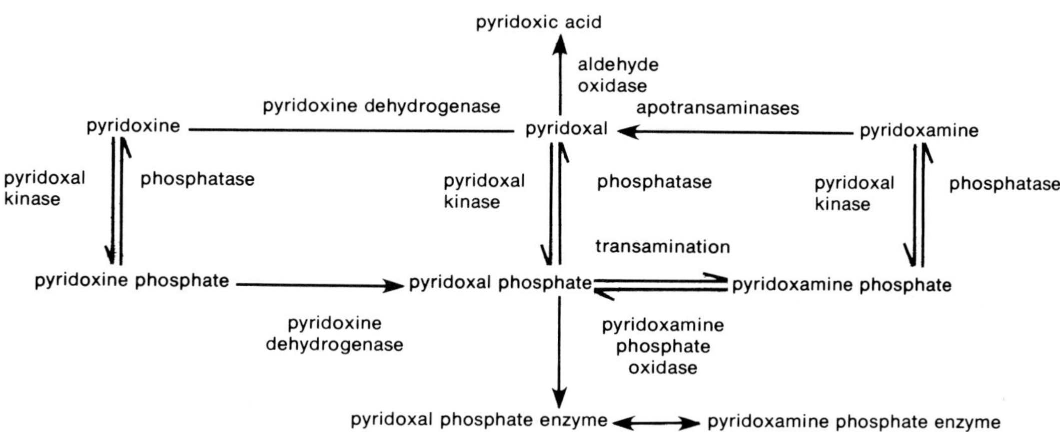

Figure 8-7. Vitamin B_6 Interconversions[23]

(1) histaminase—oxidation of histamine
(2) diaminoxidase

b. synthases
(1) serine and indole → tryptophan
(2) serine → cysteine
(3) serine + methanethiol → methlycysteine

c. decarboxylases
(1) histidine → histamine
(2) tyrosine → tyramine
(3) dopa → dopamine
(4) hydroxytryptophan → serotonin

d. deaminases—for many amino acids

e. desulfurases
deamination and desulfuration of cysteine and homocysteine

f. threonine aldolase—threonine → glycine + acetaldehyde

g. racemases—d-amino acid ⟷ 1-amino acid

h. serine hydroxymethyltransferase formation of 5, 10-methylene tetrahydrofolic acid

i. alpha-glucan phosphorylase phosphorolysis of glycogen

Laboratory Tests for Nutritional Status[12]

1. Measurement of plasma or serum level (protozoan assay technique):
   Normal—more than 5 μg/dl (Range: 3 to 8 μg/dl)
   Deficiency—less than 2.5 μg/dl
2. Deficiency: Urinary excretion of less than 20 μg of pyridoxine/g creatinine, with increased excretion following supplementation.
3. Determination of pyridoxal-5-phosphate (by tyrosine decarboxylase).
4. Increase in urinary excretion of tryptophan metabolites (xanthurenic acid, kynurenine and 3-hydroxykinurenine) after a 2 to 5 g loading of L-tryptophan.
5. Decrease in erythrocyte GOT (glutamine-oxaloacetic transaminase) and GPT (glutamic-pyruvic transaminase) activity and in vitro stimulation of activity by pyridoxal phosphate (E-GOT or E-GPT activation test).
6. Low urinary excretion of 4-pyridoxic acid.

Deficiency

Deficiency symptoms have been produced by deficient diet and by feeding of vitamin B_6 antagonists (deoxypyridine). Dietary sources of vitamin B_6 are listed in Table 8-14. Because many of the clinical symptoms are the same as symptoms of deficiency of other B vitamins, response to doses of pyridoxine hydrochloride is used to make the diagnosis. Vitamin B_6 products are listed in Table 8-15.

TABLE 8-14. Dietary Sources of Vitamin B_6*

Food	μg/100 g
Bananas	300
Beans, lima	450
Beef liver	800
Cabbage	290
Molasses	270
Peas	190
Peanuts	300
Pork	86-270
Sweet potato	320
Wheat germ	600

Note: This table is incomplete because there has been no intensive investigation of the vitamin B_6 content of foods. Processing may reduce availability.[25]

* Smaller amounts (25 to 100 μg/100 g) are found in apples, whole wheat, bread, canteloupe, cauliflower, cheese, chicken, halibut, oranges, potatoes, spinach, turnips.

CLINICAL SYMPTOMS

1. Increased irritability.
2. Mental depression and confusion.[13]
3. Microcytic hypochromic anemia with rise in serum iron and deposition of iron pigments in spleen and bone marrow (in infants).
4. Abnormal encephalograms and convulsions (in infants)

Use of the vitamin antagonist also produced:

1. Peripheral neuropathy.

TABLE 8-15. Vitamin B_6 Products

Brand	Manufacturer	Strength
Pyridoxine Hydrochloride		
Tablets		
Generic	Various	5, 10, 25, 50, 100, 200, 250, 500 mg
Pan-B-6	Panray	25, 50, 100 mg
Hexa-Betalin	Lilly	10, 25, 50 mg
Tablets, timed-release		
Generic	Various	500 mg
Capsules, timed-release		
Tex Six T.R.	Scherer	100 mg
*Injection**		
Generic	Various	50, 100 mg/ml
Hexa-Betalin	Lilly	100 mg/ml
Hexavibex	Parke-Davis	100 mg/ml

* By prescription only.

2. Inflammation of the mouth, tongue, and gums and seborrheic dermatitis (as produced by riboflavin deficiency). Note that vitamin B_6 therapy is rarely effective in dermatitis.

BIOCHEMICAL SYMPTOMS

Excretion of xanthurenic acid:

Xanthurenic acid forms a complex with insulin, acts as an insulin antagonist, and has a diabetogenic effect in animals.[14] This may be the cause of "gestational diabetes."

HYPERTHYROIDISM

Deranged tryptophan metabolism correctible by high-level pyridoxine administration has been reported.[15] The only clinical symptom was obvious muscular weakness in one patient. Tryptophan metabolism is shown in Figure 8-8.

DRUG-INDUCED[16]

The following drugs induce vitamin B_6 deficiency. Their use requires supplementation, frequently in large doses.

1. Isoniazid
2. Carbohydrazide
3. Cycloserine (in tuberculosis)
4. Penicillamine (in Wilson's disease and heavy metal poisoning)
5. Hydralazine (in hypertension)

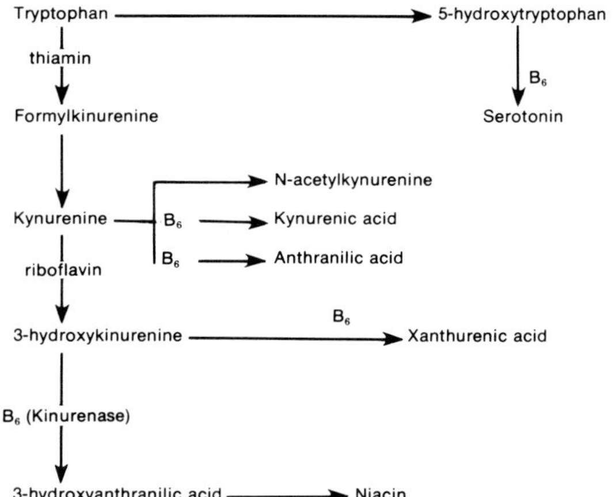

Figure 8-8. Tryptophan Metabolism and the Vitamins B[24]

6. Phenytoin
7. Succinimide (epilepsy)
8. Ethionamide
9. Pyrazinamide

GENETIC DISORDERS

1. Cystathioninuria[17]
2. Xanthurenic aciduria[18]
3. Homocystinuria (pyridoxine responsive)[19]
4. Sideroblastic anemia (pyridoxine responsive)

These genetic disorders are rare, require sophisticated techniques of diagnosis, and require therapy in addition to pyridoxine.

Toxicity

ACUTE

1. No cases of acute toxicity have been reported in humans.
2. Oral LD-50 in rats or mice is 4.0 to 5.5 mg/kg.[20]

CHRONIC[20]

1. No toxic effect at 50 to 200 mg per day pyridoxine for several months; except one patient with encephalitis had the seizures aggravated and another showed deteriorative changes in the encephalogram.
2. Transient induced dependency:
   After 200 mg per day for 33 days, three of eight subjects had abnormal encephalograms 8 days after the supplement was stopped.[21]
3. The following have been reported for one patient only
   a. aminoaciduria in a child (120 mg per day for 2 years)
   b. insomnia (100 mg per day); relieved at 50 mg per day
   c. somnolence (5 mg per day)

Uses in Therapy

1. Drug-induced deficiency anemia or neuritis:
   100 to 200 mg per day orally for 3 weeks, then prophylactically 25 to 100 mg per day.
2. Pyridoxine-dependent infants with convulsions:
   10 to 100 mg intramuscularly or intravenously generally stops seizure in 2 to 3 minutes. These infants may require 2 to 100 mg per day orally throughout life.
3. For patients on isoniazid or penicillamine:
   10 to 50 mg per day orally.
4. For patients on cycloserine:
   100 to 300 mg per day orally in divided doses.
5. Hereditary sideroblastic anemia:
   200 to 600 mg per day orally for 1 to 2 months. If ineffective, other therapy must be tried. If effective, a lifetime dose of 30 to 50 mg per day.
6. For isoniazid acute toxicity:
   Pyridoxine hydrochloride equal in amount to the isoniazid taken, plus use of other anticonvulsants. Pyridoxine is administered at 1 to 4 g intravenously, followed by 1 g intramuscularly every 30 minutes until the entire calculated dose has been given.
7. Cycloserine overdose:
   300 mg or more per day.
8. Hydrazide acute toxicity:
   25 mg/kg—one third intramuscularly, the rest by intravenous infusion over a period of 3 hours.

INADEQUATELY SUBSTANTIATED THERAPIES

1. Acne
2. Dermatosis
3. Anorexia
4. Premenstrual tension
5. Hyperlipidemia
6. Radiation sickness
7. Pernicious vomiting of pregnancy
8. Motion sickness
9. Psychosis
10. Depression associated with use of oral contraceptives
11. Tardive dyskinesia
12. Asthma
13. Petit mal epilepsy
14. Suppression of post partum lactation
15. Prevention of leukopenia due to mitomycin
16. Treatment of procarbazine neurotoxicity
17. Atopic dermatitis in children
18. Childhood bronchial asthma
19. Prevention of calcium oxalate kidney stones

Interference with Laboratory Tests

1. Urobilinogen spot test with Ehrlich's reagent: false positives at high dose levels of pyridoxine.

Drug and Nutrient Interactions

1. Patients treated with large amounts of pyridoxine for homocystinuria may develop folate deficiency.[22]
2. Diminution in the effectiveness of levodopa in treatment of Parkinsonism, due to acceleration of peripheral metabolism of levodopa when pyridoxine supplementation is 5 mg per day or more. This effect is prevented by concomitant administration of carbodopa which inhibits decarboxylase.
3. Decrease of 50% in serum levels of phenytoin and phenobarbital when 200 mg per day of pyridoxine was given for 1 month.

REFERENCES—Vitamin B_6

1. Sauberlich, H.E., Dowdy, R.P., and Skala, J.H.: Laboratory Tests for the Assessment of Nutritional Status. Cleveland, CRC Press, 1974.
2. Linkswiler, H.M.: Vitamin B_6 Requirements of Men, *In* Human Vitamin B_6 Requirements. Washington, DC, National Academy of Sciences, 1978.
3. Cleary, R.E., Lumeng, L., and Li, T.-K.: Am. J. Obstet. Gynecol., *121:*25, 1975.
4. McCoy, E.E.: Vitamin B_6 Requirements of Infants and Children, *In* Human Vitamin B_6 Requirements. Washington, DC, National Academy of Sciences, 1978.
5. Bessey, O.A., Adam, D.J.D., and Hansen, A.E.: Pediatrics, *20:*33, 1957.
6. Dempsey, W.B.: Vitamin B_6 and Pregnancy, *In* Human Vitamin B_6 Requirements. Washington, DC, National Academy of Sciences, 1978.
7. Shane, B., and Contractor, S.F.: Am. J. Clin. Nutr., *28:*739, 1975.
8. Kirksey, A., and West, K.D.: Relationship Between Vitamin B_6 Intake and the Content of the Vitamin in Human Milk, *In* Human Vitamin B_6 Requirements. Washington, DC, National Academy of Sciences, 1978.
9. Bossé, T.R., and Donald, E.A.: Am. J. Clin. Nutr., *32:*1015, 1979.
10. Donald, E.A., and Bossé, T.R.: Am. J. Clin. Nutr., *32:*1024, 1979.
11. Dixon, M., and Webb, E.C.: Enzymes. 2nd Ed. New York, Academic Press, 1964.
12. Sauberlich, H.E., et al.: Am. J. Clin. Nutr., *25:* 629, 1972.
13. Adams, P.W., et al.: Lancet, *1:*897, 1973.
14. Kotake, Y., and Murakami, I.: Am. J. Clin. Nutr., *24:*826, 1971.
15. Wohl, M.G., et al.: Proc. Soc. Exp. Biol. Med., *105:*523, 1960.
16. Roe, D.A.: NY State J. Med., *71:*2770, 1971.
17. Frimpter, G.W., Haymovitz, A., and Horwith, M.: N. Engl. J. Med., *268:*333, 1963.
18. Knapp, A.: Clin. Chim. Acta, *5:*6, 1960 (in German).
19. Carson, N.A.J.: Proc. Roy. Soc. Med., *63:*41, 1970.
20. Unna, K.R., and Honig, G.R.: Vitamin B_6 Group XII, Pharmacology and Toxicology, *In* The Vitamins, 2nd Ed. Vol. II. W.H. Sebrell, Jr. and R.S. Harris, eds. New York, Academic Press, 1954.
21. Ekelund, H., Gamstorp, I., and von Studnitz, W.: Acta Paediatr. Scand., *58:*572, 1969.
22. Wilcken, B., and Turner, B.: Arch. Dis. Childhood, *48:*58, 1973.
23. Snell, E.E.: Vitam. Horm., *22:*485, 1964.
24. Goodwin T.W.: Biosynthesis of Vitamins and Related Compounds. New York, Academic Press, 1963.
25. Gregory, J.D., and Kirk, J.R.: Vitamin B_6 in Foods: Assessment of Stability and Bioavailability, *In* Human Vitamin B_6 Requirements. Washington, DC, National Academy of Sciences, 1978.

FOLACIN

Folacin, or folate (vitamin B_9), is used as a term for substances having structures and nutritional properties similar to folic acid (pteroylglutamic acid, PGA). Necessities for activity are (1) the pteridine nucleus, (2) aminobenzoic acid residue, and (3) at least one glutamic acid residue. Many naturally occurring folates are polyglutamates, and the pteridine nucleus may be N-substituted. Folacin structures are shown in Figure 8-9.

Because of the large variety of substances with folacin activity, the content in food is measured biologically by growth of Lactobacillus casei on a defined folate-free medium to which known amounts of the test substance are added. This assay is known to understate folate because, although it responds to the greatest number of different folates, it does not respond to all of them. Polyglutamates must be hydrolyzed with conjugase before assay. The folates vary widely in bioavailability, stability, and effectiveness.

The commercial forms are folic acid and calcium leucovorin. Leucovorin is folinic acid, a reduced form of folic acid, which is an active metabolite. It is also known as "citrovorum factor."

Recommended Dietary Allowances

An extensive review has been made of folacin requirements in man.[1] Estimates of

Folic Acid

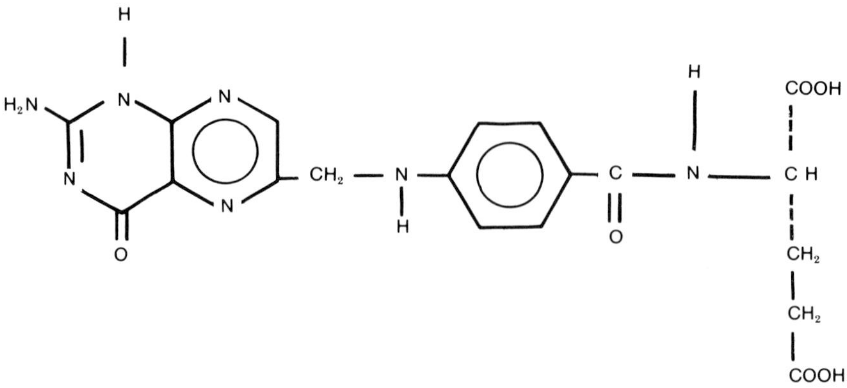

Calcium Leucovorin

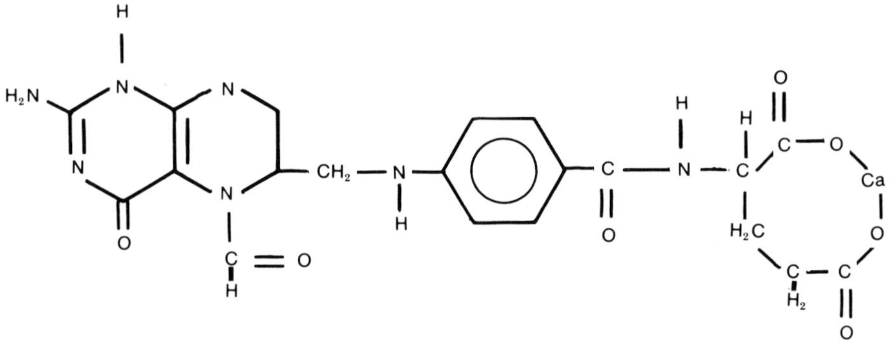

Figure 8-9. Folacin Structures

folacin needs are complicated because of synthesis of large amounts of folic acid by the intestinal bacteria. The following information is currently accepted.

1. Availability of folacin in the human diet is about 25 to 50% (ranges reported for individuals are 7 to 72%) with 10% availability from brewer's yeast.[2]
2. Body pool in the normal adult male is estimated as 5 to 10 mg[3] and may be as high as 50 mg.
3. Biologic half-life is about 100 days.[4]
4. 100 μg/per day of folic acid maintains serum folacin levels.

On the basis of maximal body pool, minimum availability, body turnover rate, and amounts in the diets of healthy humans, the RDA is set at 400 μg. This is not an unusual intake, and some diets contain 1000 to 2000 μg per day.

Requirements for infants are estimated from concentrations in human milk (20 to 40 μg/850 ml). Cow's milk would be suitable (20 to 30 μg/L) except that the folacin in cow's milk is destroyed by heating, even pasteurization. Supplementation is therefore necessary. The folacin in goat's milk is poorly available. The RDA is set at 5 μg/kg. For children between 1 and 10 years of age, the RDA supplies 8 to 10 μg of intake/kg to allow for variability in the availability from a mixed diet.

During pregnancy, an increase of 400 μg per day (800 μg total) is recommended. During lactation, an additional 100 μg per day (500 μg total) is recommended.

Note that the recommendations are for folate from dietary sources and assume not more than 50% absorption. Dietary sources of folate are shown in Table 8-16. If folic

TABLE 8-16. Dietary Sources of Folate*

Food	μg/100 g	Food	μg/100 g
Asparagus	118-280	Liver	
Bananas	95	beef	290
Beans		chicken	380
lima		pork	220
dried	330	Mushrooms	30
green		Nuts	
fresh	28	almonds	45
Bread		hazelnuts	67
whole wheat	69	peanuts	
Broccoli	100	roasted	280
Cantaloupe	130	peanut butter	60
Cheese		Oranges	83
cottage	30	Oysters	240
Eggs	86	Parsley	40
Endive	62	Pork	65-140
Fennel	100	Salmon	870
Ham	58-120	Swiss chard	62
Lentils		Watermelon	150
dried	100	Brewer's yeast	2400

Note: Availability from brewer's yeast is 10% for humans.

* Note that the values are by L. casei assay. Availability for humans may be different.

acid, which is well absorbed, is given, administration at half of the RDA is usually adequate.

Chemistry

Synthetic folic acid is yellow. It is slightly soluble in water. Its preparations are usually made by forming the sodium salt at pH 8 to 11. The solutions are incompatible with oxidizing and reducing agents and heavy metal ions, which catalyze decomposition, and decompose in the presence of light or riboflavin.

Absorption

Polyglutamates are hydrolyzed to folic acid by gastrointestinal enzymes. The folic acid is absorbed mainly in the proximal portion of the small intestine.

Distribution

After an oral dose, serum folate levels peak in 30 to 60 minutes. Low doses (1 mg) are converted in the liver to N^5-methyltetrahydrofolic acid. Large doses saturate the liver metabolic pathway and appear in the blood as folic acid. The following levels have been observed in normal healthy, well-nourished adults:

Serum—0.5 to 1.5 μg/dl
Cerebrospinal fluid—1.6 to 2.1 μg/dl (note concentration from serum)
Erythrocytes—17.5 to 31.6 μg/dl

Excretion

Trace amounts of folic acid appear in urine after doses of 0.1 to 0.2 mg. About 50% of a 2.5 to 5 mg dose and up to 90% of a 15 mg dose are excreted in the urine. In the absence of supplementation, excretion is about 0.05 mg per day by all pathways.

Pharmacology

Folic acid is converted by a series of reductions to the tetrahydrofolates which act as coenzymes in one-carbon transfer reactions. These include the biosynthesis of purines and thymidylates of nucleic acid. A defective thymidylate synthesis in deoxyribonucleic acid (DNA) is thought to be the cause of the megaloblastic and macrocytic anemias characteristic of folacin deficiency.[5]

Deficiency

Symptoms of deficiency are not apparent on gross examination. Diagnosis of deficiency is based on the examination of a blood smear.

SYMPTOMS

1. Macrocytic anemia
2. Megaloblastic anemia (fetal damage if patient is pregnant)

POPULATIONS AT RISK

1. Pregnant women
2. Infants and children
3. Patients with primary liver disease
4. Alcoholics
5. Patients with gastrointestinal disease
6. Women taking oral contraceptives have increased folate requirements, but an increased incidence of anemia in this group has not been reported. Low serum levels reported may be due to changes in protein binding.[6]

DRUG-INDUCED

1. Renal dialysis
2. Phenytoin
3. Barbiturates
4. Sulfasalizine
5. Primidone

Toxicity

No reports of toxicity associated with oral doses up to 15 mg per day.

Uses in therapy

For anemias due to folate deficiency:

Up to 1 mg per day orally. If the oral route is not possible, deep intramuscular, subcutaneous, or intravenous injection may be used. Formerly, doses up to 10 mg per day were given, but there is no evidence that doses larger than 1 mg per day are any more effective. Folic acid products are shown in Table 8-17.

TABLE 8-17. Folic Acid Products

Brand	Manufacturer	Strength
Folic acid		
Tablets		
Generic	Various	0.1, 0.25, 0.4, 1.0 mg
Folvite*	Lederle	1.0 mg
*Injection**		
Folvite	Lederle	5 mg/ml

* By prescription only.

LEUCOVORIN

(Note that folic acid does not have these effects.) Because it is readily converted to other tetrahydrofolates, it is a potent antidote for the folic acid antagonists:

1. Methotrexate
2. Pyrimethamine
3. Trimethoprim

This is the basis for the "leucovorin rescue" technique in which high doses of methotrexate are used as cancer chemotherapy in osteogenic sarcoma, head and neck cancer, lung cancer, and refractory acute leukemia. It is thought that leucovorin enters normal cells in preference to tumor cells because of a difference in cell membrane transport mechanisms, thus protecting the normal cells from the cytotoxic effect of methotrexate. The administration of leucovorin is continued for several hours after the administration of methotrexate, until the serum level of methotrexate is nontoxic.

Frequently, when methotrexate is given locally by intraarterial perfusion, leucovorin may be given orally, intramuscularly, or intravenously to prevent systemic methotrexate toxicity.

Leucovorin antagonizes the hematologic toxicity of trimethoprim without interfering with its antibacterial properties; and antagonizes the hematologic toxicity of pyrimethamine.

Leucovorin can be used in the treatment of megaloblastic anemia due to congenital deficiency of dihydrofolate reductase.

Interferences

Much has been made of the masking by folic acid of the pernicious anemia associated with vitamin B_{12} deficiency. The danger is that folate relieves the anemia but does not reverse the neuropathy of vitamin B_{12} deficiency. The *parenteral* dose required to give this effect is 0.4 mg; therefore, oral doses at the RDA level would not be expected to be significant.[7] As a matter of public policy, the rare missed diagnosis of vitamin B_{12} deficiency must be weighed against the prophylaxis of folacin deficiency.

Folic acid therapy of folate-deficient patients may increase phenytoin metabolism. This effect is usually not clinically significant, but may increase the possibility of seizures in some patients.

REFERENCES—Folacin

1. Rodríguez, M.S.: J. Nutr., *108:*1983, 1978.
2. Babu, S., and Srikantia, S.G.: Am. J. Clin. Nutr., *29:*376, 1976.
3. Herbert, V.: N. Engl. J. Med., *284:*976, 1971.
4. Krumdieck, C.L., et al.: Am. J. Clin. Nutr., *31:*88, 1978.
5. Herbert, V., Colman, N., and Jacob, E.: Folic Acid and Vitamin B_{12}, *In* Modern Nutrition in Health and Disease, 6th Ed. R.S. Goodhart and M.E. Shils, eds. Philadelphia, Lea & Febiger, 1980.
6. Shojania, A.M., Hornady, G., and Barnes, P.H.: Lancet, *1:*1376, 1968.
7. Hansen, H.A., and Weinfeld, A.: Acta Med. Scand., *172:*427, 1962.

VITAMIN B_{12}

Vitamin B_{12} is defined as those cobalt-containing corinoids, the cobalamines, which have biologic activity in humans. The commercially available form is usually cyanocobalamine; the predominant forms in plasma and animal tissue are methylcobalamin, hydroxocobalamin, and 5-deoxy-adenosylcobalamin.[1] These forms are less stable than the cyanocobalamin produced by bacterial fermentation. Vitamin B_{12} activity is also available in liver extracts.

Recommended Dietary Allowances

Nutritional deficiency of vitamin B_{12} is rare. It occurs mainly in people on a strict vegetarian diet that does not contain meat, eggs, or diary products. Data on the size of the saturated body pool range from 2 to 3 mg. Half-life estimates range from 480 to 1284 days. The variation in values may be due to loss of a definite fraction of the body pool per day.[2] An additional complication is that the fraction of the available vitamin B_{12} absorbed from an oral dose is dose-dependent but highly variable, as shown in Table 8-18.[3]

TABLE 8-18. Vitamin B_{12} Absorption from a Single Oral Dose

Dose	Percentage Absorbed	
μg	Mean	Range
0.1	77	52 to 92
0.25	75	32 to 92
0.5	71	33 to 97
0.6	63	20 to 92
1.0	56	26 to 87
2.0	46	4 to 83
5.0	28	2 to 50
10.0	16	0 to 34
20.0	6	
50.0	3	

Nutritional equilibrium can be maintained on a wide range of intakes. Average diet in the United States supplies between 5 and 15 μg per day, with individual diets ranging from 1 to 100 μg per day.[4] Vitamin B_{12} content of individual foods has not been determined, even though milk, cheese, egg yolk, meat, especially liver and kidney, fish and shellfish are considered to be good sources. On consideration of all available data, the RDA is set at 3 μg for adults.

Human milk contains 0.2 to 0.8 μg/850 ml, and parallels maternal serum level.[2] Since no clinical symptom of vitamin B_{12} deficiency occurs in human-milk-fed infants, the RDA is set at 0.5 μg, which allows a safety margin. For infants receiving commercial formulas, the Committee on Nutrition of the American Academy of Pediatrics recommends a daily intake of 0.15 μg/100 kcal.[5] On this basis, a 1-year-old child weighing 10 kg should have 1.5 μg per day. The RDA for older children and adolescents is based on the recommended average energy intake for the particular age group.

In pregnancy, fetal demand is about 0.3 μg per day.[2] In addition, there is an increased maternal need due to the increase in metabolism. This is estimated as not greater than 0.5 μg per day. To allow a margin of safety, the RDA is set at 4 μg during pregnancy and lactation. Although 10 to 15 μg per day of vitamin B_{12} are produced by microflora of the large intestine, almost none of this absorbed.

Chemistry

Vitamin B_{12} is relatively thermostable and can be autoclaved for short periods. It is incompatible with ascorbic acid.

Absorption

Vitamin B_{12} is absorbed from the distal portion of the small intestine. Protein-bound dietary vitamin B_{12} is split from the protein. Free vitamin B_{12} is bound with the glycoprotein "intrinsic factor" (IF) secreted by the gastric mucosa. The complex is retained on specific receptor sites in the presence of calcium ion and a pH of 5.4 to 8.0. The efficiency of this mechanism is about 50% for doses up to 2 μg, then decreases at higher doses.[6] This mechanism is saturated at 5 to 10 μg of vitamin B_{12}. A small percentage of free vitamin B_{12} diffuses through the walls of the intestine (about 1%). This is significant only for doses exceeding 100 μg.

Distribution

Vitamin B_{12} is removed from its complex with IF in the intestinal cell and is transported in the serum mostly bound to the beta-globulin transcobalamin II. Small amounts are bound to a storage alpha-glycoprotein, transcobalamin I, and an inter-alpha-glycoprotein, transcobalamin III. Peak serum levels are reached 8 to 12 hours after ingestion.

Vitamin B_{12} is found in liver, bone marrow, and tissues. At birth, the blood level of the newborn is 3 to 5 times that of the mother. Liver storage is 1000 to 1500 μg in the adult, with total body stores estimated as 1.0 to 11 mg.

Excretion

Normally, 3 to 8 μg per day are excreted in the bile with nearly all reabsorbed. This enterohepatic circulation, therefore, acts to conserve most of the vitamin B_{12}. The usual body stores, then, represent a 3- to 4-year supply.

Free vitamin B_{12}, not bound to liver, plasma, or tissues, is available for urinary excretion. Thus, after parenteral administration of doses above 100 μg, 50 to 90% of the dose may be excreted in the urine within 48 hours, with most excreted in the first 8 hours.

Pharmacology

Vitamin B_{12} is a cofactor and is converted into unknown coenzymes. It is required in humans for the following:

1. DNA synthesis.
2. Cell replication.
3. Synthesis of myelin.
4. Erythrocyte production.
5. 5-methyltetrahydrofolate → tetrahydrofolate (deficiency produces a functional folate deficiency). Tetrahydrofolate is necessary for synthesis of thymidine.
6. Methylmalonate ⟷ succinate[7] (in deficiency, methylmalonate appears in urine).
7. Homocysteine → methionine.
8. Maintenance of $^{-}$SH in reduced form.
9. Methylmalonyl coenzyme A → succinyl coenzyme A (degradation of some amino acids and fatty acids).

Laboratory Values

Serum cyanocobalamin activity:

Normal—20 to 90 μg/dl (average 45 μg/dl)
Megaloblastic anemia—below 10 μg/dl

Deficiency

The earliest symptom of vitamin B_{12} deficiency is usually hematopoietic inadequacy.

This is followed by gastrointestinal changes and, finally, by neuropathy.

SYMPTOMS

1. Megaloblastic anemia.
2. Megaloblastic changes in gastrointestinal epithelium.
3. Neurologic degeneration (in severe, prolonged deficiency) failure of myelin production, gradual degeneration of axon and nerve head.

DIAGNOSIS

Cyanocobalamin is studied in humans by using radioactive Cyanocobalamin Co 57 (Racobalamin-57, Abbott; Rubratope-57, Squibb) in patients who have received no cobalamin therapy for the previous 4 days and have been fasted for 12 hours.

1. Schilling Test

Administer 0.5 to 1.0 microcurie of cyanocobalamin Co 57 orally. One to 2 hours later, administer 1 mg cyanocobalamin (non-radioactive) intramuscularly; determine radioactivity in urine, making appropriate corrections for radioactive decay (half-life of Co 57 is 270 days). Excretion of less than 5% of dose indicates malabsorption. Excretion of more than 10% of dose eliminates diagnosis of pernicious anemia.

2. Fecal Excretion Test

Normal—Excretion of less than 50% of dose.

Malabsorption—Excretion of more than 70% of dose.

3. Plasma Concentration Test or Liver Uptake

Malabsorption—No significant uptake in plasma or liver. Significant uptake eliminates diagnosis of pernicious anemia.

Pernicious anemia is shown if abnormal results become normal when intrinsic factor is given with the oral dose of cyanocobalamin Co 57.

POPULATIONS AT RISK

1. Strict vegetarians (vegans), after several years, and their nursing infants. (*Note:* Ovolactovegetarians do not develop deficiency.)
2. Patients lacking intrinsic factor.
3. Loss of ileal absorption site by disease or surgery.
4. Abnormal bacterial overgrowth (tropical sprue) or presence of fish tapeworm in small intestine, due to competition for dietary vitamin B_{12}.
5. Genetic defects (very rare)
   a. abnormal synthesis of intrinsic factor
   b. abnormal ileal receptors
   c. lack of transcobalamins
   d. lack of enzymes to convert vitamin B_{12} to coenzyme form

Toxicity

1. No toxic effects from oral doses (single doses up to 100 mg, chronic doses of 1 mg per week for 5 years).
2. Idiosyncratic reactions
   a. mild transient diarrhea
   b. peripheral vascular thrombosis
   c. pruritis
   d. transient exanthema (skin eruptions)
   e. urticaria
   f. anaphylaxis → death

Uses in Therapy

Cyanocobalamin is usually used. Hydroxycobalamin produces a more sustained rise in serum cobalamin levels and less short-term urinary excretion on initial intramuscular injection, but has no advantage in long-term maintenance. The older liver extracts (crude and purified) have been largely displaced because they contain impurities which increase the risk of hypersensitivity reactions. Vitamin B_{12} products are described in Table 8-19.

1. Malabsorption (sprue, idiopathic steatorrhea, gluten-induced diarrhea, gastroenterostomy, ileal resection).

   A single 100 μg dose or 30 μg per day

TABLE 8-19. Vitamin B_{12} Products

1. **Crude liver extract** is a solution for injection of the soluble thermostable fraction of mammalian livers. It contains 2 μg of cyanocobalamin activity/ml. It is available generically from various manufacturers.

2. **Liver extract** (liver injection) is purified crude liver extract which contains 10 or 20 μg of cyanocobalamin activity/ml. It is available generically from various manufacturers. The 20 μg/ml product is available as Hyliver, Hyrex, and Pernaemon, Organon.

3. **Vitamin B_{12} with intrinsic factor** is a mixture of vitamin B_{12} and dried stomach, pyloris, or duodenum of hogs or other domestic animals. Its potency is expressed as "oral units." One unit contains not more than 15 μg of cyanocobalamin activity and not more than 300 mg of the dried material constituting the intrinsic factor concentrate. It is available in tablets containing 0.5 units as Biopar, Forte (Armour).

4. **Cobalamin concentrate** is the dried, partially purified product from the growth of selected Streptomyces species or other cobalamin-producing microorganisms. It is used as a source of cyanocobalamin activity in some preparations. It is available generically from various manufacturers as tablets containing 25, 50, or 100 μg of cyanocobalamin activity.

5. **Hydroxocobalamin**—Injection, 1 mg/ml

Brand	Manufacturer
AlphaRedisol	MSD
Alpha-Ruvite	Savage
Cobalphamead	Spencer-Mead
Codroxomin	O'Neal, Jones & Feldman
Droxovite	Kay
Hycobal-12	Canfield
Neobetalin 12 Crystalline	Lilly
Rubesol-L.A. 1000	Central
Sytobex-H	Parke-Davis

6. **Cyanocobalamin**

Brand	Manufacturer	Strength
Capsules		
Generic	Various	25 μg
Tablets		
Generic	Various	10, 25, 50, 100 μg
Tablets, soluble		
Generic	Various	25, 50, 100, 200 μg
REDISOL	MSD	500 μg
*Injection**		
Generic	Various	1 mg/ml
Berubigen	Upjohn	1 mg/ml
Betalin 12 Crystalline	Lilly	0.1, 1 mg/ml
Crystimin-1000	Reid-Provident	1 mg/ml
Dodex	Organon	1 mg/ml
REDISOL	MSD	0.1, 1 mg/ml
Rubesol 1000	Central	1 mg/ml
Ruvite	Savage	1 mg/ml
Sytobex	Parke-Davis	0.1, 1 mg/ml
Vibedoz	Blue Line	1 mg/ml

Injection, repository, 1 mg/ml in gelatin.

Note: Cyanocobalamin is slowly absorbed from intramuscular injection; repository injections offer little advantage.

Generic	Various
Cyano-Gel	Maurry

Injection, repository, 500 μg/ml as cyanocobalamin zinc tannate

Depinar	Armour

* By prescription only.

for 5 to 10 days intramuscularly or deep subcutaneously, then monthly maintenance dose of 100 to 200 μg. Adjust dosage to maintain erythrocyte count above 4.5 million/mm^3 and normal blood morphology. Avoid intravenous use because of rapid urinary excretion.

2. Genetic defects:
   Very high doses, as needed (1 to 500 mg per day).
3. Deficiency due to inadequate intrinsic factor
   a. pernicious anemia
   b. gastrectomy
   c. gastric atrophy

   Oral dosage with preparations containing intrinsic factor. Parenteral route is considered more dependable.
4. Prophylaxis of megaloblastic anemia following gastrectomy:
   100 μg once a month, intramuscularly.

CAUTIONS

1. Sensitivity reactions (test by intra-

dermal injection); sensitivity to hog protein if IF is used.

2. In treatment of megaloblastic anemia, fatal hypokalemia may be produced by increased potassium needs due to erythropoeisis. Monitor serum potassium during early stages of therapy.
3. Induction of gout in susceptible people due to increase in nucleic acid degradation.
4. In heart disease, pulmonary edema and congestive heart failure, due to increase in blood volume.
5. Hereditary optic nerve atrophy (Leber disease):
vitamin B_{12} therapy causes rapid optic nerve atrophy.
6. Vitamin B_{12} deficiency masks polycythemia vera. Therapy may unmask this condition.

Patients who have had their conditions normalized must be made aware of the need for periodic therapy. After the initial relief of symptoms, the patient has had the body stores replenished and may go for months or years without relapse. Because the maintenance doses do not seem to accomplish anything, the patient may come to view them as unnecessary.

INADEQUATELY SUBSTANTIATED THERAPIES

Because of their red color and the stinging they produce, cyanocobalamin injections have a strong placebo effect. Their use was so abused that third party insurers now refuse payment for them in the absence of proof of vitamin B_{12} deficiency.

1. Acute viral hepatitis
2. Trigeminal neuralgia
3. Various neuropathies
4. Multiple sclerosis
5. Aging
6. Anorexia
7. Thyrotoxicosis
8. Sterility
9. Fatigue
10. Psychiatric disorder (in absence of vitamin B_{12} deficiency)

Laboratory Test Interactions

Methotrexate, pyrimethamine, and most antibiotics give false low results in microbiologic tests for plasma cyanocobalamin activity.

Cyanocobalamin administration gives false positive results in tests for intrinsic factor antibodies. (These are present in about 50% of patients with pernicious anemia).

Drug Interactions

Decreased intestinal absorption

1. Aminoglycoside antibiotics
2. Colchicine
3. Extended release potassium
4. Aminosalicylates
5. Anticonvulsants (phenytoin, phenobarbital, primidone)
6. Neomycin

REFERENCES—Vitamin B_{12}

1. Linnell, J.C., et al.: Clin. Sci. Mol. Med. *46:*163, 1974.
2. Food and Agriculture Organization, World Health Organization: Requirements of Ascorbic Acid, Vitamin D, Vitamin B_{12}, Folate and Iron. Report of a Joint FAO/WHO Expert Committee, WHO Tech. Rept. Ser. No. 452, Geneva, World Health Organization, 1970.
3. Chanarin, I.: The Megaloblastic Anemias, Philadelphia, F. A. Davis Co., 1969.
4. Mangay Chung, A.S., et al.: Am. J. Clin. Nutr., *9:*573, 1961.
5. Committee on Nutrition, American Academy of Pediatrics: Pediatrics, *57:*278, 1976.
6. Herbert, V., Colman, N., and Jacob, E.: Folic Acid and Vitamin B_{12} *In* Modern Nutrition in Health and Disease, 6th Ed. R.S. Goodhart and M.E. Shills, eds. Philadelphia, Lea & Febiger, 1980.
7. Stadtman, T.C.: Science, *171:*859, 1971.

Chapter 9

Substances with No Known Essential Nutrient Functions in Man

From time to time, the notion that there are unidentified factors in food which have value as nutrients in man is publicized. Just as dramatically advertised as having remarkable properties are substances widely available in foods or found in unusual foods or parts of plants or animals not normally eaten.

No nutrient function or desirable physiologic effect has ever been reliably reported for the following in *any* species.

1. Amygdalin (vitamin B_{17}, Laetrile)
2. Chlorophyll
3. Orotic acid (uracil-6-carboxylic acid, unconfirmed growth factor for calves)
4. Pangamic acid (vitamin B_{15}, an undefined mixture from apricot kernels)[1]
5. Vitamin U (methylsulfonium salt of L-methionine, used for treatment of peptic ulcer in man)

Some substances are necessary for growth in some species but not in humans. These substances can be synthesized by human tissues. Extravagant claims for their need in human nutrition or for benefits to be derived from supplementation are made on the basis of deficiency symptoms in species other than human.

1. Bifidus factor (found in human milk; promotes growth of Lactobacillus bifidus in the intestines)
2. Biopterin (from queen bee jelly, growth factor for insects)
3. Cholesterol
4. Ubiquinone (coenzyme Q, found in most aerobic organisms)
5. Hematin (found in humans in pathologic conditions)
6. Lecithin (surfactant found in all living organisms)
7. Thioctic acid (alpha-lipoic acid)
8. Pimelic acid
9. Linolenic acid
10. Arachidonic acid
11. Taurine (found in bile)
12. Inositol (myo-inositol) (a required constituent of infant formula only because it is present in human milk)
13. Nerve growth factor
14. Carnitine (found in striated muscle and liver)
15. Para-aminobenzoic acid (anti-gray hair factor in rats only)
16. Pteridines
17. Various peptides, nucleotides, and proteins
18. Unknown material in alfalfa

Pharmacologic properties are sometimes claimed for substances found in food. Absence of these substances from human diets has not resulted in any deficiency symptoms. There is no reliable evidence of therapeutic efficacy.

1. Vitamin P factors
2. Bioflavonoids
   (1) hesperidin
   (2) rutin
3. Vitamin Q[2]
4. Amygdalin (Laetrile)
5. Pangamic acid

Of the trace elements, only cobalt has been identified as being needed by another animal species, but not by humans. Cobalt is utilized by ruminants for the synthesis of vitamin B_{12}.

Deficiency of some trace elements has been reported by only one investigator as producing pathologic changes in some species. The original reports have not been confirmed. These elements are

1. Arsenic
2. Cadmium
3. Tin

Deficiency of some elements has produced pathologic changes in two or more species. These observations have been confirmed. Production of deficiency symptoms required strict environmental controls, thus indicating a low requirement easily met by the environment. Deficiency symptoms could not be produced in humans. These elements are

1. Nickel
2. Silicon
3. Vanadium

Some substances are found in food, but there is no evidence of a dietary need for them in animals. These elements are

1. Aluminum
2. Antimony
3. Barium
4. Boron (needed by some plants)
5. Bromine
6. Gallium
7. Germanium
8. Gold
9. Lithium
10. Mercury
11. Silver
12. Strontium
13. Titanium

REFERENCES—Nonessential Substances

1. Herbert, V.: Am. J. Clin. Nutr., *32:*1534, 1979.
2. Quick, A.J.: Life Sci., *16:*1017, 1975.

Chapter 10
The Minerals

IRON

Iron is available in many foods of both plant and animal origin (Table 10-1). Many salts are available as sources of iron, including ferric ammonium citrate, ammonium phosphate, pyrophosphate, sulfate, and edetate; ferrocholinate; ferroglycine sulfate; and ferrous carbonate, citrate, fumarate, glutamate, gluconate, lactate, succinate, sulfate, and tartrate. The availability of the iron is *not* the same for each salt.

Recommended Dietary Allowances

In setting the RDA for iron, the following factors were considered.

1. Control of iron status is at the site of absorption in the intestine. Excretion of iron is relatively constant and plays little role in regulation.[1] Iron is lost by shedding epidermal and gastrointestinal cells, in bile, gastrointestinal bleeding, and urine. Additional iron is lost by menstrual bleeding.
2. Evaluation of iron absorption from various diets has become more sophisticated, allowing better evaluation of iron intake requirements.[2] The method of calculation of available iron from a given meal is given in detail. It requires computation of five variables.
   a. Total iron present (from food composition tables).
   b. Heme iron (calculated as 40% of the total iron in animal tissues).
   c. Nonheme iron (total iron minus heme iron).
   d. Ascorbic acid present in the meal.
   e. The amount of meat, poultry, and fish in the meal. The calculation is made by assuming that 23% of the heme iron is always absorbed. The fraction of nonheme iron absorbed depends on the nature of the meal. Three ranges are used.
      (1) Low-availability meals (containing less than 30 g of meat, poultry, or fish or less than 25 mg of ascorbic acid). Only 3% of the nonheme iron is absorbed.
      (2) Medium-availability meals (containing between 30 and 90 g of meat, poultry, or fish or 25 to 75 mg of ascorbic acid). About 5% of the nonheme iron is absorbed.
      (3) High-availability meals (containing more than 90 g of meat, poultry, or fish or more than 75 mg of ascorbic acid *or* 30 to 90 g of meat, poultry, and fish plus 25 to 75 mg of ascorbic acid). About 8% of the nonheme iron is absorbed.

TABLE 10-1. Dietary Sources of Iron*

Food	mg/100 g	Food	mg/100 g
Almonds	4.7	Lamb	1.8
Bacon		Lentils	2.1
fried	3.3	Lettuce	
Canadian	4.1	Boston	2.0
Barley	2.0	iceberg	0.5
Beans		Liver	
white	2.7	beef	8.8
red	2.4	calf	14.2
lima	2.5	chicken	8.5
Beef	3.0	pork	29.1
Beet greens	1.9	Molasses	
Blackeye peas	1.3	light	4.3
Bran flakes (40% bran)	4.4	blackstrap	16.1
Brazil nuts	3.4	Mussels	3.4
Bread		Oysters	8.1
pumpernickel	2.4	Peanuts	2.2
white, enriched	2.2	Peanut butter	2.0
whole wheat	2.3	Pistachio nuts	7.3
Buckwheat, whole	3.1	Popcorn	2.1
Chocolate		Pork	2.6
bittersweet	5.0	Sardines	2.9
semi-sweet	2.6	Sausages	
sweet	1.4	frankfurters	1.9
milk	1.0	liverwurst	5.4
Cashew nuts	3.8	pork sausage	2.4
Caviar	11.8	Scallops	3.0
Chicken		Shrimp	2.0
light	1.3	Soybean curd	1.9
dark	1.8	Spinach	2.1
skin	2.4	Sugar	
giblets	6.5	brown	3.4
Clams	3.4	Swiss chard	1.8
Dates	3.0	Syrup	
Eggs	2.3	soybean	12.5
Filberts	3.4	corn	4.1
Indian nuts	5.2	Veal	2.8

* Availability of iron from different foods varies as does the determination of availability. Values given are for content.

These factors are the average for women who are not iron deficient and have iron stores of approximately 500 mg. The factors are higher for iron-deficient populations and lower for populations with larger body stores.

The RDA is based on an assumption that 10% of the available iron will be absorbed. Thus, the RDA of 18 mg for adult women implies absorption of 1.8 mg of iron. If iron is available from highly absorbable sources, the target of 1.8 mg absorbed is equivalent to the 18 mg RDA.

It is hoped that in diet planning utilization of the factors rather than the RDA will lead to improved nutritional status for populations needing more iron and decrease the exposure of individuals to excessive iron absorption.

Iron is lost from the body through shedding of gastrointestinal cells, bile secretion, sweat, urinary excretion, and gastrointestinal blood loss. Iron released from old erythrocytes is mostly recycled. The obligatory iron losses are about 0.5 to 1 mg per day in adults. Thus, for adult males and postmenopausal females, the RDA of 10 mg supplies adequate replacement, assuming an absorption factor not greater than 10%. This is readily provided by the average American diet which contains 6 mg of iron/1000 kcal.

For menstruating females, menstrual losses must be added to the basal iron loss. Average menstrual blood loss is 40 ml, equivalent to 210 mg of iron or about 0.7 mg per day. For 95% of menstruating women, iron loss is 1.75 mg per day or less.[3] This gives a replacement range of 1.2 to 2.75 mg per day, or a required intake of 12 (low), 17 (average), or 27.5 (high) mg per day, assuming 10% absorption. Since this is more, on the average, than would be provided by the 2100 kcal per day of recommended energy intake for this group, the possibility of iron deficiency exists if the following assumptions are true:

1. The 10% absorbability factor is not increased as iron stores are depleted.
2. The iron stores built up prior to menarche are insufficient to last through the years of menstruation.

The RDA of 18 mg of iron for this group may be inadequate, and indeed, iron deficiency anemia may affect up to 10% of this population.[4]

In lactation, additional iron loss is 0.5 to 1.0 mg per day in the milk. Since lactation is usually accompanied by amennorhea, iron requirements are about the same as for the menstruating woman.

In pregnancy, iron requirements are greatly increased due to iron transfer to the fetus in the second half of pregnancy. In addition, maternal blood volume expands during pregnancy, and blood is lost in delivery. Since pregnancy is accompanied by amennorhea, the increased need for iron is about 500 mg for the entire process, or about 2 mg per day. Individual variabilities in iron needs require up to 5 mg per day, with an average value of 3.5 mg per day. Iron absorption is markedly increased during pregnancy, being about 30% in the second trimester and about 40% in the third trimester.

Whereas it appears that the combination of prepregnancy stores plus the increase in iron absorption from the diet should provide adequate iron for the pregnancy, the incidence of iron deficiency anemia among pregnant women varies from 10% in adequately nourished groups to 50% in poorly nourished groups with multiple, closely spaced pregnancies.[4] A daily supplement of 30 to 60 mg of iron is recommended, with continuation of supplementation for 2 to 3 months after delivery to replace depleted stores.[5]

Iron requirements for infants have been estimated by two methods.

1. Calculation of total body iron needed during the first years of life.
2. Daily intakes that provide maximal hemoglobin levels. On the basis of the second method, the RDA is set at 1 mg/kg, with a maximum of 15 mg.[6]

Surveys show that iron deficiency anemia (defined as hemoglobin levels below 10 g% or transferrin saturation below 15%) is common. Incidence was about 40% in children 1 to 2 years old from upper, middle, and lower middle class families.[7] The incidence drops as age increases. Because iron in egg yolk and the iron pyrophosphate used for cereal fortification are poorly available and the iron content of milk is low, iron supplementation with a daily dose of 10 to 15 mg of iron is recommended for children 0.5 to 5 years of age.

There is some evidence of iron deficiency in the over-60-year-old geriatric populations based on intakes, hemoglobin levels and transferrin saturation. Various surveys give different results, and the data collected are difficult to correlate and interpret. Since one product is targeted at the geriatric market, the FDA has given the manufacturer until 1984 to demonstrate transferrin saturations of less than 15% in at least 10% of this population.

Absorption

Iron is absorbed in the duodenum and upper jejunum through a complex but poorly understood process. This process has the following major steps:

1. Iron present in food as Fe^{+3} or Fe^{+2} is ingested.
2. In the stomach, the Fe^{+3} is dissolved in the gastric acid, bound by gastroferrin, and reduced to Fe^{+2}.
3. In the intestine, Fe^{+2} is oxidized to Fe^{+3}. This combines with apoferritin, which is transformed to ferritin, liberating Fe^{+2} into the blood plasma.
4. In the plasma, Fe^{+2} is oxidized to Fe^{+3} and bound to transferrin.
5. Transferrin liberates Fe^{+2} to bone marrow where it is incorporated into hemoglobin. Iron in bone marrow and iron in plasma are in equilibrium.
6. Transferrin liberates Fe^{+2} to body iron storage sites (liver, bone marrow, spleen, reticuloendoethelial system), where it is oxidized to Fe^{+3}. This is combined with apoferritin to form ferritin, which is then stored. Plasma iron is in equilibrium with the storage forms.

Ascorbic acid has been shown to increase iron absorption from food. It has a marked effect in increasing absorption from iron salts through the formation of a ferrous-ascorbate chelate. Concomitant doses of 200 mg of ascorbic acid with iron salts may increase absorption by 25 to 50%.[8]

For absorption from iron salts, ferrous sulfate is considered to be the model well-absorbed compound. Salts known to be poorly absorbed as compared with the standard[9] are the following:

1. Ferric edetate
2. Ferric citrate
3. Ferrocholinate
4. Ferric ammonium citrate
5. Iron in combination with magnesium trisilicate (retards iron absorption)

Inadequate data exist for the following salts, but they are believed to be poorly absorbed.

1. Ferrous citrate
2. Ferric ammonium phosphate
3. Ferric phosphate
4. Ferric pyrophosphate
5. Ferrous tartrate
6. Ferrous carbonate

Micronized reduced iron is well absorbed.

Surface active agents (400 mg polysorbate 20, 150 mg dioctyl sodium sulfosuccinate, 200 mg sodium lauryl sulfate, 146 mg cholic acid, 37 mg dehydrocholic acid) do not increase iron absorption significantly.[10]

Various hematinics (copper, cyanocobalamin, molybdenum, intrinsic factor) influence hematopoiesis under appropriate conditions, but do not affect iron absorption.[11]

Absorption takes place by an active transport mechanism in the duodenum and upper jejunum and by passive diffusion of Fe^{+2} in the more distal portions of the digestive tract. The amount diffused drops with increasing distance, probably in response to increasing alkalinity. The active transport mechanism is adequate for iron levels in normal diet. The passive diffusion may be of importance in large therapeutic doses.

Distribution

The average normal adult male contains about 50 mg of iron per kg of body weight; the female, about 35 mg/kg. The approximate distribution is as follows:

1. Hemoglobin—70%
2. Storage forms (ferritin, hemosiderin)—25%
3. Myoglobin—4%
4. Heme enzymes—0.5%
5. Transferrin—0.1%

Storage sites are liver, reticuloendothelial system, spleen, and bone marrow. Storage in adult women is about one half that of adult men.

Transfer across the placenta is an active process occurring against a gradient.

Pharmacology

Iron is a component of energy transfer oxidases.

1. Cytochrome oxidase
2. Xanthine oxidase
3. Succinic dehydrogenase
4. Catalase
5. Peroxidase

It is a component of compounds necessary for transport and utilization of oxygen.

1. Hemoglobin
2. Myoglobin

Deficiency

Deficiency may be produced by:

1. Inadequate intake
2. Impaired absorption (achlorhydria)
3. Gastrointestinal hemorrhage

SYMPTOMS

The chief symptom is microcytic hypochromic anemia.

Other symptoms are:

1. Sore tongue
2. Angular stomatitis
3. Abnormality in skin and nail formation

POPULATIONS AT RISK

The incidence of iron deficiency anemia based on hemoglobin and transferrin saturation levels may be overstated, as a few small scale studies show that many of the people diagnosed as anemic by these criteria do not respond to iron therapy.

Note that stores of nonhemoglobin iron play an important role. The normal iron stores in an adult provide for about 3 years of need before the hemoglobin level drops. On treatment with iron, stores are rapidly rebuilt. There seems to be no rationale for continuous high-level iron intake for any group.

Toxicity

ACUTE

Iron ingestion is the fourth most frequent cause of poisoning of children in the United States. An acute toxic dose may be as low as 150 mg/kg, with the estimated average toxic dose being 200 to 250 mg/kg. Symptoms may not appear until several hours after ingestion.

1. Lethargy → coma
2. Vomiting
3. Diarrhea
4. Abdominal cramps
5. Weak, rapid pulse
6. Low blood pressure (increased capillary permeability, reduced plasma volume)
7. Central nervous system depression
8. Shock
9. Increased cardiac output
10. Sudden cardiovascular collapse

The following symptoms may also be present.

11. Local erosion of the stomach and mucosa, allowing systemic absorption of iron, raising serum ferritin levels and even producing free ionized iron in the plasma
12. Bronchial pneumonia

Treatment

1. Induce vomiting (ipecac syrup).
2. Feed eggs and milk to form iron complex.
3. Perform gastric lavage as soon as possible with 1 to 5% sodium bicarbonate, but not after the first hour because of danger of perforation due to gastric necrosis.
4. Lavage may not remove enteric-coated tablets. These are visible in abdominal radiographs. Administer a saline laxative or consider surgical removal of the tablets.
5. Administer deferoxamine (see treatment of chronic toxicity).
6. Treat as needed.
   a. dehydration
   b. blood loss
   c. shock
   d. respiratory failure

Note: Avoid the use of dimercaprol as a complexing agent for iron. The complex formed may be toxic.

CHRONIC

Chronic overload is rare, but is more prevalent in those countries requiring high levels of iron supplementation in foods in order to meet the needs of menstruating women.

Iron overload is divided into two groups.

1. Hemosiderosis: iron accumulation without tissue damage.

When no definite causative factors are known, the condition is called "secondary," such as the secondary hemosiderosis common in alcoholics.

2. Hemochromatosis: iron accumulation causing fibrosis and organ damage.

Primary hemochromatosis is thought to be caused by a genetic defect characterized by excessive absorption of dietary iron.

Iron overload is associated with the following:

1. Portacaval shunts
2. Chronic pancreatitis
3. Hematologic disorders characterized by ineffective erythropoeisis
4. Excessive medicinal intake of iron
5. Multiple blood transfusions (rare)

Treatment. Iron overload is treated with intravenous deferoxamine (Desferal, Ciba) at a dose of 0.5 to one g per day infused at a rate not greater than 15 mg/kg/hr. Iron is removed by excretion of the iron-deferoxamine chelate. Urinary excretion of the complex may be nearly doubled by administration of 500 mg of ascorbic acid three times a day.[12]

Uses in Therapy

Oral dosing with ferrous sulfate is preferred although gluconate and lactate may be less irritating. Because iron is absorbed primarily in the upper portion of the small intestine, there is little rationale for timed release. Iron products are listed in Table 10-2.

Concurrent administration of 200 mg of ascorbic acid per 30 mg of iron increases absorption. Commercial iron plus ascorbic acid preparations have too little ascorbic acid to affect absorption. The usual dose is 50 to 100 mg of iron three times a day, or for children, 4 to 6 mg/kg three times a day.

An injectable form of iron is iron dextran injection, USP (Imferon, Merrell) 50 mg Fe/ml. It is to be used for temporary treatment of iron deficiency when oral administration of iron is not possible because of gastrointestinal disease, poor tolerance, or poor

TABLE 10-2. Iron Products of Proven Efficacy

Brand	Manufacturer	Strength mg	Fe mg
Ferrous Sulfate, USP, $FeSO_2 \cdot 7H_2O$, 20.09% Fe			
Tablets, USP			
Generic	Various	195, 300, 325	39, 60, 65
Mol-Iron	Schering	195	39
Courac Pills	Pfeiffer	300	60
Tablets, Timed Release			
Fero-Gradumet	Abbott	525	105
Capsules, Timed Release			
Generic	Various	150, 225, 250, 325	30, 45, 50, 65
Ferralyn	Lannett	150	30
Mol-Iron Chronosule	Schering	390	78
Oral Solution, USP			
Fer-In-Sol	Mead-Johnson	75/0.6 ml	15/0.6 ml
Fer-Iron	Rugby	75/0.6 ml	15/0.6 ml
Syrup, USP			
Fer-In-Sol	Mead-Johnson	90/5 ml	18/5 ml
Elixir (Oral Solution, USP)			
Generic	Various	90/5 ml	18/5 ml
Feosol	Menley and James	220/5 ml	44/5 ml
Fumarol	North American	162.5/5 ml	32.5/5 ml
Mol-Iron	Schering	195/4 ml	39/4 ml

TABLE 10-2. (continued)

Brand	Manufacturer	Strength mg	Fe mg
Dried Ferrous Sulfate, USP $FeSO_4 \cdot xH_2O$, 32.17% Fe			
Tablets			
Feosol	Menley and James	200	65
Hematinic	Mallard	200	65
Capsules			
Fer-In-Sol	Mead-Johnson	190	60
Capsules, Timed Release			
Feosol Spansules	Menley and James	167	50
Sterasol	Steri-Med	150	50
Note: Since the composition of the salt is variable, different amounts may share the same iron content.			
Ferrous Fumarate, $C_4H_2FeO_4$, 32.87% Fe			
Tablets, USP			
Generic	Various	195, 325	21, 108
Fumasorb	Marion	200	66
Fumerin	Laser	195	64
Ircon	Key	200	66
Laud-Iron	Amfre-Grant	325	108
Palmiron	Hauck	200	66
Toleron	Wallace	200	66
Tablets, Chewable			
Feostat	O'Neal, Jones & Feldman	100	33
Tablets, Timed Release			
Feco-T	Blaine	300	100
Suspension			
Feostat	O'Neal	100/5 ml	33/5 ml
Laud-Iron	Amfre-Grant	100/5 ml	33/5 ml
Toleron	Wallace	100/5 ml	33/5 ml
Ferrous Gluconate, USP, $C_{12}H_{22}FeO_{14} \cdot 2H_2O$, 11.58% Fe			
Tablets, USP			
Generic	Various	325	38
Entron	LaCrosse	325	38
Fergon	Breon	320	37
Ferralet	Mission	320	37
Capsules, USP			
Ferrous Gluconate Pulvules	Lilly	325	38
Capsules, Timed Release			
Fergon	Breon	435	50
Elixir			
Fergon	Breon	300/5 ml	35/5 ml
Ferrous-G	Kenwood	325/5 ml	38/5 ml

absorbability. It is sometimes used when the patient fails to respond to oral therapy.

The injection may cause pain and permanent discoloration. The discoloration may be avoided by use of the "Z-track" technique and by deep intramuscular injection with a needle at least 2 inches long into the upper outer quadrant of the buttocks.

Hematologic response should be monitored. If there is no response, a complicating disease should be suspected. Additional parenteral iron should not be used because of hemochromatosis similar to that produced by multiple blood transfusions.

The total dose of iron recommended is that required to restore hemoglobin to normal or near-normal levels plus a 50% excess to replenish depleted stores. The basic calculation is made from the following formula:

$$\frac{\text{mg blood iron}}{\text{lb body weight}} = \frac{\text{ml blood}}{\text{lb body weight}} \times \frac{\text{g hemoglobin}}{\text{ml blood}} \times \frac{\text{mg iron}}{\text{g hemoglobin}}$$

In this, blood volume is taken as 8.5% of body weight, the normal hemoglobin level is considered as 14.8 g/dl for persons weighing 30 lb or more or 12.0 g/dl for persons under 30 lb, and the iron content of hemoglobin is 0.34%. For practical use this rearranges to:

$$\text{mg iron} = 0.3 \times \text{lb body weight} \times [100 - (100 \times \text{g/dl hemoglobin}/14.8)]$$

Since iron dextran injection contains 50 mg of iron per ml, the volume to be injected is mg iron/50. Injections are made once a day until the total calculated dose is administered. The maximum volume to be administered on any one day is 0.5 ml for infants under 10 lb, 1 ml for children under 20 lb, 2.0 ml for patients under 110 lb, and 5 ml for others.

Prior to receiving the first dose, all patients should be given an intramuscular test dose of 0.5 ml and observed for at least 1 hour for adverse symptoms, including anaphylactic reactions, before the rest of the dose is given.

Interference with Laboratory Tests

Iron imparts black color to feces. This may give false positives in the guaiac test for occult blood but rarely affects the benzidine test.

Drug Interactions

1. Antacids decrease absorption. Dosage of iron and antacids should be spaced as far apart as possible.
2. Iron and tetracycline inhibit absorption of each other. Administer tetracycline 2 hours before or 3 hours after oral iron doses.
3. Chloramphenicol delays the hematopoietic response to iron therapy. Avoid chloramphenicol therapy, if possible, in patients with iron deficiency anemia.
4. Removal of copper by penicillamine is decreased by iron. Allow a 2-hour period between administration of penicillamine and administration of iron.

REFERENCES—Iron

1. Green, R., et al.: Am. J. Med., *45:*336, 1968.
2. Monsen, E.R., et al.: Am. J. Clin. Nutr., *31:*134, 1978.
3. Beaton, G.H.: Epidemiology of Iron Deficiency, *In* Iron in Biochemistry and Medicine. A. Jacobs and M. Worwood, eds. New York, Academic Press, 1974.
4. Wallerstein, R.O.: Clin. Haematol, *2:*453, 1973.
5. Chanarin, I., and Rothman, D.: Br. Med. J., *2:*81, 1971.
6. Committee on Nutrition, American Academy of Pediatrics: Pediatrics, *43:*134, 1969.
7. Owen, G.M., Lubin, A.H., and Garry, P.J.: Pediatr., *79:*563, 1971.
8. Brise, H., and Hallberg, L.: Acta Med. Scand., *171,* (Suppl. 376):51, 1962.
9. Brise, H., and Hallberg, L.: Acta Med. Scand., *171*(Suppl. 376):23, 1962.
10. Brise, H.: Acta Med. Scand., *171*(Suppl. 376):47, 1962.
11. Fairbanks, V.F., Fahey, J.L., and Beutler, E.: Clinical Disorders of Iron Metabolism, 2nd Ed. New York, Grune & Stratton, 1971, pp. 282-358.
12. O'Brien, R.T.: Ann. NY Acad. Sci., *232:*221, 1974.

FLUORIDE

Fluoride is present in small quantities in plants, animals, and water (Table 10-3). It is available commercially as sodium or calcium fluoride (Table 10-4).

Safe and Adequate Intake

The recommendations for intake are based on the following:

1. The major variable in fluoride intake is the fluoride in the water. Fluoride in water is available not only in water actually drunk, but also in water used in food preparation. The daily intake from food and water ranges from 1 mg in low fluoride areas to 4 mg in areas in which the water supply is fluoridated.[1]

2. Fluoride causes increased caries resistance in teeth, mainly when incorporated in tooth structure prior to tooth eruption.[2]

TABLE 10-3. Dietary Sources of Fluoride

Fluoride content of foods and vegetables reflects the fluoride content of the soil in which they were grown and of the water used to prepare them.

Food	μg/100 g	Food	μg/100 g
Apples	80	Lettuce	3
Beef	200	Liver	150
Bread		Milk	7 to 22
rye	340	Oats	70 to 170
white	64	Potatoes	20
Butter	150	Salmon	
Cheese	160	canned with bones	450
Codfish		Sardines	
raw	700	canned with bones	730 to 1250
Egg yolk	80 to 120	Spinach	46 to 63
Fish		Tomatoes	4
fresh water, raw	160	Wheat	30 to 100
Kidney	860	Wheat germ	150 to 350

Post eruptive protection is given by dietary intakes of more than 1.5 mg per day.

3. When drinking water contains more than 2 mg F^-/L, children may develop mottled tooth enamel.

4. Drinking water containing more than 4 mg F^-/L may protect against osteoporosis in adults.[3]

Recommendations for daily intake are:

Adult—1.5 to 4 mg

Adolescents—1.5 to 2.5 mg

Infants consume about 0.1 mg per day from human or cow's milk and up to 1.2 mg per day from commercial formulas. Recommended intake ranges are 0.1 to 1.0 mg from birth to 1 year and 0.5 to 1.5 mg from 1 to 3 years of age.

When drinking water contains less than 1 mg/L, these intakes are difficult to obtain. It is recommended that fluoride be added to water to bring the concentration to that level.

Absorption

Fluoride is rapidly absorbed on ingestion of soluble salts.[4] Absorption from poorly soluble salts is slow and variable.

It may also be absorbed through the lungs by workers in environments containing airborne fluoride (cryolite, use of fluorspar as a flux in metal working, brick making with fluorine-rich clays, manufacture of phosphates from fluorine-containing raw materials).

Distribution

Fluoride is found mainly in bones and teeth. Between 25 and 50% of ingested fluoride is deposited in the skeleton by simple ion exchange with the hydroxy group of hydroxyapatite.[5] This process is reversible, and has a half-life of 1 to 2 years.[6] Plasma levels are 12 to 15 μg/dl for people who drink fluoridated water.

Excretion

Renal excretion maintains plasma fluoride concentrations within a narrow range.[7] Small amounts are excreted in sweat, saliva, and milk.

Toxicity

ACUTE

Lethal dose is 2.5 to 5 g in adults.

The symptoms of acute fluoride toxicity are as follow:

1. Violent gastrointestinal irritation (nausea, vomiting, diarrhea).
2. Local paralysis of legs or face.
3. Convulsions.

TABLE 10-4A. Fluoride Products (All are by prescription only)

Brand	Manufacturer	Sodium Fluoride mg/ml	Volume (ml) Containing 1 mg Fluoride
Sodium Fluoride, USP, NaF, 45.25%F			
Sodium Fluoride Oral Solution, USP			
Fluoritab Liquid	Fluoritab	6.3	0.35
Flura-Drops	Kirkman	5.0	0.44
Karidium Drops	Lorvic	4.4	0.50
Luride	Hoyt	5.5	0.40
Pediaflor Drops	Ross	0.5	2.0

4. Stimulation of respiratory center followed by depression.
5. Shock.
6. Death in 2 to 4 hours from respiratory paralysis or cardiac depression.

CHRONIC

1. At 2 to 5 mg per day in children: enamel hyperplasia (mottling).[8]
2. At 30 mg per day for 6 weeks:[9]
   a. retinopathy
   b. optic neuritis
   c. macular edema
3. Allergic reactions:[10]
   a. atopic dermatitis
   b. urticaria
   c. pruritis
   d. edema
4. At 20 to 80 mg per day for 10 to 20 years:[8] crippling fluorosis.

TABLE 10-4B

Brand	Manufacturer	Fluoride mg/tablet
Sodium Fluoride Tablets, USP		
Karidium	Lorvic	1
Stay-Flo	Stayner	1
Sodium Fluoride Tablets, Chewable USP		
Generic	Various	1
Fluorineed	Hanlon	1
Fluoritab	Fluoritab	1
Flura	Kirkman	1
Flura-Loz	Kirkman	1
Luride 0.25 Lozi-Tabs	Hoyt	0.25
Luride 0.5 Lozi-Tabs	Hoyt	0.5
Luride Lozi-Tabs	Hoyt	1
Luride-SF Lozi-Tabs	Hoyt	1
Phos-Flur	Hoyt	1

Uses in Therapy

When the concentration of fluoride in drinking water is less than 700 μg/L (0.7 ppm), supplementation should be considered. The dose should provide enough fluoride to bring *total* intake up to 0.5 mg per day for children 2 to 3 years old and one mg per day for children over 3 years. The daily dose for older children may be calculated from a knowledge of the fluoride concentration of the water supply, by subtracting from one mg the mg/L of fluoride in the water. The dose for children 2 to 3 years old is one half this amount. The dose may be administered orally as tablets or solution.

To prevent poisoning of children, it is recommended that not more than 120 mg of fluoride (264 mg NaF) be dispensed at one time.

REFERENCES—Fluoride

1. Kramer, L., et al.: Am. J. Clin. Nutr., *27:*590, 1974.
2. Sognnaes, R.F.: Science, *150:*989, 1968.
3. Bernstein, D.S., et al.: JAMA, *198:*499, 1966.
4. Hosking, D.H., and Chamberlain, M.J.: Clin. Sci., *42:*153, 1972.
5. Smith, F.A., Gardner, D.E., and Hodge, H.C.: Fed. Proc., *12:*368, Abstract 1212, 1953.
6. Largent, E.J., and Heyroth, F.F.: J. Indust. Hyg. Toxicol., *31:*134, 1949.
7. Spencer, H., et al.: Am. J. Med., *49:*807, 1970.

8. Leone, N.C., et al.: Am. J. Roentgenol., *74*:874, 1955.
9. Anon.: Lancet, *2*:889, 1973.
10. Shea, J.J., Gillespie, S.M., and Waldbott, G.L.: Ann. Allergy, *25*:388, 1967.

IODINE

Iodine is an integral part of the thyroid hormones. It is available for use as a supplement as potassium iodide or calcium iodate. Iodine products are listed in Table 10-5.

Recommended Dietary Allowances[1]

The factors considered in setting the RDA include the following:

1. Epidemiologic studies and balance studies show that iodine requirements are probably 100 to 200 μg/per day. Wide variations exist between individuals based on age, differences in urinary excretion, sex, and ingestion of goitrogenic foods (cabbage, peaches, almonds).
2. Goiter is prevented by ingestion of 50 to 70 μg or 1 μg/kg per day.
3. No renal mechanisms exist for conserving iodine.
4. Pregnancy increases iodine needs.
5. On a weight basis, children require more iodine than adults.
6. Human milk contains 30 to 100 μg/L.[2]

In considering all factors, the RDA is set at 150 μg for adults to provide a margin of safety for those populations ingesting naturally occurring goitrogens. An additional intake of 25 μg (total = 175 μg) is recommended in pregnancy and an additional 50 μg (total = 200 μg), during lactation. The amounts recommended from birth through 10 years grow smaller on a weight basis as weight increases.

Dietary intake is highly variable, but is estimated at 240 to 740 μg/day.[3]

Household use of iodized salt is recommended for noncoastal areas of the United States. Products designed for complete nutritional maintenance should contain the RDA.

Concern is expressed that the iodine in the American diet not be increased by use of alginates, iodophor sanitizers, iodine-containing colors and iodine-containing dough conditioners.

DIETARY SOURCES

1. Iodine content of fruits and vegetables depends on the iodine level in the soil. Iodine content of animal tissue and dairy products depends on the iodine content of the feed.
2. The only consistent natural sources of iodine are seafood and seaweed (kelp), including commercial alginate thickeners.
3. Bread made by the continuous-mix process may contain calcium iodate as a conditioner. This bread contains about 500 μg of iodine/100 g.
4. Iodized salt in the United States con-

TABLE 10-5. Iodine Products

Brand	Manufacturer	Strength	Iodine Content
Potassium Iodide, USP, 76.45% I			
Potassium Iodide Oral Solution, USP (100%)			
Generic	Various	1 g/ml	765 mg/ml
SSKI	Upsher-Smith	1 g/ml	765 mg/ml
Oral Solution (not USP)			
	Philips-Roxane	500 mg/15 ml	25.5 mg/ml
Syrup (not USP)			
Pima	Fleming	325 mg/5 ml	50.0 mg/ml
Potassium Iodide Tablets, USP (enteric coated)			
Generic	Various	120, 300 mg	230 mg
Enseals	Lilly	300 mg	230 mg

tains 76.4 μg of iodine (100 μg potassium iodide)/g. Thus, the average salt use of 3.4 g, if it is iodized, provides about 260 μg per day. Bulk salt used by manufacturers, canners, and restaurants is not usually iodized.

Absorption

Free and bound iodine and iodate are rapidly converted to iodide in the gastrointestinal tract. Iodide is rapidly absorbed by fasting people. Iodine absorption is nearly complete within 1 to 3 hours when ingested with food.[4] Some iodine is absorbed from the stomach, but most is absorbed from the intestines.

Distribution

Iodide is taken up by the thyroid until total stores reach about 2 mg, but is not metabolized. Thyroid uptake is then diminished. Iodide is used as needed in the synthesis of thyroxine and triiodothyronine. This synthesis is inhibited by excessive accumulation of iodine in the thyroid.

Excretion

Urinary excretion roughly parallels intake levels. Triiodothyronine is excreted, then reabsorbed. The reabsorption is inhibited by soybean products.[1]

Deficiency

The primary symptom of iodine deficiency is simple goiter, defined as an increase in the size and number of thyroid epithelial cells, leading to thyroid gland enlargement. Deficiency does not always produce goiter. Iodine treatment does not reduce simple goiter.

The incidence of goiter in the United States has markedly decreased since the introduction of iodized salt. The residual goiters are puzzling, since endemic areas are found in Michigan and Texas. The incidence in these areas does not correlate with iodine intake as measured by urinary excretion. It has been postulated that other factors such as infection, ingestion of dietary goitrogens, or genetic deficiency in enzymes required for thyroid hormone synthesis may be responsible.

SYMPTOMS

Other symptoms are due to lowered production of thyroid hormones.

1. Cretinism
2. Lowered fertility
3. Lowered metabolic rate
4. Lowered physical activity
5. Lowered mental activity

Toxicity[5]

Safe levels of intake for adults are between 50 and 1000 μg per day.

ACUTE

1. Doses of 200 to 4000 μg per day for 4 months produced no symptoms of toxicity.
2. In sensitive people, the following are sometimes, although rarely, seen.
   a. angioderma
   b. hemorrhagic skin lesions
   c. serum sickness

CHRONIC

1. metallic taste
2. rhinorrhea
3. headache
4. parotitis
5. acne-like skin lesions
6. pulmonary edema
7. iodine-induced goiter (This may cause respiratory problems in the newborn, with goiter caused by excessive maternal ingestions.)

REFERENCES—Iodine

1. Cavalieri, R.R.: Trace elements, Iodine, *In* Modern Nutrition in Health and Disease, 6th Ed. R.S. Goodhart and M.E. Shils, eds. Philadelphia, Lea & Febiger, 1980.
2. Man, E.B., and Benotti, J.: Clin. Chem., *15:*1141, 1969.
3. Oddie, T.H., et al.: J. Clin. Endocrin. Metab., *30:*659, 1970.
4. Wayne, E.J., Coutras, D.A., and Alexander, W.D.: Clinical Aspects of Iodine Metabolism. Philadelphia, F.A. Davis, 1964.
5. Fisher, K.D., Carr, C.J.: Iodine in Foods, Chemi-

cal Methodology and Sources of Iodine in the Human Diet. Division of Nutrition, Bureau of Foods, Food and Drug Administration. Federation of American Societies for Experimental Biology, May 1974. ex. Fed. Reg. *44:*16182, Mar. 16, 1979.

SELENIUM

Selenium content of plant and animal tissues is highly variable and dependent on the selenium content of ingested food and water.[1] A commercial source of selenium for dietary supplementation is yeast grown in a medium containing selenium as selenate. Selenium behaves chemically in a manner analagous to sulfur. Many of the sulfur-containing compounds of biochemical importance occur in nature contaminated with their selenium analog; thus, naturally occurring methionine contains selenomethionine.

Safe and Adequate Intake

1. Extrapolations from animal models to humans are undependable because selenium functions and selenium requirements vary widely by species. Selenium requirements seem related to needs for the other antioxidants, vitamins C and E.

2. No symptoms of selenium excess or deficiency have been seen in studies of human populations living in areas in which other animals, usually cattle, show severe symptoms of deficiency or excess.[2] Deficiency occurs in animals at intakes of less than 0.02 μg/g of diet (dry weight). Optimal growth and reproduction occur in animals on intakes of about 0.1 μg/g of diet (dry weight). Toxic symptoms occur in animals at dietary levels of more than 2 μg/ml of water or 3 μg/g of food (dry weight). Some humans live symptom-free on balanced diets that provide more than 200 μg/day.[3]

3. Tables of selenium content of food are not available and would probably be meaningless because of the wide variations. Seafoods, kidney, and liver are good sources. Meat generally is a considerable source. Grains are highly variable, whereas fruits and vegetables contain little selenium.[1]

On the basis of available information, safe and adequate intakes are considered to be 50 to 200 μg per day for adults and proportionately less on a weight basis for infants and children.

Pharmacology

The role of selenium is largely unknown. It is known to be a cofactor for glutathione peroxidase[4] which inhibits peroxidation of fats, decomposes hydrogen peroxide, and scavenges free radicals.

Chronic Toxicity[5]

The following symptoms of chronic toxicity have been reported for humans exposed, usually occupationally, to high levels of selenium.

1. Loss of hair
2. Brittle fingernails
3. Fatigue
4. Irritability
5. Garlic odor on breath

REFERENCES—Selenium

1. Morris, V.C., and Levander, O. A.: J. Nutr., *100:*1383, 1970.
2. Griffith, N.M., and Thomson, C.D.: NZ Med. J., *80:*199, 1974.
3. Sakurai, H., and Tsuchiya, K.: Environ. Physiol. Biochem., *5:*107, 1975, ex Biol. Abstr., *60:*50655 1975.
4. Rotruck, J.T., et al.: Fed. Proc., *31:*691, Abstr. 2684, 1972.
5. Food and Nutrition Board, National Research Council: J. Am. Diet. Assoc, *70:*249, 1977.

ZINC

Zinc is widely distributed in plants and animals (Table 10-6). Some areas of the world however, notably areas of Iran and Egypt in the Middle East and the Michigan upper peninsula in the United States, have soils with a very low zinc content. People who exclusively eat food produced in those areas have a high incidence of zinc deficiency. Zinc is available as a nutritional supplement as zinc sulfate (Table 10-7).

Recommended Dietary Allowances

Older data about zinc metabolism are unreliable because of inadequate methods of

TABLE 10-6. Dietary Sources of Zinc

Food	mg/100 g
Beef	2 to 5
Beets	2.8
Clams	2.0
Egg yolk	2.6 to 4
Liver, beef	3.5 to 8.5
Milk	0.4 to 3.0
Oysters	29 to 40
Peanut butter	2
Peas	3
Wheat bran	14
Whole grains	
Oats, rolled, raw	3 to 5
Barley, raw	2.7
Corn, whole	2.5
Wheat, whole, raw	2.5 to 8.5
Rice, brown, raw	1.5

Note that the best sources are meat, liver, eggs, and seafood, especially oysters. Significant sources are milk, whole grain products (whole wheat, rye, whole corn). The content of zinc is variable, depending on the geographic origin of the dietary source. Municipal drinking waters generally contain no zinc. Availability is higher from animal sources than from vegetable sources.

analysis. In setting the RDA, only studies later than 1965 were considered. Nevertheless, there appear to be no modern studies of total zinc content and zinc distribution in the human body nor of daily zinc losses in infants. The following observations affected the setting of the RDA.

1. Human metabolic studies showed equilibrium or positive balance at dietary intakes of 12.5 mg of zinc per day, neglecting losses of zinc in sweat and through loss of epithelial cells.[1]
2. Radioisotope studies showed a daily turnover of about 6 mg per day.[2]
3. Absorption from dietary sources is about 40%.

Based on the above data and allowing for dermal losses, the RDA is set at 15 mg for adults. Intake of an additional 5 mg (total = 20 mg) is recommended during pregnancy and an additional 10 mg (total = 25 mg), during lactation. These rather high additions are calculated for diets with poor zinc availability (absorption factor of 15% in pregnancy and 30% during lactation).

The zinc content of human milk decreases during lactation from about 20 mg/L in colostrum to about 2 mg/L in mature milk. The average content is about 3 mg/850 ml. Assuming that this zinc is highly available, the RDA is set at 3 mg for infants from birth to 6 months.

The most recent study of the American diet[3] shows intakes for adults of 6 to 12.4 mg per day (average 8.6 mg per day). Careful diet planning is necessary if the RDA for zinc is to be met. The problem of diet planning is that the availability of zinc from various foods is highly variable and quantita-

TABLE 10-7. Zinc Products Known to be Efficacious

Brand	Manufacturer	mg/unit	mg Zn/unit
Zinc Sulfate, USP, $ZnSO_4 \cdot 7H_2O$, 22.74% Zn			
Tablets			
Generic	Various	44, 66, 88, 100, 132, 200, 220, 440	10, 15, 20, 22.5, 30, 45, 50, 100
Medizinc*	Medics	220	50
Zinc 20	Fibertone	88	20
Capsules			
Generic*	Various	220	50
Orazinc	Mericon	220	50
ScripZinc*	Scrip	220	50
Verazinc	O'Neal, Jones & Feldman	220	50
Zinkaps-110	Ortega	110	25
Zinkaps-220	Ortega	220	50
Zinc-220	Alto	220 ($ZnSO_4 \cdot H_2O$)	80

* Prescription only.

tively unknown. Zinc in meat and fish is more available than zinc in vegetables. Phytate and fiber reduce zinc availability[4] especially in the presence of calcium. Phosphate salts and phosphate in milk reduce availability.[5]

Absorption

Absorption is highly variable. The relationship between the dose and the amount absorbed by fasting subjects is approximately linear between doses of 25 to 50 mg. Meat had no effect on absorption but serum response was reduced by at least 43% by milk, cheese, whole wheat bread, or coffee.[5]

Distribution

Total zinc content of the normal adult male is about 2.2 g.[6] The distribution is approximately as follows:

1. Bone—20%. This is not in rapid equilibrium with plasma.
2. Muscle—63%.
3. Blood—2%.

Excretion

1. Urine—about 0.5 mg per day, average.
2. Sweat—up to 1 mg/L.[7] Average loss under normal conditions is about 2.8 mg per day.[8]
3. The pancreas contributes about 1.5 mg per day in adults.[9]
4. Menstrual losses are about 0.3 to 0.6 per menses.[10]
5. The neonate is in negative zinc balance, losing more than 1% of the body content per day.[11] It is not known whether this should be or can be reversed by supplementation.
6. Abnormally high levels of urinary zinc are found in the following:
   a. alcoholics
   b. fasting obese patients
   c. renal disease
   d. diabetes
   e. liver disease
   f. porphyria
   g. proteinuria
   h. trauma, especially burns[12]
   i. sickle cell disease

Pharmacology

1. Zinc is part of at least 18 enzymes and enzyme cofactors, including:[13]
   a. alkaline phosphatase
   b. alcohol dehydrogenase
   c. insulin
   d. carbonic anhydrase
   e. carboxypeptidase
2. It is involved in protein and nucleic acid synthesis[14] in rats and presumably in other species, since there is a consistent finding of high zinc concentrations in nucleic acids.
3. It is required for mobilization of vitamin A from the liver.[15]

Deficiency

1. No technique provides direct evidence of deficiency. The crucial test is response to supplementation under controlled conditions.[15] Techniques used to assess zinc status are:
   a. metabolic balance studies
   b. isotope turnover studies
   c. plasma zinc levels
   d. urinary zinc excretion
   e. zinc content of hair[16]
   f. taste acuity
2. Zinc depletion is associated with the use of some drugs:
   a. histidine[17]
   b. penicillamine[18]
   c. phenytoin[19]
   d. thiamazole[20]
   e. thiazides[21]
3. Malabsorption is associated with:
   a. recurrent infection
   b. hypogammaglobulinemia
   c. celiac sprue
   d. regional enteritis
   e. sickle cell disease
   f. acrodermatitis enteropathica in infants,[22] a genetically-inherited disorder

SYMPTOMS

Symptoms of deficiency remedied by zinc sulfate administration are as follow:

1. Reduced taste acuity.[23]
2. Delayed healing of ulcers.[24]
3. Short stature and delayed puberty.[25]
4. Acrodermatitis enteropathica.[26] If present in pregnant woman, it is associated with birth defects.

Toxicity

ACUTE

As an emetic, zinc sulfate has been used in doses of 1 to 2 g (225-450 mg Zn). Symptoms include the following:

1. Nausea
2. Vomiting
3. Stomach cramps
4. Diarrhea
5. Fever

Death has been reported in one case after ingestion of 6 g of zinc as zinc sulfate.[27] Complications included:

1. Hemorrhagic pancreatitis
2. Severe renal damage

In many cases of acute toxicity due to ingestion of food or drink prepared or stored in galvanized (zinc-coated) vessels, the symptoms are mental confusion and lack of muscle coordination.

Treatment. Hemodialysis or intravenous chelating agents.

CHRONIC

Reports of the symptoms of chronic toxicity all seem to be due to the interference with the metabolism of copper, iron, or calcium. The zinc/copper ratio may be critical. The chief effect of high zinc intake in relation to copper may be a predisposition to coronary heart disease.[28]

Uses in Therapy

Because even transient zinc deficiency in the mother produces defects in the fetus in animal experiments and because the zinc pool in bone is not readily available, there is some feeling that the RDA be ingested daily. On the other hand, because of the adverse effects of excess zinc intake on copper metabolism, it is recommended that chronic ingestion of zinc supplements be limited to 15 mg per day in addition to the dietary intake. It appears that much more information is necessary about zinc availability from foods, availability of body stores, and interactions with other nutrients.

For zinc deficiency, a dose of 50 mg administered orally three times a day is recommended.

REFERENCES—Zinc

1. Spencer, H., et al.: Intake, Excretion and Retention of Zinc in Man, *In* Trace Elements in Human Health and Disease. Vol. I. A.S. Prasad, ed. New York, Academic Press, 1976.
2. Engel, R.W., Miller, R.F., and Price, N.O.: Metabolic Patterns in Preadolescent Children, XIII. Zinc Balance, *In* Zinc Metabolism. A.S. Prasad, ed. Springfield, IL, Charles C Thomas, 1966.
3. Holden, J.M., Wolf, W.R., and Mertz, W.: J. Am. Diet. Assoc., *75:*23, 1979.
4. Reinhold, J.G., Ismail-Beigi, F., and Faradji, B.: Nutr. Rep. Int., *12:*73, 1975.
5. Smith, J.C., et al.: Science, *181:*954, 1973.
6. Widdowson, E.M., McCance, R.A., and Spray, C.M.: Clin. Sci., *10:*113, 1951.
7. Prasad, A.S., et al.: J. Lab. Clin. Med., *62:*84, 1963.
8. Schraer, K.K., and Calloway, D.H.: Nutr. Metabol., *17:*205, 1974.
9. Burch, R.E., Hahn, H.K.J., and Sullivan, J.F.: Clin. Chem., *21:*501, 1975.
10. Schroeder, H.A., et al.: J. Chronic Dis., *20:*179, 1967.
11. Cavell, P.A., and Widdowson, E.M.: Arch. Dis. Childhood, *39:*496, 1964.
12. Carr, G., and Wilkinson, A.W.: Clin. Chim. Acta, *61:*199, 1975.
13. Parisi, A.F., and Vallee, B.L.: Am. J. Clin. Nutr., *22:*1222, 1969.
14. Grey, P.C., and Dreosti, I.E.: J. Comp. Pathol., *82:*223, 1972.
15. Halstead, J.A., Smith, J.C., Jr., and Irwin, M.I.: J. Nutr., *104:*345, 1974.
16. Strain, H.W., et al.: J. Lab. Clin. Med., *68:*244, 1966.
17. Henkin, R.I., et al.: Arch. Neurol., *32:*745, 1975.
18. Lyle, W.H.: Lancet, *2:*1140, 1974.
19. Barbeau, A., and Donaldson, J.: Arch. Neurol., *30:*52, 1974.
20. Hanlon, D.P.: Lancet, *1:*929, 1975.
21. Cohanim, M., and Yendt, E.R.: Johns Hopkins Med. J., *136:*137, 1975.
22. Lombeck, I., et al.: Lancet, *1:*855, 1975.
23. Henkin, R.I., et al.: JAMA, *217:*434, 1971.

24. Pories, W.J., et al.: Lancet, *1:*121, 1967.
25. Ronaghy, H.A., et al.: Am. J. Clin. Nutr., *27:*112, 1974.
26. Moynahan, E.J.: Lancet, *2:*399, 1974.
27. Cowan, G.A.B.: Br. Med. J., *1:*451, 1947.
28. Klevay, L.M.: Am. J. Clin. Nutr., *28:*764, 1975.

COPPER

Copper metabolism is intimately bound with the metabolism of zinc. Copper is widely available, including copper from water carried in copper pipes. Chemical sources of copper are cupric sulfate and gluconate.

Safe and Adequate Intake

Copper requirements in humans have been estimated on the basis of balance studies. These include the following:

1. Adult males on a variety of diets required an average intake of 1.24 mg per day to maintain balance.[1]
2. Young adult females showed positive balance at intakes of 3.9 mg per day.[2]
3. Preadolescent girls were in negative balance at about 35 μg/kg per day,[3] but were in balance at 1.6 to 2.1 mg per day.[4]
4. Copper should not be considered alone but only in relation to zinc intake.[5]

The recommendation is 2 to 3 mg per day in order to allow a safety margin. The lower level may be inadequate for people with large sweat losses.[2]

5. In boys 3 to 6 years of age, 53 to 85 μg/kg per day were required to maintain balance.[6]
6. Normal children showed positive balance with intakes as low as 35 μg/kg per day.[7]
7. Requirements of infants and children have been estimated at between 50 and 100 μg/kg per day.

The recommendation is an intake of 80 μg/kg per day. For infants receiving only formula, the recommendation is 100 μg/kg per day. Copper content in human milk varies from 1050 μg/L at the beginning of lactation to 150 μg/L at the end.

The copper content of the American diet is unclear. Older data show between 2 and 5 mg per day; more recent surveys[5] show much lower intakes, sometimes well below 1 mg per day. Whether this discrepancy is due to changes in diet or to differences in analytic techniques is not known. Dietary sources of copper are shown on Table 10-8.

Absorption

About 30% of the copper content of the usual diet is absorbed.[8]

Absorption is by active transport, primarily in the stomach and upper portion of the small intestines.[9] Absorption is variable and is decreased by the presence of

1. Amino acids
2. Protein

TABLE 10-8. Dietary Sources of Copper

Food	μg/100 g
Asparagus	141
Avocado	690
Bananas	200
Beets	187
Bread, whole wheat	205
Corn	450
Eggs	250
Flour, whole wheat	435
Kale	328
Liver, beef	2450
Mackerel	230
Oats, rolled, raw	738
Oysters	3623
Prunes, dried	290
Rye, whole, raw	656
Spinach	197
Sweet potatoes	187
Wheat, whole, raw	787
Milk, human	1050 to 150, decreasing from highest value to lowest during lactation
Milk, cow's	1150 to 180

Notes: 1. Variable amounts of copper are obtained from drinking water carried in copper pipes.
2. The RDA is based on the content of copper in the normal diet. Actually, an intake of 8 μg/kg per day appears to be adequate.

3. Phytates
4. Other trace elements which may compete for absorption sites or antagonize copper metabolism (Ca, Cd, Hg, Ag, Zn, Mo)
5. Ascorbic acid

Distribution

1. The standard 70 kg adult male contains 75 to 150 mg of copper. Concentrations are highest in the brain, liver, heart, and kidney.
2. Copper stores are very low in premature infants.
3. During the first year of life, copper stores decline, then remain constant, showing adequate dietary intake and homeostasis.
4. During growth, the highest concentrations of copper are found in the rapidly developing structures.
5. Normal plasma copper levels are about 100 μg/dl, with more than 90% bound to ceruloplasmin, the rest loosely bound to albumin or amino acids.[9]
   Increased values are found in
   a. pregnancy
   b. patients taking steroid contraceptives

Excretion

The major loss of copper is in bile, with small amounts appearing in urine. Losses through sweat and menstrual fluid are usually negligible.

Pharmacology

Copper is a constituent of many enzymes.[9]

1. Cytochrome oxidase
2. Monoamine oxidase
3. Tyrosinase
4. Superoxide dismutase

Ceruloplasmin is necessary for utilization of iron in the production of hemoglobin. Copper is, therefore, involved in the following:

1. Energy metabolism
2. Development of bone
3. Development of connective tissue
4. Development of the central nervous system

Genetic Errors

There are two characteristic genetic metabolic errors.

1. Menke's steely-hair (kinky-hair) syndrome. This is produced by an X-linked recessive gene which causes impaired intestinal absorption. It is characterized by the following:
   a. peculiar hair (like steel wool)
   b. growth retardation
   c. neurologic damage
   d. convulsions
   e. bone changes
   f. lack of temperature regulation
   g. early death (usually before 3 years of age)

   Symptoms appear during the first few months of life. The disease may be treated by oral doses about 10 times the RDA (520 μg/kg per day) or preferably by intramuscular or intravenous administration of copper ion.
2. Wilson's disease, hepatolenticular degeneration, dysfunction of the lenticular area of the brain. This is a rare recessive trait. It is characterized by the following:
   a. low serum copper
   b. high urinary excretion of copper
   c. cirrhosis of the liver, due to excessive copper accumulation
   d. abnormalities in kidney excretion

Deficiency

Copper deficiency is rare in humans, although cases have been reported in unusual situations.

1. Premature infants fed low-copper formula.
2. Severely malnourished children fed milk diets (low copper content or poor absorption in presence of milk protein).
3. Long-term parenteral nutrition following bowel surgery.

Diseases such as the following may cause a lowering of serum copper levels.

1. Microbial infection
2. Viral infection
3. Rheumatoid arthritis
4. Rheumatic fever
5. Lupus erythematosus
6. Myocardial infarction
7. Acute and chronic leukemia
8. Cirrhosis of the liver
9. Many cancers
10. Thyrotoxicosis

Toxicity

ACUTE

1. Data on the level required for acute poisoning are scarce. One report of acute symptoms following ingestion of 5 to 32 mg is suspect. Ingestion of gram quantities have produced the following symptoms in the few cases reported.
   a. nausea
   b. vomiting
   c. headache
   d. diarrhea
   e. epigastric pain
   f. weakness
   g. dizziness
   h. metallic taste
   i. tachycardia
   j. hypertension
   k. jaundice
   l. hemolytic anemia
   m. uremia
   n. coma
   o. death
2. There is one report of symptoms following application of copper sulfate to a patient with extensive burns.

CHRONIC[10]

There have been rare reports of chronic toxicity. One involved a 15-month-old child ingesting water containing 79 μg/100 ml.

REFERENCES—Copper

1. Sandstead, H.H., et al.: Effect of Dietary Fiber and Protein Level on Mineral Element Metabolism, *In* Dietary Fibers: Chemistry and Nutrition. G.E. Inglett and S.I. Falkehag, eds. New York, Academic Press, 1979, ex Recommended Dietary Allowances, 9th Ed. Washington, DC, National Academy of Sciences, 1980, p. 154.
2. Butler, L.C., and Daniel, J.M.: Am. J. Clin. Nutr., *26:*744, 1973.
3. Engel, R.W., Price, N.O., and Miller, R.F.: J. Nutr., *92:*197, 1967.
4. Price, N.O., Bunce, G.E., and Engel, R.W.: Am. J. Clin. Nutr., *23:*258, 1970.
5. Klevay, L.M.: Am. J. Clin. Nutr., *28:*764, 1975.
6. Scoular, F.I.: J. Nutr., *16:*437, 1938.
7. Alexander, F.W., Clayton, B.E., and Delves, H.T.: Quart. J. Med., New Series, *169:*89, 1974.
8. Li, T.-K., and Vallee, B.L.: The Biochemical and Nutritional Roles of Other Trace Elements, *In* Modern Nutrition in Health and Disease , 6th Ed. R.S. Goodhart and M.E. Shils, eds. Philadelphia, Lea & Febiger, 1980.
9. Evans, G.W.: Physiol. Rev., *53:*535, 1973.
10. Bremner, I.: Quart. Revs. Biophys., *7:*75, 1974.

MANGANESE

Manganese is found principally in nuts and grains, with lesser amounts in fruits and vegetables, smaller amounts in dairy products and meats, and very little in seafood, (Table 10-9). Chemicals used for supplementation include manganous chloride, gluconate, and oxide.

Safe and Adequate Intake

Recommendations are based on the following considerations.

1. In adults, intakes of 0.7 mg per day lead to negative balance, whereas intakes of 2.5 mg per day produced equilibrium or positive balance.[1]
2. Intake from the average American diet is 2 to 9 mg per day.[2]
3. In the United States, manganese concentrations in human tissues show little variation.[3]

The recommended range for intake in adults is 2.5 to 5 mg per day in order to provide a margin of safety.

4. Human milk contains up to 15 μg/850 ml. During the first 6 months of life, intakes of 2.5 to 7.5 μg/kg have been reported.[4]
5. Average intakes for children from 3 to 5 years of age were 0.08 mg/kg; for 10 to 13 year-olds, 0.06 mg/kg. This is in

TABLE 10-9. Dietary Sources of Manganese

Food	μg/100 g	Food	μg/100 g
Bananas	640	Oatmeal	
Beans		raw	4945
dried	1500	Onions	363
Beans		Peas	
green, raw	325	dried	1990
Beets		Prunes	
raw	575	dried	436
Corn		Rice	
whole	680	white, raw	1010
Flour		Rye	
white	710	whole grain	3065
whole wheat	4300	Spinach	825
Kale	590	Sweet potato	405
Lettuce	1240	Wheat	
Liver	390	whole, raw	4590

agreement with balance studies.[5] These values plus a safety margin are the basis for the recommended ranges in infants and children.

Absorption[6]

Little is known about manganese absorption in humans. Animal models suggest that manganese and iron share a common absorption mechanism.

1. Manganese is absorbed in the small intestine.
2. Manganese may be absorbed by inhalation.

Distribution[6]

The standard 70 kg adult male contains about 12 to 20 mg of manganese. Absorbed manganese is transported in the trivalent form bound to a beta-1-globulin, transmanganin. Whole blood contains 1.5 to 3.0 μg/dl equally divided between the plasma and erythrocytes. High levels of manganese occur in bone, liver, kidney, pancreas, and pituitary. Levels in skeletal muscle are low. Manganese in bone is not readily mobilized.

Excretion[6]

Manganese is excreted primarily in bile. At high intakes, it is excreted in pancreatic juice. Urinary excretion is low.

Pharmacology

Manganese is a cofactor for many enzyme systems involved in protein metabolism, energy metabolism, and formation of mucopolysaccharides.

1. Isocitrate dehydrogenase (tricarboxylic acid cycle)
2. Iminodipeptidase (prolinase) (in various tissues)
3. Imidodipeptidase (prolidase) (in various tissues)
4. Leucine aminopeptidase (cathepsin III) (in many tissues, particularly kidney and gastrointestinal tract)
5. Hexosediphosphatase (kidney, liver)
6. Pyruvate decarboxylase

Deficiency

Manganese deficiency has not been observed in humans, although it can be induced readily in animals, particularly rodents and fowl. Symptoms in animals include impairment of the following:[6]

1. Growth
2. Reproduction
3. Skeletal formation
4. Central nervous system functioning
5. Glucose tolerance

Roles for manganese have been proposed in a number of diseases, but no explanations of the roles exist which might form a rational basis for therapy.

Toxicity

Few data exist about acute toxicity in humans. Chronic toxicity, manganism, is an industrial hygiene problem in the processing of manganese ores. Although the manganese is absorbed by the lungs, it is excreted mostly in the feces. Central nervous system impairment, occurs, which resembles Parkinson's disease. The effects appear long after exposure to high levels of airborne manganese and generally do not involve elevated levels of manganese in the tissue. There is no usable evidence of risk of chronic high dietary intakes.

REFERENCES—Manganese

1. McLeod, B.E., and Robinson, M.F.: Br. J. Nutr., *27:*221, 1972.
2. Underwood, E.J.: Trace Elements in Animal and Human Nutrition, 4th Ed. New York, Academic Press, 1977.
3. Schroeder, H.A., Balassa, J.J., and Tipton, I.H.: J. Chron. Dis., *19:*545, 1966.
4. McLeod, B.E., and Robinson, M.F.: Br. J. Nutr., *27:*229, 1972.
5. Engle, R.W., Price, N.O., and Miller, R.F.: J. Nutr., *92:*197, 1967.
6. Cotzias, G.C.: Physiol. Revs., *38:*503, 1958.

CHROMIUM

Chromium is available in animal (but not fish) protein, whole grain products, and brewer's yeast. Chromium in green leafy vegetables is poorly available. A chemical source is chromium trichloride.

Safe and Adequate Intake

Recommended intake levels are based on the following information.

1. Absorbable chromium, estimated from urinary loss, ranges from 0.4 to 1.8 μg per day (mean, 0.8 μg).[1]
2. Chromium balance in a patient on total parenteral alimentation was maintained by intravenous administration of 20 μg per day.[2] Positive balance was obtained at 46 μg per day.[3]
3. No toxicity was noted when 150 μg per day were added over long times to the average American diet containing 60 μg per day.[4]

A tentative recommendation of 50 to 200 μg per day is made for adults, with recommendations for infants and children made by extrapolation to expected dietary intakes. Because of the uncertainties of this recommendation, consumption of a varied diet balanced with regard to other nutrients is recommended.

Absorption

Absorption from chromium chloride hexahydrate ($CrCl_3 \cdot 6H_2O$) was between 0.5 and 0.69% of the administered dose.[5] Absorbability of organically bound chromium in food is higher.

Excretion

Chromium is excreted primarily in the urine.

Pharmacology[5]

Trivalent chromium is required to maintain normal glucose metabolism. It probably acts as a cofactor for insulin at the insulin-responsive cell membrane.[6]

Deficiency

Chromium-responsive disturbances of glucose metabolism have been reported in the United States, indicating that some people are at risk for chromium deficiency.[4,7]

REFERENCES—Chromium

1. Veillon, C., Wolf, W.R., and Guthrie, B.E.: Anal. Chem., *51:*1022, 1979.
2. Jeejeebhoy, K.N.: Am. J. Clin. Nutr., *30:*531, 1977.
3. Jacobson, S., and Wester, P.-O.: Br. J. Nutr., *37:*107, 1977.
4. Glinsman, W.H., and Mertz, W.: Metabolism, *15:*510, 1966.
5. Mertz, W., et al.: Fed. Proc., *33:*2275, 1974.
6. Hambidge, K.M.: Am. J. Clin. Nutr., *27:*505, 1974.
7. Liu, V.J.K., and Morris, J.S.: Am. J. Clin. Nutr., *31:*972, 1978.

MOLYBDENUM

Molybdenum occurs in significant amounts in meat, whole grains, and legumes.[1] The concentration depends on the concentration of molybdenum in the environment in which the food was raised.

Safe and Adequate Intake

The following information was considered in making the recommendations.

1. Deficiency states have not been reported for humans. Molybdenum is known to be a cofactor for xanthine oxidase and for enzymes involved in the production of uric acid and the oxidation of aldehydes and sulfites. Balance studies in humans show equilibrium at intakes of 2 μg/kg, corresponding to daily intakes of 100 to 150 μg for an adult; although a negative balance was obtained at 100 μg per day in some subjects.[2]
2. Ingestion of 540 μg per day caused considerable loss of copper and elevated blood levels of uric acid.[3]
3. Since no deficiency has been reported in humans, it is assumed that the mixed diet providing 100 to 460 μg per day is adequate.[1] Food tables are unreliable in diet planning because of the high variability of molybdenum content.

The recommendation is 150 to 500 μg for adults, with recommendations for other age groups based on interpolation by weight.

REFERENCES—Molybdenum

1. Schroeder, H.A., Balassa, J.J., and Tipton, I.H.: J. Chron. Dis., *23:*481, 1970.
2. Engle, R.W., Price, N.O., and Miller, R.F.: J. Nutr., *92:*197, 1967.
3. Deosthale, Y.G., and Gopalan, C.: Br. J. Nutr., *31:*351, 1974.

Chapter 11
Feeding the Normal Infant

Feeding the normal infant can be divided into two stages:

1. Human milk, or milk substitutes, as the sole source of nourishment from birth to the introduction of solids.
2. Milk plus increasing amounts of solids from about 3 to 6 months to about 1 to 2 years of age.

In the first stage, the best available criterion for estimating human needs is the quality and quantity of milk produced by humans. It would seem obvious to all that nutrition that produces a healthy child with good physical and mental development is adequate nutrition. This was recognized by the Food and Nutrition Board of the National Research Council in basing the recommended *intake* of nutrients *from milk substitutes* on the nutrient values in human milk plus an excess to allow for the poorer utilization of nutrients from milk substitutes. It is obvious, therefore, that any comparison of human milk with RDA values will show that human milk does not meet those values. Misinterpretation of this to mean that human-milk-fed infants are nutritionally deprived and require nutritional supplements demonstrates ignorance of the fact that the RDA values refer to intakes from a particular diet and not to amounts absorbed, utilized, or needed.

The actual composition of human milk is variable (Table 11-1), and the components and the ranges of quantitative composition are inadequately known. This information may be of value in the formulation of milk substitutes and for demonstrating why human milk is superior to the substitutes, but the fact remains that infants thrive over a wide range of nutrient values, so that nutrition of the human-milk-fed infant is frequently adequate even when the diet of the mother is nutritionally inadequate.

Another common error in assessing adequacy of infant nutrition is to assume that biochemical indices of nutrition such as saturation of tissues and activities of biochemical systems should be those of the adult. The argument usually advanced is that the "normal" (adult) values should be attempted to be produced by supplementation. Actually, there is little in the literature about normal values in thriving human-milk-fed infants or the actual success in changing biochemical indices by supplementation. When these have been changed, there is little information as to whether the changes are due to supplementation or normal maturation or whether there was any change in the clinical evaluation of the child's health. The most shocking example of the "little adult" approach is the routine administration of vita-

TABLE 11-1. Composition of Mature Human Milk

Data mainly from: K. Diem and C. Lentner, eds., Scientific Tables, *7th ed., Ciba-Geigy, Ltd., Basle, Switzerland, 1970, pp. 688-689.*

Substance	Units	Mean	Experimental Range
Calories	kcal/L	747	446 to 1192
Cations	mEq/L	41	—
Calcium	mg/L	344	173 to 609
Magnesium	mg/L	35	18 to 57
Potassium	mg/L	512	373 to 735
Sodium	mg/L	172	64 to 436
Anions	mEq/L	28	
Chlorine	mg/L	375	88 to 734
Phosphorus	mg/L	141	68 to 268
Sulfur	mg/L	140	5 to 300
Trace elements			
Cobalt	μg/L	trace	—
Copper	μg/L	510	—
Fluorine	μg/L	107	0.0 to 240
Iodine	μg/L	61	44 to 93
Iron	μg/L	500	200 to 800
Manganese	μg/L	trace	—
Selenium	μg/L	21	—
Zinc	μg/L	1180	170 to 3020
Protein	g/L	10.6	7.3 to 20
Casein	g/L	3.7	1.4 to 6.8
Whey protein	g/L	7	4 to 10
Alpha-lactalbumin	g/L	3.6	1.4 to 6.0
Lactoglobulin			
Lactotransferin			
Blood serum			
Albumin	g/L	0.32	0.20 to 0.47
Blood serum			
Immunoglobulin	g/L	0.09	0.02 to 0.27
sIgA			
IgE			
IgM			
Amino acids			
Total	g/L	12.8	9.0 to 16.0
Alanine	g/L	—	0.36 to 0.42
Arginine	g/L	0.43	0.28 to 0.64
Aspartic acid	g/L	—	0.89 to 0.98
Cystine	g/L	—	0.23 to 0.25
Glutamic acid	g/L	—	1.89 to 2.00
Glycine	g/L	—	0.23 to 0.24
Histidine	g/L	0.24	0.12 to 0.30
Isoleucine	g/L	0.61	0.41 to 0.92
Leucine	g/L	0.97	0.65 to 1.47
Lysine	g/L	0.70	0.36 to 0.93
Methionine	g/L	0.12	0.07 to 0.16
Phenylalanine	g/L	0.40	0.24 to 0.58
Proline	g/L	—	0.84 to 0.94
Serine	g/L	—	0.47 to 0.51
Threonine	g/L	0.52	0.30 to 0.66
Tryptophan	g/L	0.19	0.14 to 0.26
Tyrosine	g/L	—	0.46 to 0.52
Valine	g/L	0.73	0.54 to 1.14
Nonprotein Nitrogen:			
Total	mg/L	324	173 to 604
Amino acids	mg/L	50	28 to 113
Choline	mg/L	10.3	6.2 to 16.8

TABLE 11-1. (continued)

Substance	Units	Mean	Experimental Range
Creatine	mg/L	11	2 to 41
Creatinine	mg/L	11	8 to 19
Urea	mg/L	180	127 to 235
Uric acid	mg/L	22	13 to 41
Carbohydrates			
Citric acid	mg/L	—	350 to 1250
Galactosamine	mg/L	—	0 to 400
Glucosamine	mg/L	—	700 to 800
Inositol	mg/L	450	390 to 560
Lactose	g/L	71	49 to 95
Oligosaccharides	g/L	6	—
fucose	g/L	1.3	—
Fats			
Total	g/L	45.4	13.4 to 82.9
Cholesterol (total)	mg/L	139	88 to 202
free cholesterol	mg/L	106	—
Lipid phosphorus	mg/L	10.5	7 to 14
Vitamins			
Ascorbic acid	mg/L	52	0 to 112
Biotin	μg/L	2	1 to 3
Folate	μg/L	24.0	7.4 to 61.0
Niacin	mg/L	1.83	0.66 to 3.30
Pantothenic acid	mg/L	2.46	0.86 to 5.84
Riboflavin	μg/L	373	198 to 790
Thiamin	μg/L	142	81 to 227
Tocopherol	mg/L	2.4	1.0 to 4.8
Vitamin A	μg/L	610	150 to 2260
carotenes	μg/L	250	20 to 770
Vitamin B_6	μg/L	180	100 to 220
Vitamin B_{12}	—	—	trace
Vitamin D	IU/L	—	4 to 100
Enzymes			
Lysozyme	mg/L	390	30 to 3000
Acetylesterase			
Acid phosphatase			
Adenosine triphosphatase (ATPase)			
Aldolase			
Alkaline phosphatase			
Amylase			
Arylesterase			
Aspartate aminotransferase			
Catalase			
Cholinesterase			
Glucose-6-phosphate dehydrogenase			
Glucosephosphate isomerase			
Inorganic pyrophosphatase			
Lactate dehydrogenase			
Lipase			
Malate dehydrogenase			
Peptide hydrolase			
Peroxidase			
Xanthinoxidase			

min K to neonates. The neonate does have lower than adult levels of prothrombin, but without any significant change in bleeding time. The normal pattern for prothrombin levels is the following: very low at birth, increasing dramatically to a maximum at about day 3 to 5, and then declining to adult levels. For 99% of infants, the hazard of the parenteral insult of vitamin K injection is not compensated by any improvement in *clinical* status, since adult prothrombin levels are reached with or without the parenteral supplement. It would seem more logical to investigate the reason why it is advantageous to the infant to have the usual biochemical values than to assume that the vast majority of infants are "abnormal," hardly a rational concept in the context.

A third common error is to ignore the nutritional reserves of the healthy infant born of a well-nourished mother. An excess supply of nutrients that prevents normal depletion of these reserves has unknown effects. Little in the literature addresses the adequacy and advantages of the normal pattern except a recognition that children thrive with or without nutritional supplements. Little mention also is made of the advantages of supplementing the diet of the nursing mother rather than that of the infant.

There will be no discussion here of the immunologic, psychologic, economic, and societal advantages of suckling, as these have been extensively reviewed elsewhere.[1] It suffices to observe that, nutritionally, normal healthy infants physically thrive on an exclusive diet of human milk, on human milk plus supplements, on formulated milk substitutes (Table 11-2), or on modified cow's milk (Table 11-3).

NURSING

Because normal nursing infants have not been observed by many health professionals, the process of nursing will be described in detail.[2] Normal infants are born with a "snuffling" reflex. If a smooth object is placed against the cheek, the head will be turned toward that side, the mouth will open and the head will move about in search of the nipple. The technique of nursing starts with a mother at ease and comfortable. Many women find nursing while lying on a bed to be the most relaxing. When she is out of bed, a comfortably low chair with an armrest and footstool for raising the knee and resting the foot on the side that is being nursed is usually satisfactory. The baby is comfortably supported by one arm and hand while the other hand supports the breast so that the baby can reach the nipple easily without interference with the baby's breathing. The modern mother should not allow old cultural inhibitions to prevent her

TABLE 11-2. Products Used to Replace or Supplement Human Milk

Product	Manufacturer
Milk base	
Advance	Ross
Enfamil	Mead Johnson
Enfamil with Iron	Mead Johnson
Probana	Mead Johnson
Similac	Ross
Similac PM 60/40	Ross
Similac with Iron	Ross
SMA Improved	Wyeth
Hydrolyzed casein base	
Nutramigen	Mead Johnson
Pregestimil	Mead Johnson
Soy base	
Cho-Free	Syntex
Isomil	Ross
Mull-Soy	Syntex
Neo-Mull-Soy	Syntex
Nursoy	Wyeth
ProSobee	Mead Johnson
Soyalac	Loma Linda
Meat base	
MFB (Meat Base Formula)	Gerber

TABLE 11-3. Products Used to Modify Cow's Milk for Human Nutrition

Product	Manufacturer	Notes
Lactose, USP	Various	powder
Casec	Mead Johnson	calcium caseinate containing Ca, P, Na, and other minerals
LactAid	Sugario	lactase enzyme

from exposing her breast or holding it in the most comfortable position for her and her baby. When the baby's face contacts the breast, the snuffling reflex will take over and the lips will find the nipple. Usually a considerable amount of the aureola as well as the nipple will be in the baby's mouth. Note that the hand should not be used to turn the baby's head toward the nipple because when the baby's cheek is touched the reflex will cause the baby's head to turn toward the hand and away from the nipple.

For the first several days after birth, infants are usually sleepy, and although many babies nurse eagerly from the start, most infants will not suck strongly during this period. The small amount (10 to 40 ml per day, or about 1/3 to 1 1/3 ounces) of colostrum produced during about the first 4 days after delivery is adequate nourishment. Colostrum is a deep yellow, alkaline, concentrated liquid. It contains less carbohydrate and fat but more minerals and nearly three times as much protein as mature human milk. After the first few days of lactation, the milk composition gradually changes, reaching the mature milk composition about the third or fourth week. This change from yellow to white or bluish-white may be misinterpreted by the mother as the milk becoming "thin" or "weak," or inadequate. Reassurance as to its adequacy may be needed.

If the baby is not hungry it will not search for the nipple or suck. Mothers should not become anxious about this nor about the normal loss of weight about the third day. This weight loss is normal and does not imply an inadequate milk supply. Unfortunately, health personnel are too familiar with the formula-overfed, nursery-isolated infant and become alarmed at this normal occurrence.

The initially sleepy newborn will wake up and start to show some real interest in nursing about the fourth day. The baby should never be waked or forced to nurse by shaking, pinching, or slapping the feet. This is not only cruel but rarely successful.

Infants nurse at different rates. Some may empty a breast in 5 minutes, others require 20 minutes or more. The baby should be permitted to nurse until satisfied. At the end of the nursing period, the infant should be held upright over the mother's shoulder or on her lap in order to bring up swallowed air ("burping"). This may also be necessary several times during the nursing period if and when the baby stops nursing temporarily for a rest or "break." The baby should be burped again 5 to 10 minutes after being placed in a horizontal position. Ideally, the baby should remain close to the mother and in good body contact. This allows colonization of the baby's skin by normal nonpathogenic flora and prevents impetigo, the scourge of hospital nurseries. The nipple should never be disinfected with alcohol, particularly rubbing alcohol which contains a bitter nonvolatile denaturing agent, nor treated with tincture of benzoin. Washing gently with mild soap and water once a day is adequate. The desired body contact of the mother and infant and the desired lack of sterility may be a troublesome concept to some hospital personnel. Nevertheless, exposure to the normal, adult, nonpathogenic organisms is what is most desirable and beneficial for the baby.

Successful nursing is the norm. Most mothers can nurse their children if the normal spontaneous pattern is not interfered with by rigid schedules and factory assembly methods found in many hospitals. If the baby is put to the breast when it exhibits the normal hunger urge, and if the baby is satisfied, the situation is normal. Ideally, the baby should be in the same room as the mother to allow for the natural situation. The most abnormal technique is for the baby to be brought to the mother at some predetermined time after having been fed formula to still cries in the nursery or allowed to cry until exhausted.

LACTATION

The milk ejection or "let-down" reflex is necessary for successful nursing. This reflex may be inhibited if the mother is physically uncomfortable, worried, or embarrassed. In American culture, often a quiet, private place is desired

Suckling or psychologic factors associated with nursing cause secretion of oxytocin by the posterior pituitary gland. This causes contraction of the smooth muscle fiber of the alveoli (milk glands), forcing the milk into the larger ducts. This usually causes milk to flow from the opposite breast when the baby starts nursing.

Oxytocin also causes uterine contraction, thus helping the uterus to return to normal size and muscle tone. These contractions are usually not felt at all, but may be experienced as "cramps" (particularly about the time menstruation would occur) or as orgasm.

The initiation and maintenance of lactation by hormonal response to suckling is so powerful that it may be initiated in any woman of child bearing age. Adoptive mothers who wish to nurse their children may obtain information from La Leche League International, 9616 Minneapolis Avenue, Franklin Park, IL 60131.

One breast should be emptied at each nursing in order to stimulate refilling. Both breasts should be used at each nursing during the first few weeks in order to encourage maximal production. After the milk supply is well established, about the third or fourth week, the breasts may be alternated at successive nursings, since the infant will generally be satisfied by the contents of one breast.

During the first few weeks of lactation, the breasts may feel uncomfortably heavy and full. Having the baby partially empty both breasts at each nursing will reduce this feeling. The milk supply will adjust to the demand, and balance should be achieved in the first month. This balance and loss of the uncomfortable feeling may be misinterpreted as the milk supply's becoming inadequate. Reassurance may be necessary.

Adequacy of the milk supply should *never* be judged by weighing the baby before and after nursing, because of the large variations in individual nursings during a day. "Test feeding" formula from a calibrated bottle to see how much is ingested is likewise difficult to interpret. The correct criteria are the following:

1. Satisfaction of the baby at the completion of each nursing period.
2. Sleeping for 2 to 4 hours between nursings.
3. Adequate weight gain as judged by weighing at weekly or monthly intervals, with due care in interpretation and knowledge that growth curves are erratic and highly individualized and rarely conform to average values.

If the infant fails to thrive, an assumption of an inadequate milk supply should *not* be made. Inquiry should be first made into

1. Whether the technique used for nursing is correct.
2. Whether the infant had physical disturbances that interfered with feeding or weight gain.
3. Whether assumed inadequacies in the milk supply can be remedied by improvement in the maternal diet, relief of maternal emotional stress, or more maternal rest.

If nursing is normal, failure to thrive may be due to inherited metabolic errors. Special nutritional products, as given in Table 11-4, are available for the more common conditions. Special individualized formulations can be obtained, if necessary, from the manufacturers shown.

BOTTLE FEEDING HUMAN MILK

If it is necessary to provide more flexibility for the mother, after about the first 6 weeks, human milk may be fed from a bottle. The milk may be manually expressed from the breast in the following way. The whole breast is first compressed between the hands starting at the chest and moving toward the nipple. Firm, but not uncomfortable, pressure is maintained throughout this movement, which is repeated several times to bring the milk into the large ducts. The breast is then supported with one hand

TABLE 11-4. Therapeutic Formulas

Product	Manufacturer	Notes
High calorie		
Enfamil Premature Formula	Mead Johnson	24 kcal/fluid ounce
Restricted sodium		
Lonalac	Mead Johnson	1.4 mEq Na/100 ml
Similac PM 60/40	Ross	0.7 mEq Na/100 ml
Phenylketonuria		
Lofenalac	Mead Johnson	hydrolyzed casein processed to remove most of the phenylalanine
Restricted carbohydrate		
CHO-Free Formula Base	Syntex	carbohydrate 0.02 g/100 ml

while the tissue just behind the aureola is compressed repeatedly between the thumb and index finger of the other hand. The direction of pressure is backward toward the chest rather than toward the nipple. This empties the ducts. The skin over the breasts and nipples must not be rubbed. Note that this procedure may also be used if the nipples are sore or cracked. While the manual method just described is the gentlest and most effective method, some women prefer an electric breast pump. The manual breast pumps are frequently ineffective and may cause irritation and pain in congested breasts and nipples.

The milk is collected in clean (sterile?) wide-mouthed nursing bottles, each sufficient for one feeding, and refrigerated. The bottle may be warmed before being offered, although most babies have no difficulty with refrigerator-cold milk. If any temperature error is made, it is better to have the milk too cold than too hot. The traditional test is that a few drops shaken on the inside of the wrist should feel neither cold nor warm. The holes in the nipple should be adjusted so that the baby needs to exert the same amount of effort to obtain milk as would be required by suckling. This can be determined by timing the feeding. About the same amount of time should be required by bottle feeding as by nursing. If the bottle feeding becomes too easy, the baby may refuse to nurse adequately.

Using this technique, the infant may be provided with all the nutritional advantages of human milk without undue interference with maternal activities.

FEEDING SCHEDULE

Many infants in normal circumstances set up a regular schedule for themselves within the first few weeks of life. These schedules are highly individual. Many infants will give up the middle of the night feeding first and sleep through most of the night. Some may be satisfied with four or even three feedings a day, whereas others may require more frequent nursing. All these patterns are normal.

Nursing should not be used as a pacifier for crying. If the baby cries at times which are not usual feeding times, check to see that the baby is clean and dry, was not wakened by unusual noise, is not in pain, and does not have a physical ailment. The baby may be satisfied by some physical contact. Hunger, however, may be the problem. The usual schedule may not be dependable. For no apparent reason, the daily number of feedings desired by some babies may vary markedly from day to day.

TRANSITION TO OTHER FOODS

The transition from an exclusive milk or milk substitute diet to a mixed diet containing nonmilk foods and the subsequent weaning from suckling have been recognized by all communities as presenting particular hazards to the infants. There are many different practices based on age or physical development (number of teeth, ability to walk), with varying degrees of success. The problem is bridging the period in which the young human changes from a milk-drinking to a starch-and-flesh-eating organism. All cultures seem to have food classifications which limit the range of choices (foods considered particularly appropriate or completely inappropriate for particular ages). The major objective should be to use a food that is high in both protein and calories to prevent protein-calorie malnutrition (kwashiorkor, marasmus). The contribution to nutrition from continuing milk feeding before weaning should not be ignored. An adequate and preferred "first food" is a cereal grain.

In the United States, it is customary to base nonmilk feeding on weight, usually starting the feeding at weights of about 6 to 7 kg, on the assumption that the growth rate at that time cannot be sustained by milk alone. Feeding is generally not started, however, before the age of 3 months[3] to minimize problems of food intolerance or allergy, lack of neuromuscular readiness for solids,[4] and chronic overeating.

The general pattern is as follows:

1. Use single ingredient foods, feeding for at least 5 to 14 days before introducing another food. This allows identification of food sensitivities. Foods are most acceptable if fairly thin or dilute. Juices are also introduced singly (usually orange or apple), preferably from a cup.
2. Start with a small serving of 1 to 2 teaspoonsful and gradually increase to 3 to 4 teaspoonsful per serving.
3. Do not force foods that are not acceptable to the infant. However, do not mistake "spitting back" due to inadequate swallowing reflex for food rejection. The usual order of food introduction is (rice) cereal, fruits (usually banana), vegetables, meats and egg yolk, and starches. The texture should be compatible with the ability of the infant to chew and swallow. Pureed foods are suitable for early introduction, whereas finely chopped "junior" foods are generally suitable after 6 months, and increasingly coarser foods as the ability to chew increases. These may be economically prepared at home or bought in prepared form.
4. Avoid developing in the infant a taste for excessive sugar or salt, particularly by using sweet or salty items (pretzels, popcorn) as a form of "treat" or reward.
5. Gradually decrease milk intake to about three glasses (24 ounces).
6. When feeding solids is well established, use a diet plan such as the "basic four" to provide a balanced mixed diet.
7. Monitor growth and development (well-baby clinic) periodically.

The proper amount of food is that which will satisfy the baby's hunger. To avoid overfeeding, acceptance of food should not be mistaken for hunger. If the baby does not demand more food between meals and is eager to eat at meals, the correct amount has been fed.

Between 6 and 12 months, as the infant becomes accustomed to increasing quantities of solid food and to liquids taken by cup or bottle, the demand for nursing decreases. As the demand decreases, the amount of milk produced will decrease naturally and there should be no problem of discomfort. It should be noted that nursing does not permanently alter the size or shape of the breast since no new tissue is formed during nursing. If anything, nursing increases the muscle tone of the breast tissue.

Weaning

Weaning is initiated by substituting whole (not skim) cow's milk for part and then substantially all of the human milk. It is advantageous to offer this from a cup and thus avoid the transition from bottle to cup. When one of the nursings has been completely replaced, over the course of several days additional nursings are successively replaced until weaning is complete. During this time, the infant needs cuddling and attention.

Learning to Self-Feed

An infant should be allowed to participate in its own feeding before it is 1 year old. Many infants can reliably hold a bottle at about 6 months, and a cup at 8 or 9 months. Hand-held foods can be self-fed at about 7 to 8 months, and a spoon may be used at about 10 to 12 months. This learning process should not be inhibited by people who object to the messiness of learning control. By the time the child is 2 years old it should be substantially responsible for its own feeding.

NUTRITION

If excessively sweet or salty foods are not available and a reasonable range of foods is offered, a child will self-select a diet that is balanced over a period of several days. There will be days of almost exclusive eating of a single food, perhaps followed by rejection of that food for several weeks. Although pediatricians are greatly concerned about the adequacy of iron intake in infants and resort to the daily multi-vitamin or at least a vitamin D supplement as a panacea, the fact is that the normal infant can thrive well without them. Vitamin D can be obtained by daily exposure of the face to the sun even on cloudy days, since the ultraviolet light that produces vitamin D in the skin substantially penetrates clouds. The RDA values, which are daily averages over long periods of time, are generally misinterpreted (even on the nutrition labels on foods) as the recommended *daily* (rather than the correct "dietary") allowance. In addition, they are based on absorption factors for adults, which may or may not be lower than for children, and in an effort to include nearly all the population, are much more than is required by a majority of the population. Body reserves of most nutrients are sufficient for several weeks, so that the normal pattern of balance over several days is adequate. The routine use of nutritional supplements may produce physical dependency on high intakes which will make subsequent adequate nutrition by normal foods difficult. As in the adult, nutritional supplements should be used for infants only when there is a clear clinical indication of deficiency. Prophylactic use of supplements should be based on a careful analysis of *monthly* diet and should not exceed the RDA on a monthly basis.

Analysis of the monthly diet may show it does not quite meet the criterion of 30 × RDA. For those who mistakenly interpret the RDA as a minimum value, it may be psychologically important that the value be achieved. Since the RDA provides an excess of nutrients for more than half the population, the need to achieve RDA values for infants who are clinically healthy is questionable.

Food should be offered only to satisfy hunger. Infants should not be given a bottle of formula, milk, juice, or water to suck intermittently before going to sleep. In the same category, between meal snacks of milk or juice and crackers offered midmorning in the nursery school and kindergarten are suspect, as is the after school snack of older children. The criteria for appropriate feedings between meals are the following:

1. Does the child feel hungry enough to ask for food?
2. After snacking, is there an increase in activity and enthusiasm for play?
3. Is the child reasonably hungry for the meal following the snack?

The fundamental purpose of the snack is to raise blood glucose levels if they have dropped because the previous meal has been substantially digested. Thus, small quantities of sugars and complex carbohydrates such as provided by fruit are probably the most desirable. Fats, such as chocolate or potato chips, which prolong stomach-emptying time are probably undesirable because of their interference with hunger at the next meal.

Eating habits formed in the first 2 years impact on the rest of the person's life. Eating should not be a cause of stress nor a response to stress. Some of the things that should be avoided are over-concern about the amount of food ingested, confused mealtimes, inadequate time for eating, offering disliked, poorly prepared, or unattractive food, and uncomfortable chairs. Mealtimes should be happy family times and an opportunity for conversations of interest to the entire family.

REFERENCES—Infant Feeding

1. Jelliffe, D.B., and Jelliffe, E.F.P.: Human Milk in the Modern World. London, Oxford University Press, 1978.
2. Nelson, W.E., et al. (eds.): Nelson Textbook of Pediatrics, 11th Ed. Philadelphia, W.B. Saunders, 1979, pp. 190-210.
3. Committee on Nutrition: Pediatrics, *21:*685, 1958.
4. Gesell, A., and Ilg, F.L.: Feeding Behavior of Infants. Philadelphia, J.B. Lippincott, 1937.

Chapter 12

Weight Reduction and Maintenance

The poor success rate in the treatment of obesity may be due to a lack of complete understanding of the mechanisms that cause it. In the normal person, adult weight does not vary by more than 2% over long intervals of time, indicating a precise energy balance mechanism. Obesity is obviously a failure of this mechanism.

FACTORS IN FOOD INTAKE

1. **Perception of hunger.** This is an innate unconditioned physiologic response to the need for food. It involves blood levels of glucose and amino acids and gastric contractions. Animal studies indicate this mechanism is controlled by the ventrolateral nucleus of the hypothalamus.

2. **Perception of satiety.** This is a signal that at the particular moment enough food has been consumed. Animal studies indicate that this mechanism is controlled by the ventromedian nucleus of the hypothalamus.

3. **Appetite.** In contrast to hunger, this is a learned response involving pleasurable anticipation. It is used to deal with emotional needs rather than nutritional needs, so that food is eaten in the absence of a nutritional need for it. It is postulated that the mechanism involves the cerebral cortex.

Of these three, appetite, the psychogenic factor, is usually the most important in weight control.

Theories, Myths, and Facts

Many theories have been proposed about the causes of obesity based on supposed differences between normobaric and obese people. These theories have not been substantiated.

1. Differences in adipocyte size and number between obese children and adult-onset obesity.
2. "Brown fat."
3. Genetic predisposition.
4. Obesity theories based on animal models.

The following myths about obesity are current.

Myth: Food is diverted to fat in an abnormal manner.

Myth: The diet of obese people has an abnormal caloric distribution.

Myth: Thermogenic response to food is abnormal.

Fact: Obese people have a normal or slightly increased lean weight.

Fact: Obese children have slightly accelerated structural growth. They grow taller and have an increase in lean body mass roughly proportional to the degree of obesity. This is evidence of nutritional adequacy and proper hormone balance.

Fact: Obese people lose weight predictably on dietary restriction.

Psychogenic Factors

The psychogenic factors in obesity can be divided into two groupings.

SITUATIONAL OBESITY

Situational obesity develops in relation to the following:

1. Social situations and expectations.
2. Use of food as reward.
3. Cultural approval of the obese child.
4. Response to immediate stresses.

The cure requires an understanding of the problem, reassurance, and support. The various group behavior modification organizations and individual therapies work well for some people. Note that there are no groups available for the obese child.

DEVELOPMENTAL OBESITY

A long established pattern of compulsive eating, caused by psychologic stresses and usually coupled with low physical activity, is the overt symptom. Attempts at forcing weight loss are unsuccessful and may cause serious emotional disturbance. Psychotherapy is usually indicated and weight loss may be contraindicated.

DIET PLANNING

In devising plans for weight reduction and weight maintenance, the following principles should be kept in mind.

1. The *only* way to lose weight is to absorb fewer calories than are utilized by the metabolism.

2. Weight reduction is only part of the solution. After the desired weight is reached, how is it to be maintained? In answering this question, it should be obvious that quick-weight-loss diets without a permanent change in eating habits will be followed by quick weight gain and a perpetual cycle is produced. Note also that the caloric needs of the smaller normal body mass are less than those of the larger obese body. Because severe caloric deficit produces a rise in serum triglyceride, the cycle may actually impair health.

3. An extreme change in diet generally produces loss of water for the first 7 to 10 days. Thus "lose 10 pounds in the first week" is true for nearly any diet, including some that actually contain an excess of calories. Results of weight loss diets cannot readily be judged before the third week.

4. It is nearly impossible to obtain needed nutrients on caloric intakes of less than 1200 kcal per day. Severe dieting should be kept up for periods not to exceed 2 weeks and should not be repeated within 4 weeks. Thought should be given to the use of supplements. It is obvious that single-food or highly restricted diets will not be balanced and are so monotonous that long term compliance is low.

5. The diet plans that have been most successful in obtaining a "cure" for obesity (as measured by 5 years of successful maintenance of weight) are those which

   a. provide motivation for weight loss and weight maintenance. This can be group support such as in "Weight Watchers" and "TOPS"[1].
   b. initially have the objective of behavior modification and do not expect weight loss until the behavioral problem is solved.
   c. do not have the patient "count calories."
   d. do not urge consumption of particular foods and "forbid" others.
   e. do not use drugs as a crutch.
   f. educate the patient in nutrition and food choices.
   g. provide for a moderate increase in physical activity.

Weight Reduction with No Provision for Maintenance

Before going on to suggestions for weight reduction and maintenance, a number of diets that do not lay a foundation for continued weight maintenance will be discussed in groups according to their common characteristics.

FASTING OR STARVATION

This produces no serious problems if of short duration.[2] Prolonged fasting, however, produces the following:[3]

1. Loss of lean body mass.
2. Increase in serum bilirubin (indicates hepatic dysfunction).
3. Anemia.
4. Hyperuricemia.
5. Postural hypotension.
6. Ketosis (reduces feeling of hunger).
7. Electrolyte imbalance.
8. Death, due to cardiac complications.

Fasting is contraindicated in patients with a history of heart failure (may lead to ventricular fibrillation and cardiac arrest) and in patients with clinical signs of atherosclerosis.

In a 7-year study of 121 patients, the following were found.[4]

1. Reduced weight was maintained for 12 to 18 months.
2. Weight was regained within 2 to 3 years by 50% of the patients.
3. Only 7 of the 121 patients (5.8%) had maintained reduced weight over the full 7.3 years of the study.

PROTEIN-SPARING MODIFIED FAST (PSMF)

This diet provides 400 to 600 kcal per day and 1.0 to 1.5 g protein/kg of desired body weight, water, and supplementary vitamins and minerals. This diet must be closely supervised by knowledgeable people. Popular versions of the PSMF are the following:

1. 9 to 12 ounces of lean meat or fish a day with black coffee or tea.
2. Protein powders to be reconstituted with water, soda, fruit juice, or other liquid.
3. Liquid protein solutions.
4. The "Last Chance" diet.

Many of these do not supply a complete spectrum of nutrients and have produced the following problems:[5]

1. Nausea.
2. Vomiting.
3. Constipation.
4. Electrolyte imbalance.
5. Dehydration.
6. Hyperuricemia, due to destruction of body muscle to obtain glucose.
7. Postural hypotension.
8. Thrombophlebitis of legs.
9. Pulmonary embolism.
10. Sudden cardiac death (50/100,000 in 25 to 44 year olds as compared with a rate of 2/100,000 in this age group for nondieters).

Because of the potential for harm, the Food and Drug Administration requires warning labels on protein products sold for use as foods.[6] These warnings include the following:

1. "Very low calorie protein diets (below 800 calories per day) may cause serious illness or death. Do not use for weight reduction without medical supervision. Use with particular care if you are taking medication. Not for use by infants, children, or pregnant or nursing women."
2. If promoted for weight reduction as part of a nutritionally balanced diet plan:
   "Use only as directed in the diet plan (location of plan). Do not use as the sole or primary source of calories for weight reduction."
3. If promoted as a food supplement:
   "Use this product as a food supplement only. Do not use for weight reduction."

The diet is unsuitable for people with heart disease, diabetes, liver problems, or gout, and for those wanting to lose less than 50 pounds.

ONE-FOOD DIETS

1. Grapefruit or Mayo (not Mayo Clinic) diet is based on the hypothesis that grapefruit contains a substance that increases fat breakdown. No food is known which does this.[7]
2. Candy diet ("lollipop breaks" and hard candy between meals) is based on the hypothesis that calories are saved by candy displacing snacks with an even higher caloric content. (Ayds, a chewy candy, requires use of a balanced, calorically deficient 1100 kcal per day diet.)

3. Ice cream diet, for every meal except breakfast *but* total intake is not to exceed 1000 kcal per day.
4. Yogurt diet of 5 to 6 pints of *plain* yogurt daily (about 1500 kcal).
5. Skim milk and bananas.
6. Rice diet (Walter Kempner, M.D.), designed for patients with kidney disease. It consists of cooked rice, fruit, sugar, and tea. There are many popular modifications.

Weight is lost on all these diets because they are calorically inadequate. They are, however, nutritionally inadequate as well and include no provision for weight maintenance.

LOW CARBOHYDRATE DIETS

1. Banting Diet (1870's)
2. Dupont Diet
3. Drinking Man's Diet (Robert Wernick)
4. Air Force Diet
5. Airline Pilot's Diet
6. Astronaut's Diet
7. Thinking Man's Diet (Ed McMahon)
8. "Carbo-cal" diets (Sidney Petrie)
9. Miracle Diet (Sidney Petrie—6 meals a day)
10. McCall's Snack Diet
11. Wisconsin Diet

All of these produce weight loss because the diet plan provides about 1000 kcal per day. They share the following problems:

1. Low carbohydrate intake produces water and salt loss. The initial weight loss of salt and water is regained when the diet is stopped.
2. Frequent complaints of fatigue accompanying diets containing less than 30 g per day of carbohydrate.
3. *Zero* carbohydrate intake causes ketosis.
4. Frequent complaints of postural hypotension.
5. No provision is made for weight maintenance after the desired weight is reached.

HIGH PROTEIN DIETS

1. Does-It Diet (Gayelord Hauser), high protein, low calorie vegetables and vitamin supplement.
2. Lazy Lady Diet (Sidney Petrie), 1000 kcal per day of protein and fats plus 150 kcal per day of carbohydrate.
3. Doctor's Quick Inches Off Diet (Irwin Maxwell Stillman, M.D., Stillman Diet, Water Diet, Quick Weight Loss Diet; Scarsdale Diet, Herman Tarnower, M.D.). The general plan of the Stillman diet will be given to aid recognition of diets of this type. Others follow the Stillman plan with various modifications.
   a. The diet is to be used for 14 consecutive days.
   b. Eat until no longer hungry from the following list:
      (1) lean meat and poultry
      (2) lean fish and seafood
      (3) eggs
      (4) low fat cheeses (cottage, pot, farmers, ricotta)
   c. Nothing else may be eaten: no bread, pastry, alcohol, whole milk, cream, or drinks with sugar.
   d. Prepare foods without addition of fat.
   e. Drink at least 8 glasses of water a day (tea, diet soda, black coffee).
   f. Take a daily vitamin supplement.
   g. Sleep not more than 8 hours a day.
   h. Only if fatigued, drink a small amount of orange juice.

These diets share the following characteristics:

1. Monotony
2. Frequent urination
3. Fatigue
4. Cyclic weight gain and loss as people go on and off the diet ("yo-yo" effect)
5. Hypercholesterolemia[8]

HIGH FAT–HIGH PROTEIN–LOW CARBOHYDRATE DIETS

1. Calories Don't Count (Herman Taller, M.D., 1971)

2. Dr. Atkins Diet Revolution (Robert C. Atkins, 1972). The general plan of the Atkins diet will be given to aid recognition of diets of this type.
   a. For the first 7 days, a zero carbohydrate intake. No fruits, vegetables, bread, sweets, ice cream, catsup, etc.
   b. After the first week, add 5 g of carbohydrate each day until urinary ketones are no longer present (Keto-Diastix, Ames; Chemstrip, Bio-dynamics) then drop back 5 g. The presence of urinary ketones shows that fat is being incompletely metabolized.
   c. Add low calorie foods gradually: grapefruit, cantaloupe, tomatoes, peapods; then wine, cottage cheese, alcohol, etc., check for presence of ketones.

These diets have the following characteristics:

a. The maintenance of ketosis saves about 100 kcal per day.
b. The high fat may produce elevation of serum lipids.
c. The diet may cause diarrhea with loss of water and electrolytes.
d. Serum nitrogen (BUN) is increased.
e. The accompanying low blood glucose may produce brain damage in the fetus if the mother is on this diet.
f. Fatigue, as is common in low carbohydrate intake.

ZEN MACROBIOTIC DIET

This diet is a graded reduction in food variety until the "perfect" diet of brown rice and tea is reached. The directions for each diet require that food be chewed slowly, 50 to 150 times, until it is completely liquified before it is swallowed. The first three stages of the diet (-3, -2, -1) appear nutritionally adequate for adults, and the first two stages are suitable for growing children. The "more advanced" stages are nutritionally inadequate.

BALANCED LOW CALORIE FOOD SUBSTITUTES

(Dietene, Doyle; Metrical, Drackett; Slender, Carnation)

These provide 900 kcal per day and a low sodium diet. They are effective in producing initial weight loss, but do not provide for maintenance on normal foods.

USE OF DRUGS

Human Chorionic Gonadotropin (HCG)—Simeons Diet.[9] The claim was made that chorionic gonadotropin makes "abnormal" fat deposits readily available so that obese people can live comfortably on 500 kcal per day for several days. No claim was made that HCG in itself reduces weight. After much controversy about the role of HCG (there never was any doubt about the weight loss produced by the 500 kcal per day diet), two well-controlled studies showed:[10]

1. HCG was no more effective than a placebo in preventing feelings of hunger on a 500 kcal per day diet.
2. HCG does not cause preferential mobilization of any "abnormal" fat.

Thyroid.[11] Drugs with thyroid activity must be labeled with the following warning:

"Drugs with thyroid hormone activity, alone or together with other therapeutic agents, have been used for the treatment of obesity. In euthyroid patients, doses within the range of daily hormonal requirements are ineffective for weight reduction. Larger doses may produce serious or even life-threatening manifestations of toxicity, particularly when given in association with sympathomimetic amines such as those used for their anorectic effects."

Digitalis.[11] Digitalis and related drugs must be labeled with the following warning:

"Digitalis alone or with other drugs has been used in the treatment of obesity. The use of digoxin or other digitalis glycosides is unwarranted. Moreover, since they may cause potentially fatal arrhythmias or other adverse effects, the use of these drugs in the treatment of obesity is dangerous."

Sympathomimetic Amines Used as Anorectants. These are thought to suppress hunger (but not appetite) by action on the hypothalamus. They may have some short-term use as an adjunct to a calorically restricted diet, but tolerance to the anorexic effect develops in not more than 6 weeks. Since overeating is a learned response rather than a response to hunger, the use of these drugs delays the establishment of the desired behavior. Side effects include the following:

1. Central nervous system excitation
   a. nervousness
   b. restlessness
   c. insomnia
   d. headache
   e. nausea
2. Cardiovascular stimulation: elevation of blood pressure. Phenylpropanolamine hydrochloride in doses of 25 mg every 4 hours (not more than 150 mg per day) is considered safe for use up to 12 weeks. Although the FDA Advisory Panel considers it an effective anorectant in that dosage, many previous evaluations do not agree.

Bulk Producers. The hypothesis is that filling the stomach reduces the desire to eat. The effectiveness of these substances (methylcellulose, carboxymethylcellulose, psyllium hydrophilic mucilloid, agar, karaya gum), however, has not been demonstrated. In general, stomach emptying time is 30 minutes after ingestion, followed by increased intestinal peristalsis.

STAPLE PUNCTURE

Small metal staples are placed in the ears at "acupuncture points." In addition, a diet providing 400 kcal per day is needed. Hunger is eliminated, supposedly, when the patient wiggles the staple.

The diet works because it is calorically inadequate. It is also nutritionally inadequate and makes no provision for weight maintenance.

SURGICAL TREATMENT

1. For those morbidly obese people who do not respond to attempts at dietary control, jejunoileal bypass surgery may be performed. The benefits of such surgery are as follow:[12]
   a. weight loss
   b. improved psychosocial interactions
   c. reduction of serum cholesterol in the hyperlipidemic
   d. decreased blood pressure in the hypertensive
   e. decreased serum glucose

The complications of such surgery are the following:

   a. mortality from the surgery
   b. postoperative complications
      (1) liver failure
      (2) cardiac failure
      (3) pulmonary embolism
      (4) pancreatitis
      (5) suicide
   c. gastrointestinal complications
      (1) "bypass enteritis"
      (2) hemorrhage
      (3) intractable diarrhea
      (4) malabsorption
         (a) severe mineral loss (calcium, potassium)
         (b) hypoproteinemia
         (c) anemia (vitamin B_{12} deficiency)
   d. renal complications
      (1) hyperoxaluria
      (2) nephrolithiasis
   e. loss of lean muscle mass (up to 50% of the total weight loss)

These complications are treated as needed by appropriate medication and dietary supplementation.

2. It has been suggested that a more nearly normal digestion and absorption of food may be obtained with gastric bypass. This also seems to avoid the hepatic and metabolic complications of jejunoileal bypass.
3. In 1981, an experimental surgical procedure of wrapping the stomach in medical grade plastic so as to limit its

TABLE 12-1.

	g Carbohydrate	g Protein	g Fat	Kcal
1. Milk (skim) exchanges	12	8	Trace	80
2. Vegetable exchanges	5	2	Neg	25
3. Fruit exchanges	10	Neg	Neg	40
4. Bread exchanges (bread, cereal, crackers, dried peas, beans and lentils, starchy vegetables)	15	2	Neg	20
5. Meat exchanges	Neg	7	3	55
6. Fat exchanges	Neg	Neg	5	45

The values for nutrients are approximate.

ability to expand, and hence its capacity, was reported informally. This procedure was thought to eliminate the metabolic complications of the other surgical techniques. Not enough patients nor sufficient follow-up yet exist to evaluate this procedure.

FOOD EXCHANGES

Weight reduction and maintenance can be achieved through the use of a six-group (actually seven, with the extra group consisting of foods and portions with negligible dietary effects) list of interchangeable foods[13] (Table 12-1). These lists may be extended to include commercially processed foods[14] (Table 12-3).

The diet plan allows the choice of a calorie-deficient diet initially, followed by a calorie increase for weight maintenance. If weight is gained on the increased diet, a lower calorie diet is tested. Weight maintenance is ultimately achieved. The daily food plans are shown in Table 12-2.

The 1100 and 1300 kcal diets may not provide the RDA for each nutrient. Weight reduction is started by using one of the lower calorie diets to produce weight loss. When the desired weight is attained, caloric intake is increased. If weight gain begins, the next lower caloric intake diet is used. Because there are no dramatic changes in diet, it is possible to finally determine the caloric intake that produces weight maintenance.

SUGGESTIONS FOR APPROACH TO WEIGHT CONTROL

In planning for weight reduction and lifelong weight maintenance the following hints may be helpful.

1. You must have a commitment to weight control. Without the commitment, the attempt is futile.
2. Start with a medical check-up.
3. Obtain information about nutrition from a qualified dietician or nutritionist.

TABLE 12-2. Number of Exchanges Per Day

	kcal								
Food Exchange	1100	1300	1400	1600	2000	2200	2500	2700	3000
1. Milk	2	2	2	3	3	3	3	3	3
2. Vegetable	2	3	3	3	4	4	4	5	5
3. Bread	6	7	7	8	11	12	15	16	18
4. Meat	2	2	3	3	3	4	5	6	7
5. Fruit	1	1	2	3	3	3	3	3	3
6. Fat	7	9	9	10	14	15	19	17	19

TABLE 12-3. Food Exchange Lists[15]

The following lists have been adapted from Exchange Lists for Meal Planning.[13]

List 1—Milk Exchanges

Carbohydrate, 12 g	Protein, 8 g	Calories, 80

Nonfat fortified milk (Fat, trace)	
Skimmed milk	1 cup
Powdered milk, dry powder	⅓ cup
Canned evaporated skim milk, undiluted	½ cup
Buttermilk, made from skimmed milk	1 cup
Yogurt, plain, unflavored, made from skimmed milk	1 cup
1% fat fortified milk (Fat, 2.5 g, omit ½ fat exchange)	1 cup
2% fat fortified milk (Fat, 5 g, omit 1 fat exchange)	1 cup
Whole milk (Fat, 10 g, omit 2 fat exchanges)	
Whole milk	1 cup
Canned evaporated whole milk	½ cup
Yogurt, plain, unflavored, made from whole milk	1 cup

List 2—Nonstarchy Vegetable Exchanges

Carbohydrate, 5 g	Protein, 2 g	Calories, 25

The following *raw* vegetables may be used as desired:

Chicory	Escarole	Radishes
Chinese cabbage	Lettuce	Watercress
Endive	Parsley	

For the following, one exchange is ½ cup cooked:

Asparagus	Greens	Rhubarb
Bean sprouts	beet	Rutabaga
Beets	chard	Sauerkraut
Broccoli	collard	String beans
Brussel sprouts	dandelion	Summer squash
Cabbage	kale	Tomatoes
Carrots	mustard	Tomato juice
Cauliflower	spinach	Turnip
Celery	turnip	Vegetable juice cocktail
Cucumber	Mushrooms	Wax beans
Green pepper	Onion	Zucchini

List 3—Bread, Cereals and Starchy Vegetables

Carbohydrate, 15 g	Protein, 2 g	Calories, 70

The following have little or no fat:

Bread

White	1 slice	Bagel, 2 oz	½
French	1 slice	English muffin, 2 oz	½
Italian	1 slice	Plain roll, 1 oz	1
Pumpernickel	1 slice	Kaiser roll, 2 oz	½
Raisin	1 slice	Frankfurter roll	½
Rye	1 slice	Hamburger bun	½
Whole wheat	1 slice	Dried bread crumbs	3 tbs
Brown, canned	¼ slice	Tortilla, 6 in	1

Crackers

Animal (Nabisco)	5	Ry Krisp	3
Arrowroot	3	Soup and Oyster (Nabisco)	20
Goldfish (Pepperidge Farm)	24	Toasted Thins (Nabisco)	5
Graham 2½ in sq	2	Matzo 4 × 6 in	½

TABLE 12-3. (continued)

Cooked Dried Legumes

Beans		Lentils	½ cup
baked	½ cup	Peas	½ cup
canned, no pork	¼ cup		

Starchy Vegetables

Corn	⅓ cup	Pumpkin	¾ cup
on cob	1 small	Squash	
Lima beans	½ cup	winter or acorn	½ cup
Parsnip	⅔ cup	Yam or sweet potato	
Green peas	½ cup	mashed	¼ cup
Potato			
white	1 small		
mashed	½ cup		

Commercial Products

About 1 g Fat		About 2.5 g Fat (omit ½ fat exchange)	
Biscuits	1	Cookies	
Ballard		Arrowroot	3
Buttermilk		Mallomars	1
Oven Ready		Nilla Wafers	4
Pillsbury		Nutter Butter	1
Buttermilk		Oatmeal Raisin	1
Country Style		Muffins	
Extra Light		Blueberry (Morton)	1
Fig Newtons	1	Corn, small	1
Gingersnaps (Nabisco)	2	Potatoes	
Graham Crackers	2	frozen fried	10
Scones (Wonder)	½		
Zwieback	2		

List 4—Meat and Meat Substitute Exchanges

Protein, 7 g	Calories, 55
Fat, 3 g	
Beef	
Baby beef (very lean), chipped beef, chuck, flank steak, tenderloin, plate ribs, skirt steak, bottom round, top round, rump, spare ribs, tripe	1 oz
Lamb	
Leg, rib, sirloin, loin chops, loin roast, shank, shoulder	1 oz
Pork	
Leg, rump, center shank; ham (center slice)	1 oz
Veal	
Leg, loin, rib, shank, shoulder, cutlets	1 oz
Fish	
Any fresh or frozen	1 oz
Canned salmon, tuna, mackerel, crab, lobster	¼ cup
Clams, oysters, scallops, shrimp	1 oz
Sardines, drained	3
Poultry	
Chicken, turkey, cornish hen, guinea fowl, pheasant—meat without skin	1 oz
Cottage cheese	
2% fat, dry	¼ cup
Dried beans	
Lentils, peas—cooked (omit 1 bread exchange)	½ cup

TABLE 12-3. (continued)

Fat, 6 g (omit ½ fat exchange)	
Beef	
Ground, ground round, canned corn beef, rib eye	1 oz
Pork	
Loin, shoulder arm (picnic), shoulder blade, Boston butt, Canadian bacon, boiled ham	1 oz
Liver, heart, kidney, sweetbreads (high in cholesterol)	1 oz
Cottage cheese	
Creamed	¼ cup
Cheese	
Mozzarella, ricotta, farmer, Neufchatel	1 oz
Parmesan, grated	3 tbs
Egg	1
Fat, 8 g (omit 1 fat exchange)	
Beef	
Brisket, corned beef brisket, hamburger, ground chuck, rib roast, club steak, rib steak, frankfurter	1 oz
Lamb	
Breast	1 oz
Pork	
Spare ribs, back ribs, ground pork, deviled ham	1 oz
Veal	
Breast	1 oz
Poultry	
Capon, duck, goose	1 oz
Cheese	
Cheddar and other full-fat hard cheeses	1 oz

Note: Sometimes 2 tbs of peanut butter is suggested as a meat substitute exchange. This amount contains about 16 g of fat and 190 calories. If used, omit 2½ fat exchanges.

List 5—Fruit Exchanges

Carbohydrate, 10 g — Calories, 40

Apple	1 small
juice	¼ cup
Applesauce	
no sugar	½ cup
Apricot	
fresh	2 medium
dried	2 halves
Banana	½ small
Berries	
blackberries	½ cup
blueberries	½ cup
raspberries	½ cup
strawberries	¾ cup
Cherries	10 large
Cider	⅓ cup
Figs	1
Grapefruit	½
juice	½ cup
Grapes	½ cup
juice	¼ cup
Mango	½ small
Melon	
cantaloupe	¼ small
honeydew	¼ medium
watermelon	1 cup
Nectarine	1 small
Orange	1 small
juice	½ cup
Papaya	¾ cup
Peach	1 medium
Pear	1 small
Persimmon	1 medium
Pineapple	½ cup
juice	⅓ cup
Plum	2 medium
Prune	2 medium
juice	¼ cup
Raisins	2 tbs
Tangerine	1 medium

TABLE 12-3. (continued)

List 6—Fat Exchanges

Fat, 5 g | Calories, 45

Primarily polyunsaturated fat		*Primarily monounsaturated fat*	
Avocado		Oil	
4 inch	1/8	olive	1 tsp
Margarine		Olives	5 small
from unhydrogenated listed oils	1 tsp	*Primarily saturated fat*	
Nuts		Margarine	
almond	10	hydrogenated	1 tsp
pecan	2 large	Butter	1 tsp
peanuts		Bacon	
Spanish	20	fat	1 tsp
Virginia	10	crisp	1 strip
walnuts	6 small	Cream	
Oils	1 tsp	light	2 tbs
corn		heavy	1 tbs
cottonseed		Sour cream	2 tbs
safflower		Cream cheese	1 tbs
soy		Salad dressing	
sunflower		liquid	1 tbs
Salad dressings		mayonnaise-type	2 tsp
liquid from listed oils only	1 tbs	mayonnaise	1 tsp
mayonnaise-type	2 tsp	Salt pork	
		3/4 in cube	1
		Lard	1 tsp

4. Eat three meals a day, starting with a good breakfast. If you like an evening snack, plan it as part of the daily diet.
5. Follow the "Basic Four" food group eating pattern (Chapter 1), if you cannot stay with the more elaborate six-group plan.
6. Avoid purchasing high calorie foods. If you do not have them, you cannot eat them.
7. Be sure to have a varied diet that includes foods you like and avoids foods you dislike. Occasional use of small amounts of high calorie foods may help you stay on the diet. No foods are forbidden, but note the following:
   A baked potato has about 100 kcal. In the form of potato chips it has about 550 kcal.
8. Use veal, fish, and poultry which have less fat and therefore fewer calories than equal weights of beef and pork.
9. Cook without added fat.
10. Season with vinegar, lemon, pepper, paprika, herbs and spices.
11. Substitute lower calorie foods such as fresh or unsweetened canned fruits for desserts to replace pies, pastry, or cake.
12. Substitute tomato juice (with lemon or Worcestershire sauce) or other vegetable juices for alcoholic drinks whenever possible. Make an effort to decrease alcohol consumption if you do not want to eliminate it.
13. Gradually decrease the use of sugar until you use no sugar in foods (coffee, tea, cereal). Drink unsweetened fruit juices. Do not rely on saccharin-sweetened foods to replace sugar, but try to modify your food habits. Recognize sugars in all of their forms: corn syrup, invert sugar, dextrose, maltose, honey, fructose, sorbitol, molasses, whey solids.
14. Keep a supply of low calorie "munchies" on hand. Crisp vegetables and pickles may provide the

TABLE 12-4. Approximate Calories Used in Activity

Activity	kcal/min	kcal/hour
Sitting	0.77	46
Standing	0.78	47
Bathing and dressing	1.30	78
Bowling	2.20	132 (only when you are bowling, not when you are sitting)
Walking (3.5 mph)	2.50	150
Bicycling	3.50	210
Running	5.42	325
Swimming	5.75	345

"crackle" satisfaction of higher calorie snacks. Their water content contains no calories.

15. Look at the calorie content of your most frequently eaten foods. You may be surprised by the actual calorie content as opposed to popular opinion. Know those with very high and very low calories per serving; then forget about calories.
16. Weigh yourself not more than once a week, without clothes, on the same scale and preferably at the same time of day.
17. Exercise moderately. Exercise burns some calories, makes you feel better, and perhaps, reduces hunger. Tables 12-4 and 12-5 may be encouraging.
18. Plan your diet daily. You will find you can eat in restaurants and attend parties.
19. Chew a lot. It not only utilizes calories but reduces swallowing, which increases caloric intake. Foods high in fiber help.

TABLE 12-5. Sex and Calories

Kissing—0.6 to 1.2 kcal each

Sexual Activity	kcal/HOUR Weight (lbs) 110	150	200
Foreplay	80	100	115
Intercourse			
Active	235	300	350
Passive	105	135	155

20. Watch for added fats, such as butter or margarine on bread, salad dressing and mayonnaise. They contain about 100 calories per tablespoon. Substitute apple butter on bread, lemon juice on vegetables, low fat yogurt for salads.
21. Don't eat if you're not hungry.
22. Try not to eat by yourself. Table conversation seems to slow down eating and reduce food intake.
23. Think before you eat, "Do I really want this?"

REFERENCES

1. Jordan, H.A., and Levitz, L.S.: A Behavioral Approach to the Problem of Obesity, *In* Obesity: Its Pathogenesis and Management. T. Silverstone, ed. Acton, MA, Publishing Sciences Group, 1975.
2. Stunkard, A.J., and Rush, J.: Ann. Intern. Med., *81:*526, 1974.
3. Vertes, V., Genuth, S.M., and Hazelton, I.M.: JAMA, *238:*2151, 1977.
4. Johnson, D., and Drenick, E.J.: Arch. Intern. Med., *137:*1381, 1977.
5. Roberts, J.J.: N. Engl. J. Med., *298:*165, 1978.
6. Federal Register, *45:*22904-14, April 4, 1980.
7. White, P.L.: Today's Health, *49:*59, 1971.
8. Rickman, F., et al.: JAMA, *228:*54, 1974.
9. Simeons, A.T.W.: Lancet, *2:*946, 1954.
10. Federal Register, *39:*42397, December 5, 1974.
11. Federal Register, *43:*22007-10, May 23, 1978.
12. Bray, G.A., et al.: Am. Fam. Physician, *15:*111, 1977.
13. American Dietetic Association: Exchange Lists for Meal Planning. New York, Chicago and American Diabetes Association, 1976.
14. Carper, J.: The Brand Name Nutrition Counter. New York, Bantam Books, 1975.
15. O'Brien, D., and Chase, H.P.: Diabetes, *In* Pediatric Nutrition Handbook. P.O. Box 1034, Evanston, IL, 60204, American Academy of Pediatrics, 1979.

Chapter 13

Drug–Food Interactions

Much has been written in the past decade about interactions between drugs. Of more recent interest, however, has been the elucidation and evaluation of interactions between drugs and food. The drug–food interactions may be grouped into two broad categories:

1. The effects of dietary intake on drug therapy.
2. The effects of drugs on nutritional status.

The clinical significance of drug–food interactions as they relate to patient therapy and nutritional status are reviewed in this chapter.

EFFECT OF FOOD ON THE BIOAVAILABILITY OF DRUGS

The magnitude of pharmacologic response to an orally administered drug is directly related to the extent and rate of gastrointestinal absorption of that drug. The drug must be sufficiently water soluble to enable dissolution in the gastrointestinal (GI) tract and must possess sufficient lipoid properties to allow passage across the lipoidal epithelial lining of the GI tract.

While drug product formulations must adhere to stringent criteria of dissolution, stability, and bioavailability, it must be remembered that food may influence the absorption of drugs from the GI tract, irrespective of dosage formulation. Physical or chemical interactions may occur between the food and the drug molecules. Some drug–food interactions may reduce or delay drug absorption, others may actually increase drug absorption.

Most GI absorption occurs directly from the lumen of the GI tract, across the epithelial cell lining into the adjacent capillary network of the circulation. The rate of blood flow through the splanchnic capillary bed, therefore, will have a marked effect on the absorption of drugs. It has been demonstrated that high-protein liquid meals increase the rate of splanchnic blood flow, whereas high-glucose liquid meals produce small, transient decreases in splanchnic blood flow.[1]

Gastric emptying time may also affect the absorption of drugs. The optimal site of absorption for many drugs is the small intestine. Delaying gastric emptying time, therefore, is likely to delay drug absorption. In addition, delaying emptying time could produce deleterious effects on drugs that are acid labile or unstable to gastric enzymes.

It has been demonstrated that gastric emptying time is delayed by hot meals,[2] high fat content,[3] and by high viscosity solutions.[4] Both protein and carbohydrate meals delay gastric emptying time to a lesser extent than fat.[3] In addition to affecting splanchnic blood flow and gastric emptying time, food may also combine with drug molecules as well as form a physical barrier against passage of the drug across the mucosal surface of the GI tract. All these factors affect the absorption of orally administered drugs.

Drugs Whose Absorption May Be Reduced by Food

Penicillin G
Penicillin V
Phenethicillin
Nafcillin
Ampicillin
Amoxicillin
Tetracyclines
  (except Doxycycline)
Erythromycin stearate
  (but not the base
  if enteric coated)
Lincomycin
Levodopa
Aspirin
Theophylline

Most penicillins produce both delayed and somewhat lowered peak serum levels following postprandial administration.[5–9] In 16 subjects given a single dose of penicillin G, penicillin V, phenethicillin, or phenylmercaptomethylpenicillin 15 minutes after breakfast, somewhat delayed and lower peak serum levels were obtained than when the subjects were given the dose while in the fasting state.[5]

Absorption of phenethicillin and penicillin V is retarded in the presence of foods.[6,7] Lower peak levels, but somewhat prolonged activity, were produced when these penicillins were administered with food. Reduced absorption of penicillin V and penicillin G from tablets has been reported.[9]

Studies of the absorption of oral suspensions of penicillin G, penicillin V, and cephalexin, administered to children who were fasted or given to them with milk or formula, showed about a 40% decrease in the 6-hour "area under the curve" blood levels for each of the three antibiotics.[8] Erratic absorption of oral doses of nafcillin has been demonstrated. Serum levels were higher, were achieved more quickly, and were more predictable in the fasted subjects.[10]

Ampicillin or amoxicillin was given to various groups of patients: fasting, fasting except for small volume (25 ml) of water, fasting except for large volume (250 ml) of water, various test meals, test meals plus small volume of water, test meals plus large volume of water. Serum levels of the drugs were reduced in all groups receiving food, as compared with the fasting, or fasting plus water, groups. The reductions were independent of the components of the meal. In the fasted subjects, serum levels of ampicillin were only slightly affected by fluid volume. Amoxicillin levels, however, were significantly reduced when the dose was taken with a small volume of water as compared with a large volume of water.[11]

Decreased absorption of tetracyclines due to chelation with heavy metal ions or binding to macromolecules has been well documented.[12–15] The absorption of tetracyclines is reduced by the presence of milk, dairy products, eggs, cereals, and divalent and trivalent ions such as Mg^{+2}, Ca^{+2}, Al^{+3} or Fe^{+2}, due to the formation of insoluble combinations in the GI tract. Iron has been shown to decrease the serum levels of tetracyclines by 40 to 60% after a single dose and by 80% after 4 days of concomitant therapy.[16] Ingestion of 8 oz or more of milk with tetracycline has been shown to reduce serum concentration of the antibiotic by 50% or more.[17] Doxycycline absorption is less affected by the presence of food, milk, or dairy products, but serum levels are reduced by iron salts.[18]

An overall postprandial reduction in the absorption of erythromycin stearate from orally administered film-coated tablets has been shown.[19] In fasted subjects, drug absorption was reduced 47 to 60% by food and 43% by small volumes of water. The absorption of erythromycin base from enteric coated tablets, however, was not inhibited by the presence of food.[20] The reduced bioavailability of erythromycin stearate and erythromycin estolate when the drugs were administered in the presence of food has been confirmed by one study[21] but refuted for the estolate salt in a more recent study.[22]

The absorption of lincomycin after ingestion of food has been shown to be erratic, delayed, and decreased.[23] It has been recommended that nothing be given orally except water for 1 to 2 hours before and after oral administration of lincomycin.[24] The absorption of clindamycin is only slightly delayed by ingestion of food.[25]

The clinical response of eight patients with parkinsonism who received levodopa while on controlled diets providing 0.5 g, 1 g, or 2 g of protein per kg of body weight, or a total of 10 g per day, showed that high-protein diets inhibit the therapeutic effect of levodopa.[26] The effects of food and fluid volumes on the absorption of aspirin (ASA) has been studied in healthy volunteers.[27] Peak ASA levels were reduced by 40 to 50% by food, and the rate of absorption was also significantly reduced. Serum ASA levels were somewhat reduced by limiting fluid volume to 25 ml.

A 30% increase in clearance of theophylline in subjects who ate charcoal-broiled meat as compared with subjects not given this food has been reported.[28] The effect was attributed to stimulation of hepatic microsomal enzymes by the polycyclic hydrocarbons produced by charcoal broiling.

Drugs Whose Absorption May Be Delayed by Food

Cephalosporins Digoxin Sulfonamides

The absorption of most cephalosporins and sulfonamides is delayed in the presence of food. A comparison of the absorption of cephradine and cephalexin after oral doses administered to fasted subjects and to the same subjects 30 minutes after breakfast showed that the serum-drug profile was delayed in the nonfasted state.[29] These findings were confirmed in a study of the absorption characteristics of cephalexin, in both suspension and capsule dosage forms, in children in the fasting state and after a standard meal.[30] The rate of absorption was faster from suspension than from capsules. The presence of food delayed the absorption of the drug from both dosage forms. A generally delayed absorption of sulfonamide when the drug was taken after a meal has been reported.[31] Somewhat more prolonged serum levels, however, suggest a clinical advantage to the administration of sulfonamides with meals.

It has been reported that the rate of absorption of digoxin from tablets was depressed in nonfasted subjects during the first 2 to 3 hours after dosing but not at later times. No difference in serum levels of fasted and nonfasted subjects was observed for digoxin elixir.[32] Since there is no simple relationship between the peak pharmacologic activity of digoxin and its peak plasma level, it may be advisable to administer digoxin tablets with food in order to decrease the side effects without compromising the therapeutic efficacy of the drug.

Drugs Whose Absorption is Increased by Food

Griseofulvin Propranolol
Erythromycin Estolate Metoprolol
Nitrofurantoin Phenytoin
Methoxsalen

Griseofulvin is lipophilic. Its dissolution in and absorption from the GI tract is expected to be accelerated by the presence of fat. Serum levels of griseofulvin have been shown to be about double when the drug is taken with fatty meals as compared with ingestion in the fasting state.[33]

The increased absorption of nitrofurantoin in the presence of food has been attributed to delayed stomach emptying time, permitting greater dissolution of the drug.[34] The presence of food may also decrease the local GI side effect produced by nitrofurantoin.

The absorption of methoxsalen (8-methoxypsoralen) used in the treatment of psoriasis was increased over the value obtained in the fasting state when it was taken after breakfast.[35] The absorption of both propranolol and metoprolol was increased in subjects who received the drugs following a standard breakfast.[36] Concurrent intake of food enhances the absorption of phenytoin.[37,38] The presence of food may increase the dissolution and dispersion of this poorly water-soluble compound.

The clinical significance of altered drug bioavailability is necessarily a function of the specific drug. Drugs with narrow therapeutic indices, with steep dose-response relationships, with serious dose-related side effects, with short biologic half-lives or with well-defined blood or tissue levels required for therapeutic activity are most likely to be affected by delayed or reduced absorption. This may produce significant clinical consequences.

FOODS THAT MAY ALTER URINARY EXCRETION RATES OF DRUGS

Excretion of drugs can be significantly affected by changes in urinary pH. Drug moieties in the ionized form are more readily excreted in the urine, whereas the nonionized forms are more readily reabsorbed into the circulation. Although normal dietary intake alone does not produce the urinary pH changes necessary to effect changes in drug excretion, concomitant consumption of excessive amounts of acid or alkaline ash diets with drugs that acidify or alkalinize the urine may produce unexpected and untoward results in drug therapy. Examples of acid ash and alkaline ash foods follow. An extensive list is given by Krause and Mahan.[39]

Foods producing acid residue include:

Bacon	Macaroni
Bread (all types)	Meats
Cheeses	Nuts (except almonds)
Corn	Oatmeal
Eggs	Puffed wheat
Lentils	Shredded wheat

Foods producing alkaline residue include:

Almonds, Chestnuts
Dairy products (milk, cream, ice cream)
Fruit (except cranberries, plums, prunes)
Vegetables (except corn, lentils)

DRUGS THAT MAY AFFECT NUTRITION

A number of drugs have been implicated in the production of nutritional deficits through malabsorption of vitamins, increased excretion of vitamins or minerals, and altered nutrient metabolism. The following are the most commonly encountered deficits.

1. Alcohol. Chronic abuse of alcohol produces deficiencies of thiamin, vitamin B_{12} and folate.[40]

2. Antibiotics. Chronic use of antibiotics can decrease absorption of vitamin B_{12} and intestinal synthesis of vitamin K.[40,41]

3. Cholestyramine. Causes malabsorption of vitamin B_{12}.[40]

4. Clofibrate. Causes malabsorption of vitamin B_{12}.[40]

5. Corticosteroids. Lower serum calcium levels, impair calcium transport, and have caused osteoporosis, particularly in postmenopausal women.[41] They also decrease uptake of amino acids and promote excretion of amino acids, thus producing a negative nitrogen balance and muscle wasting.[42]

6. Cytotoxic Agents. Methotrexate causes folate deficiency and may interfere with vitamin B_{12} absorption.[43]

7. Griseofulvin. May produce altered or unpleasant taste sensation which decreases appetite, thus decreasing food intake and producing weight loss.[44]

8. Isoniazid. Causes pyridoxine deficiency, resulting in peripheral neuropathies. It has been successfully treated with a daily supplement of 50 mg of pyridoxine.[41]

9. Mineral Oil. Traditionally has been thought to decrease the absorption of the fat-soluble vitamins A, D, E, and K, even though it is commonly taken at bedtime. A review of the literature failed to yield any report of clinically significant deficiency[45] associated with its use.

10. Neomycin. Decreased absorption of fat, cholesterol, vitamin B_{12}, and iron. Has caused steatorrhea.[46]

11. Oral Contraceptives. Implicated in riboflavin, vitamin B_6, vitamin B_{12}, and folate deficiencies[47] and in the acceleration of ascorbic acid breakdown.[48]

12. Phenytoin. Has been shown to cause folate deficiency in at least 40% of the patients taking the drug.[49]

PHARMACOLOGICALLY ACTIVE FOOD CONSTITUENTS

A number of foods have been shown to evoke unexpected and untoward effects in patients who ingested these foods while medicated with monoamine oxidase inhibitors (MAOI).

Monoamine Oxidase Inhibitor Antidepressants

Isocarboxazid
Nialamide
Pargyline hydrochloride
Phenelzine sulfate
Tranylcypromine sulfate

Acute hypertensive reactions were reported in patients taking MAOI who ate aged cheeses.[50] Monoamine oxidase (MAO) is the enzyme responsible for intracellular degradation of catecholamines. Tyramine, found in many foods, can produce an increase in blood pressure by causing release of norepinephrine at the presynaptic neuron. Tyramine in food is usually metabolized by intestinal and hepatic MAO. When a patient is taking MAOI or has a genetic deficiency of MAO, however, the tyramine escapes degradation and is able to provoke an acute rise in blood pressure. As little as 6 mg of tyramine is deleterious[51] and 25 mg may be dangerous.[52] Severe pounding occipital headache within one-half to 2 hours after ingestion of tyramine-containing food heralds a hypertensive crisis. It is often accompanied by arrhythmia, tachycardia, anxiety, tremors, chest pain, flushing, hyperpyrexia, and vertigo.[53] The prolonged duration of action of MAOI requires a period of about 14 days between the last dose of the drug and the ingestion of a tyramine-containing food.

Foods with Significant Tyramine Content[51,54–58]

Beer
Broad bean pods
Cheese, cheddar
Herring, pickled
Meat extracts
Sausage, dried
Wine, chianti
Yeast extracts
Liver, chicken

It should be noted that hypertensive crisis occurring in patients taking MAOI who ate broad beans (Vicia faba) involved eating the whole sliced bean.[58,59]. The active agent, dihydroxyphenylalanine (dopa) is found in higher concentration in the pods than in the commonly eaten bean portion.

Bananas are often included in the list of foods that should not be eaten by patients taking MAOI. Although they do contain 5-hydroxytryptamine (5 HT), dopa and norepinephrine, these substances are mainly in the peel and only small amounts are in the pulp.[60,61] The tyramine content of raspberries is highly variable, but significant concentrations are found in some samples.[62] Oranges, avocados, and plums have appeared in lists of foods with significant amounts of tyramine. Since oranges contain about 10 mg/kg,[63] plums about 6 mg/kg, and avocados about 23 mg/kg,[64] a patient would have to consume unusually large amounts of these to elicit an adverse reaction.

Two cases of hypertensive episodes after consumption of large quantities of cream in patients taking MAOI have been reported.[65] A liter of milk, however, contains about 23 mg of tyramine.[66] It is evident that unusually large amounts of dairy products must be consumed to produce adverse effects.

Chocolate also has been listed as a food to be avoided by patients taking MAOI. A severe hypertensive episode after ingestion of 60 g of milk chocolate occurred in a patient taking pargyline hydrochloride.[67] Although chocolate does not contain tyramine, it does contain about 1.5 mg/oz of phenylethylamine.[68] Phenylethylamine is an effective releaser of vasoactive substances in isolated lung preparations.[69] Since degradation of phenylethylamine includes deamination by MAO, it is plausible that it may precipitate adverse reactions in patients taking MAOI.

Tyramine is found in significant concentrations in products of bacterial fermentation. The major source is produced by the action of bacterial decarboxylases on tyrosine.[51] Ingestion of chicken liver by patients taking MAOI has been reported to precipitate hypertensive episodes.[57] Since liver does not ordinarily contain appreciable amounts of tyramine, it was postulated that the aging of chicken liver to enhance flavor promotes the decarboxylation of tyrosine to tyramine.

The tyramine content of 24 different varieties of dry, fermented sausage varied from 10 to 150 mg/g.[55] The variability was attributed to different ripening conditions, including the specific bacteria in the sausage. Hard salami was reported to contain an average of 210 μg/g, pepperoni from 0 to 195 μg/g, genoa salami from 0 to 1237 μg/g, summer sausage 184 μg/g, farmer salami 314 μg/g, and lebanon bologna from 0 to 333 μg/g. The variability was attributed to differences in ripening time and moisture content.[70] Assuming that ingestion of 25 mg of tyramine produces dangerous pressor response in patients taking MAOI, it is obvious that relatively small servings of these products could produce adverse reactions in these patients.

Some cheeses contain concentrations of tyramine that can be dangerous to patients taking MAOI. Cheddar cheese can contain up to 1.5 mg/g, Camembert up to 2 mg/g, blue cheese 2 mg/g, Gouda 0.6 mg/g, mozzarella 0.4 mg/g and Swiss cheese from 0 to 1.8 mg/g.[71]

A hypertensive episode after eating pickled herring was reported for a patient taking tranylcypromine sulfate.[56] Pickled herring contains about 3 mg of tyramine per g of fish.[71]

Yeast extracts are ingredients of some sauces, canned soups, relishes, and meat spreads; some are sold in Britain as sandwich spreads, and some are used in beverages. The process used for producing Marmite, Bovril, gives a product containing 0.1 to 1.6 mg of tyramine per g, enough to produce reaction in some patients taking MAOI.[54]

Treatment of hypertensive crisis caused by ingestion of pressor amines by patients taking MAOI consists of administering 5 mg intravenously of the adrenergic blocking agent phentolamine, repeated if necessary.

Members of the Brassica genus (cabbage, brussel sprouts, mustard greens, turnip, kale, rutabaga) contain thioglycosides. On hydrolysis these yield thiocyanates which have goitrogenic activity.[72] Excessive ingestion, particularly of the raw leaves, could produce goiter.

Ingestion of raw or cooked broad beans (fava bean, Vicia faba) by persons suffering from glucose-6-phosphate dehydrogenase (G6PD) deficiency will produce favic crisis. Hemolysis of the red blood cells may be rapid and abrupt, but more usually occurs 5 to 24 hours after ingestion of the bean. The condition is usually self-limiting in adults, with the acute phase lasting 24 to 48 hours. The mortality rate in untreated children under 6 years of age is about 7%. Use of transfusion has greatly reduced the mortality rate. The causative agent is the nucleoside vicine, which yields divicine on hydrolysis.[73] The highest incidence is found in the Mediterranean area in which the beans are a staple in the diet (Sardinia, Sicily, southern Italy, Greece, Turkey, Israel, Spain).[74]

Ingestion of natural licorice or swallowing saliva from chewing tobacco which contains natural licorice produces classic symptoms of mineralocorticosteroid excess. The glycyrrhizic acid in licorice has mineralocorticoid activity. Daily ingestion of 100 to 200 g of licorice (0.7 to 1.4 g of glycyrrhizic acid) can produce sodium and water retention, hypertension, hypokalemia, and depressed renin level.[75,76]

Ingestion of monosodium glutamate (MSG) by susceptible people produces the characteristic symptoms of burning sensations of the face, neck, shoulder, forearms, back, or abdomen; facial pressure; and chest pain. Headache occurs in a small percentage of people. Experimentally, oral ingestion of 1.5 to 12 g was required to produce symptoms. They occurred 15 to 25 minutes after ingestion and lasted approximately for 1 hour.[77] There was no apparent relationship between threshold dose and body weight, sex, or age.[62]

Inhibition of the hypothrombinemic effect of coumarin-type anticoagulants (but not of heparin) may occur with excessive intake of food high in vitamin K.[78] High vitamin K content is found most often in the Brassica genus (brussels sprouts, broccoli, cabbage, cauliflower) and in spinach and other dark green leafy vegetables. The content of individual samples is highly variable.

Hypertension is a predisposing factor in coronary heart disease, congestive heart failure, cerebrovascular accident, and renal impairment. Fundamental to the treatment of hypertension is weight reduction of the obese patient, restriction of sodium intake, and diuretics. Patients on restricted sodium diets must be aware of the sodium content of the foods eaten. A comprehensive listing is given in P.L. White and S.C. Crocco: Sodium and Potassium in Foods and Drugs, 2nd Ed. Monroe, WI, American Medical Association, 1981.

Patients on chronic diuretic therapy are often told to increase their dietary intake of potassium in order to prevent hypokalemia. Patient instructions for this purpose can be found under the section on potassium.

DRUG EXCRETION IN HUMAN MILK

Problems that may occur in a nursing infant because of drugs ingested by the nursing mother have been extensively reviewed.[79] Virtually any substance in the maternal bloodstream can appear in milk. One must evaluate the clinical significance of drug levels in human milk and the potential for production of adverse effects in the nursing infant. Among the considerations are the variable fat content of milk and the lag time between peak serum levels and peak milk levels. Drug levels peak earlier in serum than in milk, but milk levels may not decline as fast as serum levels. If an attempt is made to correlate plasma levels with milk levels, spuriously high or low predictions may be made. Fat content of milk varies throughout the day, with the highest fat concentration occurring about midmorning. Depending on the time of dosing, a spurious relationship may be found for lipid-soluble drugs if a midmorning milk sample is used. Data obtained by sampling without consideration of maternal dosing and peak level times or using single doses without consideration of the cumulative effects of the drug are difficult, if not impossible, to interpret. The following have been reported.

1. Alcohol milk levels reach 90 to 95% of maternal blood levels. Although moderate consumption of alcohol appears to produce no effects in infants, chronic intake of large amounts may be detrimental.

2. Oral anticoagulants have produced bleeding episodes in nursing infants after trauma or surgery. These drugs should be used cautiously. Heparin does not pass into milk.

3. Nursing is generally contraindicated for women receiving antineoplastic agents.

4. Barbiturates may stimulate metabolism in the infant. High doses appear to have the potential for causing infant drowsiness.

5. Chloral hydrate has produced drowsiness and sedation in nursing infants.

6. Chloramphenicol at levels found in milk may cause bone marrow suppression in the infant. Nursing is probably contraindicated during the course of therapy.

7. Most sources advise against nursing by women taking corticosteroids.

8. High doses of diazepam have caused lethargy and jaundice in nursing infants.

9. Diuretics can cause a decrease in milk production.

10. Many ergot derivatives can suppress lactation. Of infants who nursed from women who were taking ergot preparations, 90% showed signs of ergotism.

11. Gold therapy has the potential for causing rashes and idiosyncratic reactions in nursing infants.

12. Many consider iodides to be contraindicated because of the possibility of thyroid suppression in the nursing infant.

13. Laxatives of the anthraquinone group (aloe, cascara, danthron, phenolphthalein, senna) may cause problems in high doses.

14. Nursing is contraindicated for patients taking lithium.

15. Metronidazole is contraindicated for nursing women because of the possible carcinogenicity of the drug.

16. Narcotic and non-narcotic analgesics

administered in therapeutic doses to nursing women usually do not attain milk levels high enough to cause problems. Excessive use of narcotics in nursing women, however, is contraindicated.

17. Nalidixic acid has produced hemolytic anemia in the nursing infant. Use this drug cautiously and with close observation of the infant.

18. Nitrofurantoin should be used with caution in nursing women when the nursing infant is G6PD-deficient.

19. Two cases of breast enlargement in male infants whose nursing mothers were taking oral contraceptive agents have been reported.

20. Penicillins appear in human milk in trace quantities which could lead to allergic sensitization. Nursing is not absolutely contraindicated, but temporary discontinuation might be considered.

21. Phenytoin has been implicated in one case of methemoglobinemia in a 4-day old nursing infant.

22. Nursing should be done cautiously by women receiving therapy with radiopharmaceuticals.

23. Sulfonamides attain sufficient levels in milk to cause hemolytic anemia and neonatal jaundice in infants with G6PD deficiency. Caution should be used in the administration of the drug. Careful observation of the infant is mandatory, especially in the first few weeks of life.

24. Tetracyclines can cause mottling of teeth and retardation of skeletal growth in children. Although the calcium in the milk probably chelates with the tetracycline, thereby significantly decreasing absorption, it seems advisable not to administer tetracyclines to nursing women.

25. Many consider thiouracils contraindicated in nursing women because of the possibility of thyroid suppression in the nursing infant.

Rashes and allergic manifestations in the nursing infant caused by the diet of the nursing mother seem plausible because of the small amount of allergen required to provoke a reaction. Eggs, chocolate, beans, celery, cotton seed, and wheat have been implicated.

It seems obvious that caution and prudent judgment is needed when deciding on administration of drugs to nursing women. When necessary, nursing should be discontinued.

REFERENCES—Drug–Food Interactions

1. Brandt, J.L., et al.: J. Clin. Invest., *34:*1017, 1955.
2. Davenport, H.W.: Physiology of the Digestive Tract, 4th Ed. Chicago, Year Book Medical Publishers, 1977, p. 194.
3. Bachrach, W.H.: Ciba Clin. Symp., *11:*3, 1959.
4. Levy, G., and Jusko, W.: J. Pharm. Sci, *54:*219, 1965.
5. McCarthy, C.G., and Finland, M.: N. Engl. J. Med., *263:*315, 1960.
6. Cronk, G.A., et al.: Am. J. Med. Sci., *240:*219, 1960.
7. Cronk, G.A., et al.: Antibiotics Annual 1959-1960. NY, Antibiotica, Inc., 1960, p. 133.
8. McCraken, G.H., Jr., et al.: Pediatrics, *62:*738, 1978.
9. Welling, P.G.: J. Pharmacokinet. Biopharm., *5:*291, 1977.
10. Watanakunakorn, C.: Antimicrob. Agents Chemother., *11:*1007, 1977.
11. Welling, P.G., et al.: J. Pharm. Sci., *66:*549, 1977.
12. Neuvonen, P.J., et al.: Br. Med. J., *4:*532, 1970.
13. Chin, T.-F., and Lach, J.L.: Am. J. Hosp. Pharm., *32:*625, 1975.
14. Price, K.W., et al.: Antibiot. Chemother., *7:*689, 1957.
15. Braybrooks, M.P., Barry, B.W., and Abbs, E.T.: J. Pharm. Pharmacol., *27:*508, 1975.
16. Neuvonen, P.J.: Drugs, *11:*45, 1976.
17. Rosenblatt, J.E., et al.: Antimicrob. Agents Chemother., *1966:*134, 1966.
18. Welling, P.G., et al.: Antimicrob. Agents Chemother., *11:*462, 1977.
19. Welling, P.G., et al.: J. Pharm. Sci., *67:*764, 1978.
20. Rutland, J., Berand, N., and Marlin, G.E.: Br. J. Clin. Pharmacol., *8:*343, 1979.
21. Hirsch, H.A., and Finland, M.: Am. J. Med. Sci., *237:*693, 1959.
22. Welling, P.G., et al.: J. Pharm. Sci., *68:*150, 1979.
23. McCall, C.E., Steigbigel, N.H., and Finland, M.: Am. J. Med. Sci., *254:*144, 1967.
24. Lincocin, Upjohn: Product Information. Physicians Desk Reference, 35th Ed. Oradell, NJ, Medical Economics, 1981.
25. De Haan, R.M., Vanden Bosch, W.D., and Metzler, C.M.: J. Clin. Pharmacol., *12:*205, 1972.
26. Gillespie, N.G., et al.: J. Am. Diet. Assoc., *62:*525, 1973.
27. Koch, P. A., et al.: J. Pharm. Sci., *67:*1533, 1978.
28. Kappas, A., et al.: Clin. Pharmacol. Ther., *23:*445, 1978.
29. Harvengt, C., et al.: J. Clin. Pharmacol., *13:*36, 1973.

30. Tetzlaff, T.R., McCracken, G.H., Jr., and Thomas, M.L.: J. Pediatr., *92:*292, 1978.
31. MacDonald, H., et al.: Chemotherapy, *12:*282, 1967.
32. Greenblatt, D.J., et al.: Clin. Pharmacol. Ther., *16:*444, 1974.
33. Crounse, R.G.: J. Invest. Dermatol., *37:*529, 1961.
34. Bates, T.R., Sequeria, J.A., and Tembo, A.V.: Clin. Pharmacol. Ther., *16:*63, 1974.
35. Ehrsson, H., et al.: Clin. Pharmacol. Ther., *25:*167, 1979.
36. Melander, A., et al.: Clin. Pharmacol. Ther., *22:*108, 1977.
37. Melander, A., et al.: Eur. J. Clin. Pharmacol., *15:*269, 1979.
38. Sekikawa, H., et al.: Pharm. Bull., *28:*2443, 1980.
39. Krause, M.V., and Mehan, L.K.: Food, Nutrition and Diet Therapy. Philadelphia, W.B. Saunders, 1979, p. 901.
40. Faloon, W.W.: NY State J. Med., *70:*2189, 1970.
41. Roe, D.A.: Life Sci., *15:*1219, 1974.
42. Hethcoe, J.M., and Stanaszek, W.F.: Hosp. Pharm., *9:*373, 1974.
43. Reynolds, E.H., et al.: J. Clin. Pathol., *18:*593, 1965.
44. Pierpaoli, P.G.: Drug Intell. Clin. Pharm., *6:*89, 1972.
45. Cohen, H.: J. Med. Soc. NJ, *67:*111, 1970.
46. Faloon, W.W., et al.: Ann. NY Acad. Sci., *132:*879, 1966.
47. Adams, P.W., et al.: Lancet, *1:*759, 1976.
48. Rivers, J.M.: Am. J. Clin. Nutr., *28:*550, 1975.
49. Labadarios, et al.: Br. J. Clin. Pharmacol., *5:*167, 1978.
50. Asatoor, A.M., Levi, A.J., and Milne, M.D.: Lancet, *2:*733, 1963.
51. Horwitz, D., et al.: JAMA, *188:*1108, 1964.
52. Blackwell, B., and Mabbitt, L.A.: Lancet, *1:*938, 1965.
53. Goldberg, L.I.: JAMA, *190:*456, 1964.
54. Blackwell, B., Mabbitt, L.A., and Marley, E.: J. Food Sci., *34:*47, 1969.
55. Vandekerckhove, P.: J. Food Sci., *42:*283, 1977.
56. Nuessle, W.F., Norman, F.C., and Miller, H.E.: JAMA, 192:726, 1965.
57. Hedberg, D.L., Gordon, M.W., and Glueck, B.C., Jr.: Am. J. Psychiatry, *122:*933, 1966.
58. Hodge, J.V., Nye, E.R., and Emerson, G.W.: Lancet, *1:*1108, 1964.
59. Blomley, D.J.: Lancet, *2:*1181, 1964.
60. Waalkes, T.P., et al.: Science, *127:*648, 1958.
61. West, G.B.: J. Pharm. Pharmacol., *10:*589, 1958.
62. Coffin, D.E.: J. Assoc. Offic. Anal. Chem., *53:*1071, 1970.
63. Wheaton, T.A., and Steward, I.: Phytochem., *8:*85, 1969.
64. Udenfriend, S., Lovenberg, W., and Sjoerdsma, A.: Arch. Biochem. Biophys., *85:*487, 1959.
65. Bethune, H.C., et al.: Am. J. Psychiatry, *121:*245, 1964.
66. Ough, C.S.: U.S. Pharmacist, *5:*52, 1980.
67. Krikler, D.M., and Lewis, B.: Lancet, *1:*1166, 1965.
68. Sandler, M., Youdim, M.B.H., and Hanington, E.: Nature, *250:*335, 1974.
69. Bakhle, Y.S., and Smith, T.W.: Br. J. Pharmacol., *46:*543P, 1972.
70. Rice, S., Eitenmiller, R.R., and Koehler, P.E.: J. Milk Food Technol., *38:*256, 1975.
71. Rice, S.L., Eitenmiller, R.R., and Koehler, P.E.: J. Milk Food Technol., *39:*353, 1976.
72. Michajlovski, N., and Langer, P.: Z. Physiol. Chem., *312:*26, 1958.
73. Lin, J.Y., and Ling, K.H.: Toxicants Occurring Naturally in Foods. Washington, DC, National Academy of Sciences, 1967, p. 48.
74. Mager, J., Razin, A., and Hershko, A.: Favism, *In* Toxic Constituents of Plant Foodstuffs. I.E. Liener, ed. NY, Academic Press, 1969.
75. Epstein, M.T., et al.: Br. Med. J., *1:*488, 1977.
76. Blachley, J.D., and Knochel, J.P.: N. Engl. J. Med., *302:*784, 1980.
77. Schaumburg, H.H., and Byck, R.: N. Engl. J. Med., *279:*105, 1968.
78. Fletcher, D.C.: JAMA, *237:*1871, 1977.
79. Anderson, P.O.: Drug Intell. Clin. Pharm., *11:*208, 1977.

Part II

Parenteral and Enteral Nutrition

In April 1979, The American Journal of Intravenous Therapy & Clinical Nutrition prepared and published a series of articles concerning parenteral and enteral nutrition. Permission has been given by the publisher and authors of this material for publication in this text. It is with extreme pleasure, satisfaction, and gratitude that we present this material.

SALVATORE J. TURCO

MURRAY M. TUCKERMAN

Chapter 14

Nutritional Assessment—Diagnosis of Malnutrition and Selection of Therapy

Mitchell V. Kaminski, Jr., M.D.
Clinical Professor of Surgery
University of Health Sciences/Chicago Medical School
Director, Midwest Nutrition Education and Research Foundation
Chicago, Illinois

Khursheed N. Jeejeebhoy, M.D.
Professor of Medicine
University of Toronto
Ontario, Canada

Nutritional support has become a vital component of the medical treatment of millions of Americans. It is considered by some to be one of the greatest medical advances in recent decades.[1]

Because protein synthesis, resistance to infection, and wound healing depend on the maintenance of adequate levels of protein and other nutrients, no other form of medical or surgical therapy can ultimately be effective if the patient suffers from severe nutritional deficits. Treating the nutritionally debilitated patient without treating the nutritional impairment will predictably result in less than optimal recovery. Patients may be dying not primarily as a result of their disease states, but rather, as a result of the malnutrition brought about by those disease states. Thus, a total program of therapy sufficient for patient recovery must include nutritional support to repair nutritional deficits as well as medical or surgical treatment of the disease state.

Despite recent advances in nutritional support therapy, up to 50% of all hospitalized patients can be shown to be suffering some degree of malnutrition, and 5 to 10% are literally dying of starvation.[2] These patients develop malnutrition as a result of the body's response to trauma or disease. Nutritional support can prevent the development of severe malnutrition or can reverse severe and life-threatening deficits.

Severe deficits are referred to as protein-calorie malnutrition, a deficiency involving protein in addition to a general inadequacy of energy sources (i.e., calories). Protein-calorie malnutrition, a disease in itself, complicates the recovery of many hospitalized patients.

Nutritional support should be routinely employed whenever a patient has a high probability of developing a severe nutritional deficit or is already suffering from malnutrition. Certain categories of patients are considered to be "high risks" for the development of malnutrition. They include the following:

1. Postsurgical patients not expected to receive oral intake for 7 days.
2. Emaciated or obviously debilitated patients prior to undergoing nonemergency surgery.
3. Patients with disorders of the gastrointestinal tract.
4. Patients with massive burns or severe trauma.
5. Cancer patients receiving chemotherapy or radiation therapy.
6. Infants suffering from idiopathic diar-

rhea, malabsorption, respiratory difficulties during feeding, and long-standing failure to thrive.

NUTRITIONAL SUPPORT (Figure 14-1)

A growing recognition of nutritional requirements in disease and trauma has led to many clinical studies of the benefits of available nutritional regimens. The oral route is preferred when intake is adequate, but patients who cannot maintain positive nitrogen balance and nutritional and physiologic homeostasis by voluntary oral intake require nutritional support by other methods of administration or by peripheral or central vein. Anorexia is part of the normal stress response, but anorexia ends at the oral cavity. In general, if the gastrointestinal tract is functioning, it should be used; if normal oral intake is inadequate, enteral feeding should be employed. Intravenous routes should be used only when enteral feeding is impossible, inadequate, or unsafe.

Several types of intravenous nutritional support may be employed, including protein-sparing nutrition by peripheral vein, total parenteral nutrition (TPN) by either peripheral or central vein, and intravenous hyperalimentation (IVH) by central vein. In much of the professional research and literature, the terminologies IVH and TPN are used interchangeably; however, definitions of each form of nutritional therapy are provided here.

Protein-Sparing Nutrition

Protein-sparing nutrition is the peripheral administration of essentially isotonic amino acids as a 3 to 5% solution mixed with other carbohydrate-free fluids and vitamins, minerals, and electrolyte additives. This hypocaloric solution provides approximately 400 to 600 kcal per day.

Blackburn and his colleagues[3] demonstrated that the infusion of near-isotonic crystalline amino acids with appropriate cofactors and micronutrients can contribute to the preservation of lean body mass. Protein-sparing nutrition provides few calories, decreases insulin levels, and mobilizes the body's own fat as an energy source. Normal

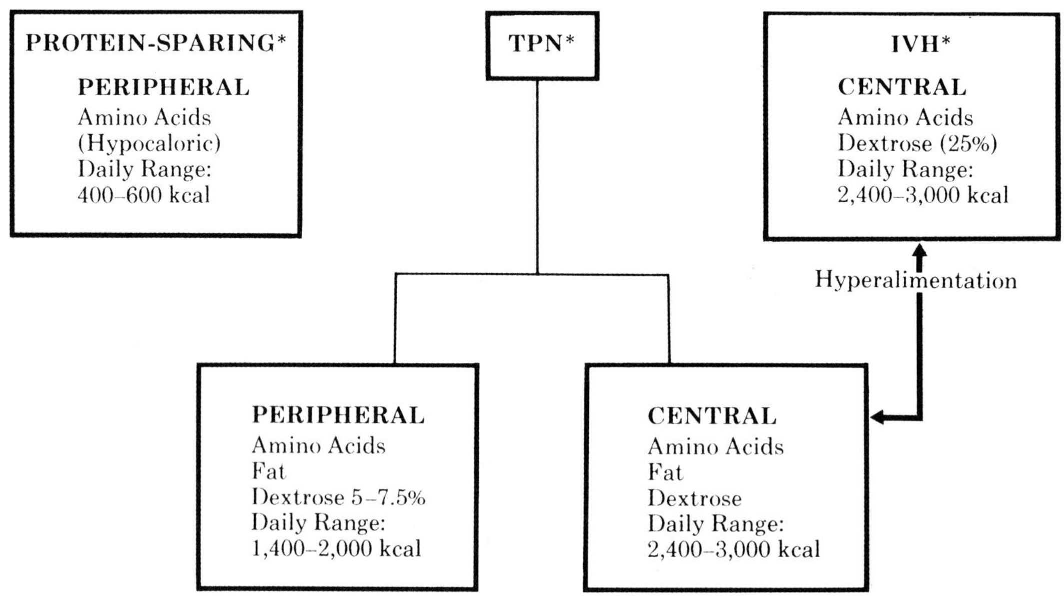

* All solutions contain appropriate vitamins, minerals, and electrolyte additives.
The caloric contribution of amino acids is traditionally excluded from the total calories provided.

Figure 14-1. Description of various forms of parenteral nutrition.

response to inadequate intake of nutrients to meet the body's energy requirements is a utilization of stored energy reserves—mainly fat. The body adapts to the use of nonprotein calories, free fatty acids, and ketone bodies as fuel substrates. Hypocaloric feeding as 5% dextrose does not provide essential amino acids required for preservation of protein synthesis and, at the same time, does not meet the energy requirements of the patient. Hence, long-term hypocaloric feeding with only dextrose will result in significant loss of muscle mass and reduction in visceral protein synthesis.[3]

In selected patients who have minimal protein deficits and adequate adipose tissue stores, and especially in markedly obese patients, it is desirable to maintain body protein stores without increasing obesity. The use of peripheral amino acids alone may provide a way of reducing the loss of body protein stores and enhancing visceral protein synthesis without contributing to obesity, provided the patient is free of renal and/or hepatic disease.

Protein-sparing nutrition can be of significant value in the treatment of the patient in whom significant protein deficits have not developed.[4] By maintaining protein synthesis, protein-sparing nutrition can contribute to the prevention of deficits in most surgical patients who have no complications.

Total Parenteral Nutrition

Total parenteral nutrition is the administration of amino acids, glucose, and fat through the peripheral or central vein. Peripheral TPN solutions which contain amino acids and fat combined with 5 to 7.5% dextrose provide approximately 1400 to 2000 kcal per day. Peripheral TPN is appropriate for the patient who has only minor nutritional deficits and who requires more calories than can be provided by protein-sparing nutrition. However, the ability to utilize this system depends on the availability of peripheral veins and the patient's ability to handle the added volume (500 ml) of fluid to be infused.

Fat emulsions, now available in the United States, have been shown to promote nitrogen retention in cases of malnutrition[5,6] and to compare favorably with glucose, even in the presence of sepsis.[7] It is now possible to supplement amino acids peripherally with nonprotein calories as a fat and carbohydrate mixture to meet the energy requirements of patients. Hence, in selected patients with good peripheral veins, it is possible to provide a spectrum of protein-calorie support from protein-sparing nutrition to TPN. Furthermore, evidence from experimentally infected animals suggests that an amino acid-fat mixture is likely to maintain albumin synthesis more effectively than glucose alone.[7]

Central TPN is the intravenous administration, through a central vein, of hypertonic dextrose, amino acids, and fat. In central TPN, fat emulsions mixed with glucose to provide 30 to 50% of calories are given by Y-connector into a central venous line. This system reduces the total carbohydrate concentration delivered to the patient, as finally mixed in the Y-connector, to a 12.5% dextrose solution. The central TPN system has several metabolic advantages.[8,9] It is lower in osmolality, does not cause rebound hypoglycemia, and greatly reduces the need for any exogenous insulin during administration. It maintains a normal substrate hormone profile, and provides enough essential fatty acids to maintain normal membrane composition. Since recent evidence suggests that fat oxidation may contribute a significant amount of energy, even if nonprotein calories are provided as glucose,[10] it appears that fat is an obligatory metabolite.

Fat emulsions can be used, therefore, both as a means of enhancing protein-sparing nutrition—peripheral TPN—or as one source of nonprotein calories in therapy designed to repair severe nutritional deficits—central TPN.

Intravenous Hyperalimentation

Intravenous hyperalimentation is the intravenous administration of nutrients in concentrated form sufficient not only to maintain metabolic homeostasis and an uncompromised response to stress, but also to promote and repair tissue synthesis when enteral feeding is either impossible or inadequate. In professional research and related literature, IVH has been referred to as TPN; however, we have differentiated between IVH (in which amino acids and hypertonic glucose are administered through a central vein) and TPN (in which amino acids, glucose, and *fat* are administered either peripheraly or centrally).

Dudrick originally described "hyperalimentation" as the delivery of high concentrations of dextrose and amino acids mixed as a hypertonic solution into the superior vena cava through a central catheter placed via the subclavian vein. The substrate calorigenic bases of IVH solutions are amino acids and glucose in water to which vitamins and electrolytes are added. This solution is prepared to meet the specific needs of the individual patient, with the purpose of repairing deficits in the somatic and visceral protein compartments. Central venous cannulation is performed by a surgeon using strict aseptic technique. In most patients, an infraclavicular approach to the left subclavian vein is initially employed.

INDICATIONS FOR PARENTERAL NUTRITION

Certain specific disease states or conditions frequently require hyperalimentation to achieve positive nitrogen balance, along with the restoration of the somatic and visceral protein compartments. These are indicated by the achievement of normal weight, creatinine height index, work tolerance and serum albumin transferrin levels, normal unimpaired cell-mediated immunity, and wound healing.

Preoperative Patients

Nutritionally debilitated or emaciated patients frequently require hyperalimentation prior to undergoing surgical procedures in order to increase their chances of recovery and survival. If possible, elective surgery should be delayed in those patients suffering from severe nutritional deficits. Generally, these patients are in a poor-risk category, and their risk factors can usually be improved by parenteral support. If the results of the patient's nutritional assessment profile are less than 85% of standard or the patient is anergic, nonemergency surgery should be withheld until the nutritional deficits can be repaired. Nutritional deficits reflect the patient's inability to withstand additional stress, resist infection, repair tissue, and generally, to recover. If adequate nutritional levels are not achieved and deficits are not repaired, patient recovery and survival will be significantly reduced.

There is a significant increase in mortality in patients found to be anergic.[11–14] One cause of anergy is malnutrition, and use of central TPN or IVH to provide sufficient calories and protein preoperatively is a desirable goal to correct this aspect of anergy. However, in the very sick and septic patient, other factors may prevent infused nutrients from improving the nutritional status of the patient, because of poor utilization of nutrients in the face of severe continuing sepsis. In such patients, necessary surgical treatment should not be withheld pending nutritional improvement by central TPN or IVH alone.

Postoperative Patients

Any postsurgical patient from whom oral intake has been withheld for seven days should be evaluated and considered for hyperalimentation. In addition, certain patients with postoperative surgical complications may require IVH or central TPN. Oral intake may be unduly delayed by complications such as prolonged ileus, peritonitis, anastomotic leak, and biliary and pancreatic fistulas. If nutritional support is not provided, these complications may lead to protein-calorie malnutrition. Any patient suffering from a chronically debilitating illness in which surgical intervention is mandatory is a candidate for parenteral nutrition.[1] A nutritional assessment, as will be described, should be performed on any patient suffering from a surgical complication that places him at risk for developing significant nutritional deficits.

Disorders of the Gastrointestinal Tract (Table 14-1)

Hyperalimentation has proven valuable in treating patients with disorders of the gastrointestinal tract that make ingestion of food impossible or impair digestion and absorption. Patients suffering from such disease processes as gastrointestinal obstruction, painful deglutition, esophageal cancer, obstructive peptic ulcer disease, and superior mesenteric artery syndrome may be unable to obtain adequate calories and protein orally. Other patients may not be allowed to ingest nutrients. Bowel rest is particularly important in the treatment of inflammatory bowel disease and gastrointestinal fistulas.[15,16]

Patients with bowel fistula appear to improve significantly when the flow of gastrointestinal contents is reduced by giving nothing by mouth. This reduces drainage through the fistula and allows it to close spontaneously. Central TPN or IVH maintains nutrition while the patient is given nothing by mouth. Prior to the regular use of central TPN or IVH for patients with GI fistulas, 40 to 60% of these patients died from fluid and electrolyte imbalance and malnutrition. Central TPN or IVH provides adequate nutrition to restore fluid and elec-

TABLE 14-1. Gastrointestinal Disease

Clinicians	Indications	Results	No. of Patients
Dudrick, et al.[a]	Bowel disease	In 55% of severe cases, disease became quiescent; surgery not required; patients tolerated relatively normal diet.	52
MacFadyen	Gastrointestinal fistulas	Nonsurgical closure rate, 71%; overall closure rate, 94%; mortality, 6%.	62
Aguirre, et al.[b]	Enterocutaneous fistulas	Operative success rate of 70%.	38
Dudrick[b]	Inflammatory bowel disease	85% of 70 patients with Crohn's colitis or enteritis and 50% of 30 patients with ulcerative colitis had temporary remissions.	100
Dudrick[a,b]	Fistulas	71% of fistulas closed during an average of 35 days of bowel rest and IVH; 23% successfully closed by surgery.	100 (126 fistulas)
Reilly[c]	Regional enteritis	75% of patients experienced weight gain. If surgery was not required, sense of well-being and relief from abdominal pain and diarrhea achieved. Low incidence of surgery required.	15
	Granulomatous colitis	7 ultimately required surgery, 7 did not; 65% of patients experienced weight gain.	14
	Ulcerative colitis	Low incidence of postoperative complications and morbidity; no wound infections or ileostomy problems.	12
Zohrab, et al.[d]	Inflammatory gastrointestinal diseases	TPN with 40-50% of calories supplied by lipid was associated with closure of fistulas, subsidence of symptoms, and apparent avoidance of complications associated with all-glucose TPN infusions.	48

[a] Dudrick, S.J., Copeland, E.M., III, and MacFadyen, B.V., Jr: Long-term parenteral nutrition: Its current status. Hosp. Pract., *10*:47, 1975.
[b] According to Fleming, C.R., et al: Subject review: Total parenteral nutrition. Mayo Clin. Proc., *51*:187, 1976.
[c] Reilly, J: Inflammatory Bowel Disease, *In* Total Parenteral Nutrition. J.E. Fischer, Ed. Boston, Little, Brown and Co, 1976.
[d] Zohrab, W.J., McHattie, J.D., and Jeejeebhoy, K.N.: Total parenteral alimentation, with lipid. Gastroenterology, *64*:583, 1973.

trolyte balance as well as to reverse malnutrition. Fleming and his colleagues[17] conclude that IVH appears to decrease the volume and modify the content of upper gastrointestinal secretions, thereby contributing to the spontaneous closure of enterocutaneous fistulas. Also, IVH may facilitate closure by correcting protein depletion, thus facilitating healing. Dudrick and his colleagues[18] achieved a spontaneous closure rate of better than 70%; among those who eventually underwent surgery, the great majority achieved successful closure. The overall success rate was nearly 95%.

Burns/Trauma

"Thermal injury results in the most accelerated rates of tissue breakdown, loss of protoplasmic mass, and erosion of available metabolic reserves associated with any disease process. Because of the relentless nature of the catabolic reaction following major injury, the lethal limit of protein and caloric loss may be approached in the hypermetabolic, starved burn patient in only 3 or 4 weeks."[21]

Hyperalimentation can provide the greatly increased levels of protein and nonprotein calories needed in the hypermetabolic state accompanying severe burn injury or severe trauma to prevent the development of severe nutritional deficits and frank catabolism, and to contribute to uncompromised wound healing.

Dudrick and his colleagues[18] conclude that burn patients receiving IVH are stronger, develop less respiratory disease (a common complication in the burn patient), show less infection and sepsis, and demonstrate accelerated healing. Also, IVH contributes to earlier granulation, which in turn, allows earlier skin-grafting. In addition, graft survival rates approach 100% in patients receiving IVH. Graft survival rates of only 50% would be expected in similar patient groups not receiving IVH. Table 14-2 summarizes recent clinical experiences.

Cancer

Hyperalimentation is used in the treatment of cancer patients as an adjunct to chemotherapy and radiation therapy, and serves two purposes: (1) to treat the malnutrition which often affects the cancer patient (and thus to improve the patient's quality of life); (2) to increase tolerance for higher levels of chemotherapy and radiation therapy, and thus, perhaps, enhance response to therapy.[17]

The cancer patient provides one of the most dramatic examples of successful nutri-

TABLE 14-2. Burns

Clinicians	Indications	Results	No. of Patients
Dudrick, et al.[a]	Burns over 50% of total body surface	Of 8 patients receiving IVH, 5 survived; of 8 not receiving IVH, all died. Patients given IVH stronger, less respiratory disease, less infection and sepsis, accelerated healing, and grafts of 100%.	16
Wilmore, et al.[b]	Extensive burns	Maintenance of pre-burn weights.	26
Liljedahl and Birke[c]	Burns over 75% of total body surface	Losses of only 5-7% of initial body weight.	—
Wilmore, et al.[c]	Average of 56% body surface burns	Maintenance of body weight.	14
	Critically ill burn patients	Nitrogen sparing.	10

[a] Dudrick, S.L., Copeland, E.M., III, and MacFadyen, B.V., Jr: Long-term parenteral nutrition: Its current status. Hosp. Pract., *10:*47, 1975.
[b] According to Fleming, C.R., et al.: Subject review: Total parenteral nutrition. Mayo Clin. Proc., *51:*187, 1976.
[c] According to Wilmore, D.W., and Pruitt, B.A.: Parenteral Nutrition in Burn Patients, *In* Total Parenteral Nutrition. J.E. Fischer, ed. Boston, Little, Brown and Co., 1976.

tional therapy. It is generally recognized that many cancer patients become anorectic and, therefore, lose weight rapidly. From the nutritional standpoint, hyperalimentation has been successful in helping patients to achieve or maintain normal weight levels. Chemotherapy and radiation therapy compound anorexia and affect the patient's immune competence, which, in turn, affects the patient's ability to withstand both the disease and the treatment. Cell-mediated immunity is an important defense mechanism, and its depression weakens and eventually eliminates the body's ability to distinguish self from non-self proteins and to withstand either therapy or disease. Hyperalimentation frequently reverses this trend by providing the protein necessary for the body to rebuild cell-mediated immunity.

Researchers[22] at the University of Texas Medical School studied 406 patients suffering from various malignant diseases; 47 were studied to determine the relationship between malnutrition and cell-mediated immunity in oncologic therapy. It was found that "those patients who are immunocompetent at the beginning of oncologic therapy have better regression of malignant disease and survive longer free of disease than do those patients who are immunologically incompetent."

These researchers reached the conclusion that immunodepression attributed to chemotherapy might be, in part, secondary to malnutrition. They noted that only patients with positive skin tests responded to chemotherapy; that skin test reactivity was depressed during radiation therapy, even though nutritional repletion was considered adequate; and that surgical or supportive-care patients with positive skin tests had an uncomplicated treatment period, whereas 4 of 7 patients with negative tests died.

Of the 406 patients studied, 39 received hyperalimentation during radiation therapy. During the course of radiation treatment without nutritional support, patients often become anorectic and experience pain on deglutition, crampy abdominal pain, nausea, and diarrhea. Radiation may cause bowel wall edema and obstruction of an already partially compromised gastrointestinal lumen. The patient ingests less food, and digestion and absorption are impaired. Malnutrition may be disabling, and therefore, the therapy often must be discontinued before an adequate tumor dose has been administered. Of the 39 patients receiving IVH, 95% were able to complete their planned courses of radiation therapy, and anorexia, nausea, and vomiting disappeared; 54% responded to radiation with a greater than 50% reduction in tumor volume.[22]

Schwartz and his colleagues[23] studied the effects of IVH on 12 patients with symptomatic, advanced malignant disease. All 12 were considered poor-risk candidates for chemotherapy. These workers concluded that, by adding hyperalimentation to chemotherapy, they were able "to convert this small group of 'poor risk' candidates to a better risk with a marked absence of gastrointestinal toxicity and a rapid reversal of marrow depression when it occurred." Intravenous hyperalimentation promoted a sense of patient well-being, increased appetite and oral intake, improved performance status, decreased analgesic requirements, and produced positive weight changes.

Copeland, MacFadyen, and Dudrick[24] point out that no scientific background exists to support the supposition that intravenous nutritional support might possibly stimulate malignant growth. Clinical results of the uses of IVH in conjunction with chemotherapy document patient gains in strength, lean body mass, and in some cases, fat deposition; the cancer did not have grossly altered growth characteristics. They further conclude that "the use of antitumor drugs with marked gastrointestinal and hematopoietic toxicity was made possible by the anabolic effect of intravenous hyperalimentation. Marked reduction in anorexia, nausea, vomiting and diarrhea during chemotherapy was observed." In addition, the tolerance to the drug employed,

5-fluorouracil, was increased, and a 40% objective response rate occurred. Table 14-3 summarizes the results observed in treating cancer patients with hyperalimentation.

Infants

In infants, IVH is an effective therapeutic measure. It can maintain or restore normal weight gain and growth in cases ranging from surgery involving the gastrointestinal tract to idiopathic failure to thrive. A major problem in infant feeding is the patient's proportionately great need. Nutrition must be adequate not merely to maintain homeostasis but also to sustain growth. As Dudrick and his associates[17] point out, this adds up to a requirement two to three times the adult level, "and when to this is superadded the additional caloric requirement posed by disease and surgery, the seriousness of the problem becomes manifest, especially if GI function has been compromised."

Parenteral nutrition can be used in the premature to sustain growth and nutrition during the phase when a complication such as apnea prevents adequate oral nutrition. Even though the average neonate requires 120 kcal/kg per day, the premature in the incubator needs only 60 to 80 kcal/kg per day to grow and thrive. With this lower

TABLE 14-3. Cancer

Clinicians	Indications	Results	No. of Patients
Copeland, et al.[a]	Chemotherapy	Reduction in anorexia, nausea, vomiting, and diarrhea; increased drug tolerance.	175
	General surgery	Weight gain, increased strength, significant rise in serum albumin, return of immunocompetence, fewer surgical complications.	100
	Head and neck surgery	Weight gain; acrominoclavicular flaps healed; skin grafts healed over a radiated base; pharyngocutaneous fistulas did not occur; early ambulation and rehabilitation in elderly.	39
	Radiation therapy	Reduction in anorexia, nausea, vomiting; completed therapeutic program; tumor reduction.	39
	Enteric fistulas	Weight gain, rise in serum albumin, spontaneous closure.	25
	Supportive care		28
Copeland, et al.[b]	Chemotherapy, radiation therapy, surgery	Reduction in anorexia, nausea, vomiting, diarrhea, tumor; increased drug tolerance and strength; completed therapy program; weight gain; significant rise in serum albumin; return of immunocompetence; fewer surgical complications.	120
Schwartz, et al.[c]	Chemotherapy	Weight gain, no anorexia, increased appetite and oral intake, decreased analgesic requirements, improved performance status, absence of gastrointestinal toxicity.	12
Blackburn, et al.[d]	Malnourished cancer patients	Weight gain, improved lymphocyte count, improved albumin and serum transferrin levels.	35

[a] Copeland, E.M., et al.: Intravenous Hyperalimentation and Cancer. University of Texas Medical School at Houston.

[b] Copeland, E.M., MacFadyen, B.V., Jr., and Dudrick, S.J.: Intravenous hyperalimentation in cancer patients. J. Surg. Res., *16:*241, 1974.

[c] Schwartz, G.F., et al.: Combined parenteral hyperalimentation and chemotherapy in the treatment of disseminated solid tumors. Am. J. Surg., *121:*169, 1971.

[d] Blackburn, G.L., et al.: Manual for nutritional metabolic assessment of the hospitalized patient. Presented at the 62nd Annual Clinical Congress of the American College of Surgeons, Chicago, Oct. 11-15, 1976.

calorie input and amino acid infusion of 3 g/kg per day, reasonable growth without complications can be achieved. In this age group, nutrients should be used with extreme care, since hyperglycemia, hyperammonemia, and acid base disturbances are common. Heird and his colleagues[25] have clearly shown a need for intravenous fats in this group of patients in order to ensure that the fatty acid content of the myelin in the central nervous system is normal. Indeed, nerve conduction defects have been found with fat-free TPN.

Intractable diarrhea is a relatively common problem among neonates and is usually unresponsive to standard treatment; it was formerly associated with a 90% mortality rate.[26] It leads to malnutrition through malabsorption of nutrients, coupled with failure to replace such losses through oral intake. This, in turn, adversely affects the gastrointestinal tract, so that the diarrhea is perpetuated.[27,28] In severe diarrhea with malnutrition, a condition ensues similar to celiac disease with a "flat" biopsy. The vicious cycle can be broken by hyperalimentation. Greene and his colleagues[29] have shown that bowel villi will regrow with hyperalimentation and the malabsorption will be corrected.

Hyperalimentation is useful, if not essential, in the following pediatric conditions: congenital atresia of the small bowel, choledochal cyst, tracheoesophageal fistula, malrotation with volvulus, ruptured omphalocele, gastroschisis, and diaphragmatic hernia.

Idiopathic diarrhea, malabsorption, respiratory difficulties during feeding, and longstanding failure to thrive have yielded to IVH. In most cases, results have been described as excellent, with the pediatric patient attaining or maintaining normal growth while the body's natural healing and

TABLE 14-4. Infants

Clinicians	Indications	Results	No. of Patients
Dudrick, et al.[a]	Surgery for ruptured omphalocele or congenital gastroschisis	Zero mortality; without IVH, would expect 60-80% mortality.	18
Lloyd-Still, et al.[b]	Protracted diarrhea	Survival of all 16 infants.	16
Avery, et al.[c]	Intractable infantile diarrhea	55% survival.	20
Winters[d]	Low birthweight	Ideal body weight; regained more rapidly with TPN; positive nitrogen balance.	14
	Surgery due to major anomalies of GI tract	15 had normal GI function; 2 on special diets.	17
Golden, et al.[e]	Disorders of GI tract, enterocutaneous fistulas, prolonged ileus or obstruction, or cachexia from disseminated malignancy	Weight gain; fistula closure; 61% survival rate.	18
Keating[f]	Chronic diarrhea	15 survived (follow-up study one year later); normal GI function.	16

[a] Dudrick, S.J., Copeland, E.M., III, and MacFadyen, B.V., Jr: Long-term parenteral nutrition: Its current status. Hosp. Pract., *10:*47, 1975.
[b] According to Fleming, C.R., et al.: Subject review: Total parenteral nutrition. Mayo Clin. Proc., *51:*187, 1976.
[c] Avery, G.B., et al.: Intractable diarrhea in early infancy. Pediatrics, *41:*712, 1978.
[d] Winters, R.W.: Total parenteral nutrition in pediatrics: The Borden Award address. Pediatrics, *56:*1, 1975.
[e] Golden, G.T., et al.: Parenteral alimentation in infants and children with life-threatening illness. Am. J. Surg., *126:*619, 1973.
[f] According to Heird, W.C., MacMillan, R.W., and Winters, R.W.: Total Parenteral Nutrition in the Pediatric Patient, *In* Total Parenteral Nutrition. J.E. Fischer, Ed. Boston, Little, Brown and Co., 1976.

homeostatic mechanisms correct the underlying problem.[11] Table 14-4 summarizes recent studies in infants.

BODY'S RESPONSE TO STRESS

Patients with disorders of the GI tract, burns/trauma, and cancer, infants with impaired digestion and absorption, and debilitated pre- and post-operative patients require hyperalimentation because their disease states or medical conditions have contributed to a predictable response to stress. Blackburn[30] summarizes the body's response in these disease states and the importance of providing nutritional support: "Dysfunction of the gastrointestinal tract and anorexia are frequent occurrences in many disease states. The ensuing periods of semistarvation will lead to wasting of body cell mass. These important tissues are involved in the function of host survival by sustaining immune function, phagocytosis, acute phase reactant protein synthesis, and tissue repair. Appropriate nutrient intake can substantially improve these processes, whereas inadequate support can result in serious protein depletion states and produce serious malnutrition."

Substrates

Three substrates of the human body—carbohydrates, fat, and protein—are capable of metabolic utilization to produce energy. This energy is stored and transferred in the form of high-energy phosphate bonds. It is expended during the biochemical and mechanical activities of daily living and is, of course, an important factor in the body's response to disease and trauma.

CARBOHYDRATES

The adult patient has approximately 1200 carbohydrate kcal stored as glycogen—25% in the liver and 75% in muscle. During stress, or trauma, glycogen is mobilized from the liver as glucose and from muscles as lactate. But these stores are only enough to meet approximately one short-term period of stress. If disease or trauma is prolonged, or if a second period of stress closely follows the first, the body must convert endogenous protein into glucose via hepatic gluconeogenesis in order to meet obligatory glucose needs.

FAT

Under stress conditions, only an inconsequential portion of the fat molecule (10%) can be converted to carbohydrate. Fat is mobilized as free fatty acids (FFA) which may be utilized by tissues per se. A portion of FFA is oxidized to ketones in the liver. Both FFA and ketones are excellent sources of energy.

PROTEIN

During the stress of trauma, disease, or sepsis, the body's metabolic response involves a mobilization of both visceral and somatic protein to ensure an adequate supply of substrates for energy production and biosynthesis.

All protein is functional. Fat and carbohydrate can be mobilized and used for energy with no adverse effect, but when protein is burned for energy, patients lose the ability to function and respond to challenges.

Antibodies are proteins and are synthesized through a reorganization of the patient's existing protein compartments. When patients suffer a protein deficit they are frequently lymphopenic. Lymphocytes comprise the essence of the patient's immune response system.

The somatic protein compartment—particularly the intercostal muscles, the diaphragm, and the accessory muscles of respiration—facilitates the patient's ability to cough and perform respiratory toilet, thus helping to prevent pneumonia. The list of essential functions dependent on protein is prodigious. As protein is lost, the patient measurably functions at levels farther and farther below optimum.

Nutritional Needs

The substrate calorigenic bases of hyperalimentation solutions are amino acids and glucose in water, to which vitamins and appropriate amounts of intra- and extracellular electrolytes—sodium, chloride, potassium, magnesium, calcium, phosphate, zinc, and copper—are added. Caloric requirements may be met by carbohydrates supplied by glucose or by glucose and fat. Nitrogen requirements are met by synthetic crystalline amino acid solutions.

CALORIC REQUIREMENTS

The caloric requirement of a normal healthy adult approximates 30 to 35 kcal/kg per day, depending on physical activity or the amount of energy expended. This is equivalent to 2100 to 2450 kcal per day. In moderate stress, this increases by 50%, and in burns, by 100%. The metabolic requirements for victims of major burns, severe trauma, and sepsis may approach 10,000 kcal per day. Medical complication or changing clinical conditions may make normal caloric intake either impossible or inadequate. If a caloric deficit develops, it is quickly filled by mobilization and conversion of protein to glucose and urea. When essential body proteins are converted to carbohydrate to be used for energy, a protein (nitrogen) deficit develops.[2]

The average patient receiving nutritional support requires 30 to 35 kcal/kg of body weight per day to maintain his weight and higher caloric levels to achieve a weight gain.

PROTEIN REQUIREMENTS

The recommended dietary allowance of protein for an average 22-year-old adult is approximately 0.9 g/kg of body weight to maintain nitrogen equilibrium. This is equivalent to approximately 10.5 g of nitrogen for a 70-kg man. The majority of patients receiving IVH require a minimum of 12 to 15 g of nitrogen daily to promote positive nitrogen balance.[31] Patients who require intravenous hyperalimentation are obviously atypical in terms of nitrogen requirement, and significantly higher levels may be required.

ELECTROLYTES AND TRACE ELEMENTS

The requirements for electrolytes and trace elements vary widely, depending on the volume and type of fluid loss; preexisting deficits; cardiopulmonary, renal, hepatic, and endocrine status; and the types and amounts of nutrients given.

Potassium, magnesium, and phosphate are absolutely essential for protein synthesis. Rudman, et al.[32] has clearly shown the need for these elements in promoting nitrogen retention.

Zinc is essential for wound healing and for promoting positive nitrogen balance and increasing insulin response. The requirements are enhanced by gastrointestinal fistula losses and diarrhea. Copper is required for hematopoietic integrity and chromium is needed to improve glucose utilization and insulin action.

Sodium and chloride are the chief extracellular electrolytes and are normally included in all hyperalimentation solutions.

Vitamins are necessary for the body to assimilate the amino acids, glucose, and micronutrients it receives into useful metabolic products. Essential fatty acids (EFA) are absolutely necessary for synthesis of normal cell membranes and cannot be provided by glucose. In man, arachidonic, linolenic, and especially linoleic acids are required to maintain the pliability of membranes and normal prostaglandin synthesis. In their absence, hypermetabolism occurs, the incidence of infections is increased, and a fatty liver develops. The characteristic sign of EFA deficiency is a cracked, flaky, "riverbed bottom" rash on the lower extremities.

Stress Response

Starvation or the stress of disease and trauma enhances glycolytic and proteolytic catabolism; in combination with limited nutrient intake, a significant loss of body cell mass results.[33] When caloric and protein requirements are not being met, the body mobilizes its substrate reserves: fat (triglycerides) stored in adipose tissue and a limited amount of carbohydrates (glycogen) stored in liver and muscle. During periods of negative caloric balance, energy reserves are mobilized to provide the body's energy requirements. Adenosine triphosphate (ATP) is the major "energy molecule" of the cell. A normal ratio of adenosine triphosphate to adenosine diphosphate (ADP) must be maintained for the cell to function; otherwise, it will die. This energy requirement is supplied by endogenous or exogenous carbohydrate or fat.

Unfortunately, during starvation, an obligatory conversion of amino acids to glucose occurs to meet the needs of the central nervous system. This may amount to 10 g of nitrogen per day initially, but falls (as the CNS adapts to using ketones) to about 3 to 5 g of nitrogen per day. This loss is the main cause of the undesirable results of starvation: depletion of liver cellular protein, bone marrow protein, and muscle protein, which in turn, cause a fall in albumin synthesis, immune dysfunction, and muscle weakness. The only way to offset this loss appears to be to give protein; hence, this is the central role of amino acid replacement in all situations of starvation. With endogenous mobilization of fat to provide energy, the utilization of exogenous protein does occur; and amino acid infusions are more advantageous than glucose infusions alone, which do not provide nitrogen. However, in the starved patient, amino acids are utilized inefficiently unless nonprotein calories are added; hence, exogenous calories are needed to obtain optimal protein synthesis.

To this background of starvation, the occurrence of injury, sepsis, and fever appears to enhance the mobilization of all energy substrates, both glucose and fat, and to increase mobilization of amino acids for energy.

The body's increased energy requirements in the presence of stress, infection, trauma, and burns are often accompanied by a total or partial inability to ingest nutrients via the gastrointestinal tract. Anorexia in the short run is a normal part of the stress response. By promoting the catabolic state, anorexia facilitates mobilization of endogenous substrates necessary to manufacture acute-phase protein. If an illness or injury is chronic or severe, however, anorexia will be prolonged and essential endogenous protein will be used to fulfill energy requirements. The mobilization of the body's resources to meet this prolonged stress can progress until the measurable deficits produced become as life-threatening as the stress itself. Physiologic deficits are multiplied, resulting in impaired stress response and increased morbidity and mortality.

NUTRITIONAL ASSESSMENT

The basis for the institution of therapy in any disease process is recognition and correct diagnosis. Effectiveness of therapy is ascertained by repetition of this process to demonstrate favorable change.

Prior to implementing hyperalimentation, it is important to evaluate the degree of nutritional impairment; that is, to what extent has the body's response to stress, starvation, injury, trauma, or disease affected the patient's nutritional level? The diagnosis of malnutrition is based on objective measurements of the patient's protein compartments. A screening nutritional assessment or anergic/metabolic profile should be performed to ascertain the need for nutritional support and the form that support should take. Following institution of therapy, dynamic or repeat assessment should be performed weekly to determine the efficacy of therapy.

Initial indications of nutritional deficits, such as:

- a recent loss of 7 to 10% of body weight,
- having recently undergone surgery or chemotherapy,
- recent illness lasting for more than three weeks,
- a serum albumin less than 3.5 g/dl, or
- a lymphocyte count of less than 1500/mm^3

point to the need for a more in-depth nutri-

ANERGIC METABOLIC PROFILE

PATIENT ______ ROOM ______ DATE ______

	PARAMETERS	VALUE	DEFICIT: SEVERE	DEFICIT: MOD	DEFICIT: MILD	DEFICIT: ADEQUATE
	SOMATIC PROTEINS					
MARASMUS	WEIGHT/HEIGHT					
MARASMUS	TRICEP SKINFOLD (mm)					
MARASMUS	ARM MUSCLE CIRCUMFERENCE (cm)					
MARASMUS	CREATININE/ HEIGHT INDEX					
KWASHIORKOR	**VISCERAL PROTEINS**					
KWASHIORKOR	ALBUMIN					
KWASHIORKOR	TRANSFERRIN					
KWASHIORKOR	TOTAL LYMPHOCYTE COUNT					
KWASHIORKOR	**CELL-MEDIATED IMMUNITY**					

NITROGEN IN (g/day) ______

NITROGEN OUT (g/day) − ______

NITROGEN BALANCE (g/day) ______

NUTRITIONAL STATUS	DEGREE
□ ADEQUATE	□ NONE
□ MARASMUS	□ MILD
□ KWASHIORKOR	□ MODERATE
□ MARASMUS-KWASHIORKOR MIX	□ SEVERE

STANDARDS	SEVERE	MODERATE	MILD
SOMATIC PROTEINS—% DEFICIT	>30%	>15–30%	>5–15%
ALBUMIN (g/dl)	<2.5	<3.0–2.5	<3.5–3.0
TRANSFERRIN (mg/dl)	<160	<180–160	<200–180
LYMPHOCYTE COUNT (No./mm^3)	<900	<1500–900	<1800–1500
CELL-MEDIATED IMMUNITY (mm)	<5–0	<10–5	<15–10

Figure 14-2.

tional/metabolic assessment.[3] In addition, any patient included in the disease categories previously discussed—disorders of the GI tract, burn/trauma, cancer/chemotherapy—should be considered "high-risk" and referred for complete nutritional assessment and evaluation for the need for therapy.

A complete anergic/metabolic profile includes a battery of tests and measurements used to evaluate the patient's nutritional condition, including somatic and visceral protein levels and cell-mediated immunity. The patient's condition in terms of protein depletion cannot be determined with only a single test. Each evaluation contributes to the overall assessment of nutritional depletion conducted by the physician.

Figure 14-2 outlines the individual components of the anergic/metabolic profile.

Visceral Proteins

Because every molecule of protein in the body performs a vital function, the depletion of protein levels indicates a nutritional impairment. Visceral or all nonmuscle protein levels are assessed by a series of laboratory tests: the adequacy of two liver secretory proteins (serum albumin, and transferrin or total iron-binding capacity) and total lymphocyte count.

ALBUMIN

The normal blood value of serum albumin, the principal contributor to the intravascular oncotic pressure, is 4.5 g/dl. If cardiac function is normal, the patient is prone to edema when albumin falls below 2.8. A mild impairment is considered to be between 3.5 and 3.0 g/dl; moderate, between 3.0 and 2.5; and severe, less than 2.5.

TRANSFERRIN

Serum transferrin has been estimated from the total iron-binding capacity (TIBC), utilizing this formula:

$$\text{Serum Transferrin} = (\text{TIBC} \times 0.8) - 43$$

A result between 200 and 180 mg/dl is considered a mild impairment; between 180 and 160, moderate; and less than 160, severe.

TOTAL LYMPHOCYTE COUNT

The total lymphocyte count is derived from a differential blood count, using the following formula:

$$\text{Total Lymphocyte Count} = \frac{\%\ \text{lymphocytes} \times \text{WBC}}{100}$$

A lymphocyte count between 1800 and 1500/mm^3 indicates a mild impairment; between 1500 and 900, moderate; and less than 900, severe.

Somatic Proteins

WEIGHT/HEIGHT

These initial measurements are important indicators of the somatic status and the need for more in-depth testing and patient evaluation. Generally, if a patient has lost over 10% of his body weight during the previous 6 months or weighs less than 90% of his ideal weight, he may be a candidate for nutritional support. However, because such conditions as edema and obesity may distort the accuracy of the weight/height measurements, additional measurements of the lean body mass and the fat stores are imperative.

$$\%\ \text{ideal body weight} = \frac{\text{actual weight}}{\text{ideal weight}} \times 100$$

$$\%\ \text{usual weight} = \frac{\text{actual weight}}{\text{usual weight}} \times 100$$

$$\%\ \text{weight change} = \frac{\text{usual weight} - \text{actual weight}}{\text{usual weight}} \times 100$$

Ideal body weights are ascertained from Table 14-5.

TRICEPS SKINFOLD

Fat reserves are estimated by measuring the triceps skinfold. A fold of skin on the posterior aspect of the nondominant arm,

TABLE 14-5. Urinary Creatinine per Centimeter of Body Height for Men and Women of Ideal Weight for Height

Height		Medium Frame Ideal Weight		Total Mg Creatinine/ 24 Hours	Mg Creatinine/ Cm Body Height/ 24 Hours
FOR MEN—Creatinine coefficient: 23 mg/kg of body weight					
5′ 2″	157.5 cm	124 lb	56 kg	1288	8.17
5′ 3″	160	127	57.6	1325	8.28
5′ 4″	162.6	130	59.1	1359	8.36
5′ 5″	165.1	133	60.3	1386	8.40
5′ 6″	167.6	137	62	1426	8.51
5′ 7″	170.2	141	63.8	1467	8.62
5′ 8″	172.7	145	65.8	1513	8.76
5′ 9″	175.3	149	67.6	1555	8.86
5′10″	177.8	153	69.4	1596	8.98
5′11″	180.3	158	71.4	1642	9.11
6′ 0″	182.9	162	73.5	1691	9.24
6′ 1″	185.4	167	75.6	1739	9.38
6′ 2″	188	171	77.6	1785	9.49
6′ 3″	190.5	176	79.6	1831	9.61
6′ 4″	193	181	82.2	1891	9.80
FOR WOMEN—Creatinine coefficient: 18 mg/kg of body weight					
4′10″	147.3 cm	101.5 lb	46.1 kg	830	5.63
4′11″	149.9	104	47.3	851	5.68
5′ 0″	152.4	107	48.6	875	5.74
5′ 1″	154.9	110	50	900	5.81
5′ 2″	157.5	113	51.4	925	5.87
5′ 3″	160	116	52.7	949	5.93
5′ 4″	162.6	119.5	54.3	977	6.01
5′ 5″	165.1	123	55.9	1006	6.09
5′ 6″	167.6	127.5	58	1044	6.23
5′ 7″	170.2	131.5	59.8	1076	6.32
5′ 8″	172.7	135.5	61.6	1109	6.42
5′ 9″	175.3	139.5	63.4	1141	6.51
5′10″	177.8	143.5	65.2	1174	6.60
5′11″	180.3	147.5	67	1206	6.69
6′ 0″	182.9	151.5	68.9	1240	6.78

Ideal Weight and Creatinine Height Index Table. These height/weight and creatinine values may serve as standards for calculating present weight in terms of percent of ideal and calculation of CHI which serves as a valuable estimate of the status of lean body mass. Since this muscle mass component is extremely important in the redistribution of amino acids to support visceral protein synthesis and maintenance of core temperature through work of gluconeogenesis, this calculation of CHI is valuable to a nutritional assessment profile. An adequate mean ideal height for men and women and appropriate creatinine excretion per day provides a valuable estimate of the status of lean body mass.

Adapted from Blackburn, G.L., et al.: Nutritional and metabolic assessment of the hospitalized patient. JPEN, *1*:11, 1977.

midway between the shoulder and elbow, is grasped and gently pulled away from the underlying muscle. Calipers are applied to measure the skinfold.[34]

Figure 14-3 illustrates how this measurement is performed and outlines both standard and substandard values.

MID-ARM CIRCUMFERENCE

One determination of the patient's lean body mass or degree of somatic protein depletion is the mid-arm circumference. First, the midpoint of the upper arm is located as illustrated in Figure 14-4. The midpoint is

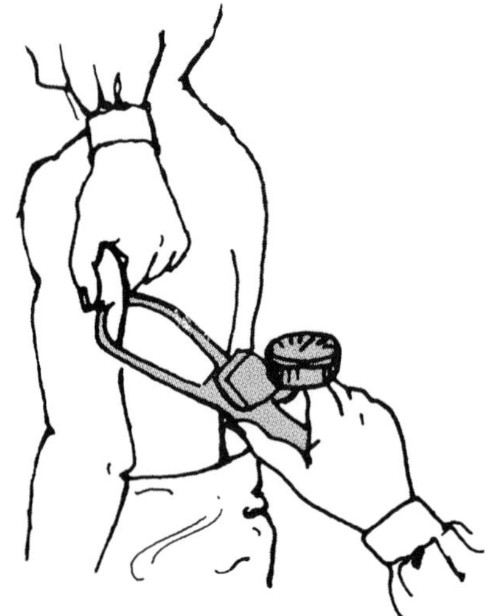

Figure 14-3. The triceps skinfold is measured to estimate the patient's fat reserves. This measurement is compared with a standard set of values to determine the level of patient depletion.

Measurement of Triceps Skinfold with Calipers

	Standard	90% Standard	80% Standard	70% Standard	60% Standard
Male	12.5 mm	11.3 mm	10.0 mm	8.8 mm	7.5 mm
Female	16.5 mm	14.9 mm	13.2 mm	11.6 mm	9.9 mm

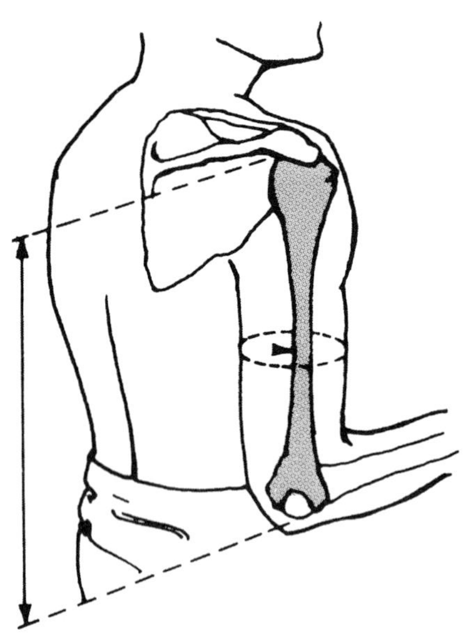

Figure 14-4. The midpoint of the upper arm is located halfway between the acromial process of the scapula and the olecranon process of the ulna.

located halfway between the acromial process of the scapula and the olecranon process of the ulna.

Next, the mid-upper arm circumference is measured. Figure 14-5 demonstrates this measurement and provides an outline of standards for evaluation.

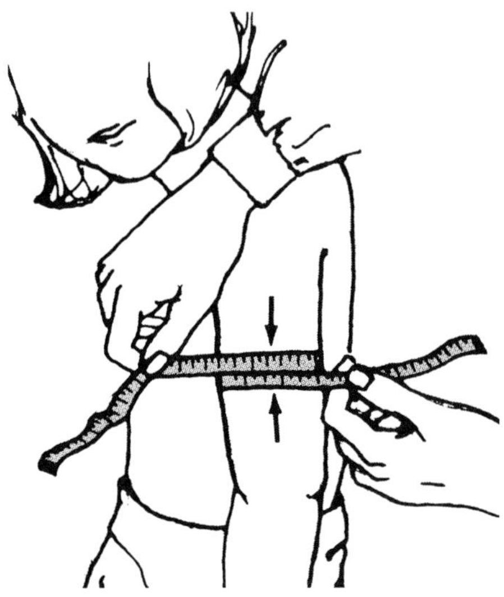

Figure 14-5. The mid-upper arm circumference is measured and compared with values in a standard table.

	Standard	90% Standard	80% Standard	70% Standard	60% Standard
Male	29.3 cm	26.3 cm	23.4 cm	20.5 cm	17.6 cm
Female	28.5 cm	25.7 cm	22.8 cm	20.0 cm	17.1 cm

ARM MUSCLE CIRCUMFERENCE

Another important indicator of the level of somatic protein deficits is the arm muscle circumference. This is calculated, utilizing the mid-arm circumference and the triceps skinfold.

Arm Muscle Circumference (cm) = mid-arm circumference − (0.314 x triceps skinfold in mm)

This is illustrated in Figure 14-6.

CREATININE/HEIGHT INDEX

Creatinine is elaborated from active muscle at a constant rate in proportion to the amount of muscle a patient has.

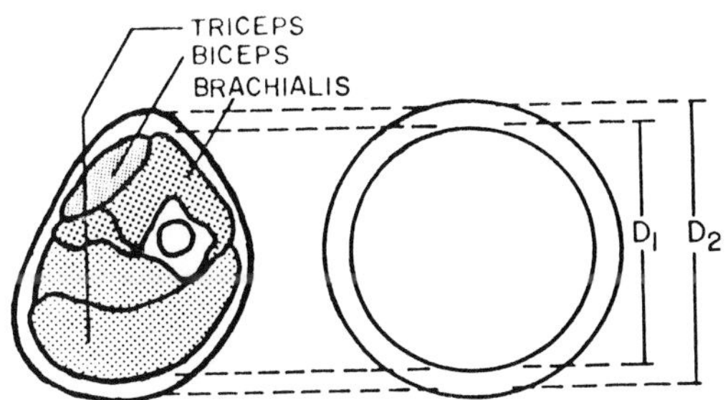

Figure 14-6. The arm muscle circumference is calculated to determine the degree of impairment of the somatic protein compartment.

	Standard	90% Standard	80% Standard	70% Standard	60% Standard
Male	25.3 cm	22.8 cm	20.2 cm	17.7 cm	15.2 cm
Female	23.2 cm	20.9 cm	18.6 cm	16.2 cm	13.9 cm

The creatinine/height index, therefore, is a more sensitive and more accurate indicator of the level of functional somatic protein (and, hence, the degree of somatic protein depletion) than are anthropometric measurements.[2] If renal function is normal, a 24-hour collection of urine can be assayed for the number of milligrams of creatinine; the percentage deficit is calculated, and this reflects the percentage of muscle deficit. The creatinine/height index is calculated by first measuring the actual urinary creatinine for a 24-hour period, determining the ideal urinary creatinine from Table 14-5, and utilizing the following equation:

$$\text{Creatinine/Height Index} = \frac{\text{actual urinary creatinine}}{\text{Ideal urinary creatinine}} \times 100$$

The patient's index is then compared to the standard to determine the degree of impairment.

Cell-Mediated Immunity

Cell-mediated immunity is an important host defense system against infection, and its depression is clearly associated with increased morbidity and mortality from disease and infection.[2,11–14] Adequacy of the cellular immune system is estimated by delayed cutaneous hypersensitivity to common recall antigens—streptokinase-streptodornase (SK/SD), mumps, candida, and purified protein derivative (PPD). Skin tests are read at 24 and 48 hours. Normal response is a wheal at least 15 mm in diameter 24 to 48 hours after administration of any one of the antigens. A result between 10 and 15 mm indicates a mild deficiency; between 5 and 10 mm, moderate; and less than 5 mm, severe immune incompetency or anergy.

Estimated Nitrogen Balance

True nitrogen balance calculation requires careful analysis of total collections, but for clinical use, an estimate of needs is satisfactory and readily made. Estimated nitrogen balance prior to the institution of therapy is extremely important in determining what approach to nutritional support should be employed, because it reflects the degree of hypermetabolism. Furthermore, nitrogen balance continues to be important throughout the nutritional therapy of a patient, serving as a monitor of progress toward the patient's therapeutic goals. Regardless of the type of therapy initially selected, if the patient remains in a negative nitrogen balance, this indicates that the selection of therapy was inappropriate. However, if the patient is in a significantly positive nitrogen balance, repair of identified protein deficits can be anticipated.

Nitrogen balance is estimated by a formula based on urine urea nitrogen (UUN) excreted during the previous 24 hours.[35] An aliquot of a 24-hour urine collected over 2 ml of N/6 HC1 is sent to the laboratory for determination of UUN. The result will be reported as mg/dl. This value is then converted into g/L by moving the decimal point two places to the left. The total volume of urine excreted in that 24-hour period is multiplied by this value to give grams of UUN excreted. A constant of 3 is added to cover the excretion of non-urea nitrogen and of that lost through skin and intestinal gas. To this value, a constant of 1 may be added for each stool.

The following example thus notes the computation.

24-hour urine output = 2 L
Urine urea nitrogen = 500 mg/dl
= 5 g/L
5 g/L × 2 L = 10 g 24-hour urea nitrogen loss
Constant non-UUN loss = 3
Estimated total nitrogen loss = 13 g

Nitrogen intake can be estimated by dividing grams of protein consumed by 6.25. Nitrogen balance is then obtained using the following formula.

$$\text{Nitrogen balance} = \text{nitrogen in} - \text{nitrogen out} = \frac{\text{protein intake in g}}{6.25} - (\text{UUN} + 3)$$

A good estimate of the sufficiency of the amount of substrate being provided is determined by calculating the nitrogen balance. Repair of significant protein deficits can occur only if the nitrogen balance is significantly positive. If severe deficits exist, the goal of therapy is the achievement of a nitrogen balance of +4 to +6, that is, the estimated nitrogen loss should be 4 to 6 g less than the estimated nitrogen intake. A near neutral or 0 balance indicates that no change in the patient's nutritional status is likely to occur. If no deficit exists, maintaining a 0 nitrogen balance is desirable as a goal of therapy. However, if deficits do exist, a 0 nitrogen balance probably indicates that the deficits are not being repaired. A large negative nitrogen balance parallels a continuing and increasing deficit in the protein compartments, indicating the inadequacy of the form or level of nutritional support to that point.

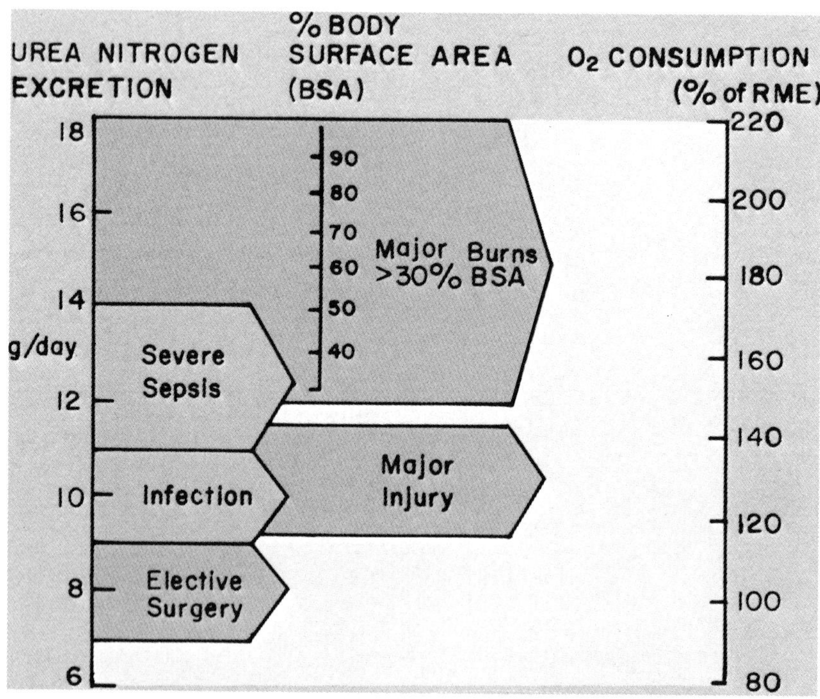

Figure 14-7. Rates of hypermetabolism estimated from urinary urea nitrogen excretion. Energy expenditure can be estimated from 24-hour urea nitrogen excretion. This relationship is based on the determination that, during stress, including infection, 12 to 16% of caloric expenditure is provided by amino-acid oxidation when the diet is protein-free. Adapted from Blackburn, G.L., et al.: Nutritional and metabolic assessment of the hospitalized patient, JPEN, E11-22, 1977.

Rate of Metabolism (Based on Urea Nitrogen Excretion)

As discussed earlier, one of the body's responses to stress is a rapid mobilization, reorganization, and utilization of body composition. This catabolism varies directly with the severity of the stress—surgical, traumatic, or infectious. Elective surgery produces little change in metabolic rate; whereas, in infection, sepsis, and peritonitis, energy demands may be 20 to 30% greater than normal. Severe stress, whether traumatic or infectious, induces a hypermetabolic state; the demands on body tissue may easily be double that of a person in health.

The amount of urea nitrogen excreted per 24 to 48 hours is a valuable indicator of the severity of hypermetabolism in stress conditions.[3] The direct relationship between UUN output and O_2 consumption is shown in Figure 14-7.

The complete patient assessment documented by the anergic/metabolic profile provides a guideline to the physician as to the need for nutritional support and the type of therapy to be employed. If the anergic/metabolic profile points to severe protein-calorie malnutrition, IVH or central TPN is obviously in order. If no nutritional deficits exist, but the patient is hypermetabolic, IVH or central TPN is also the recommended therapy. If the patient is nutritionally sound and nonhypermetabolic, but his disease state indicates a deficit is likely to develop, or if oral intake is being withheld for over 7 days, protein-sparing nutrition may well meet the patient's nutritional needs. Careful patient monitoring will indicate if protein-sparing nutrition is accomplishing its goal. If, however, the patient seems to be "sliding" toward the development of deficits, peripheral TPN may be necessary.

Figure 14-8 graphically describes which patients are candidates for protein-sparing

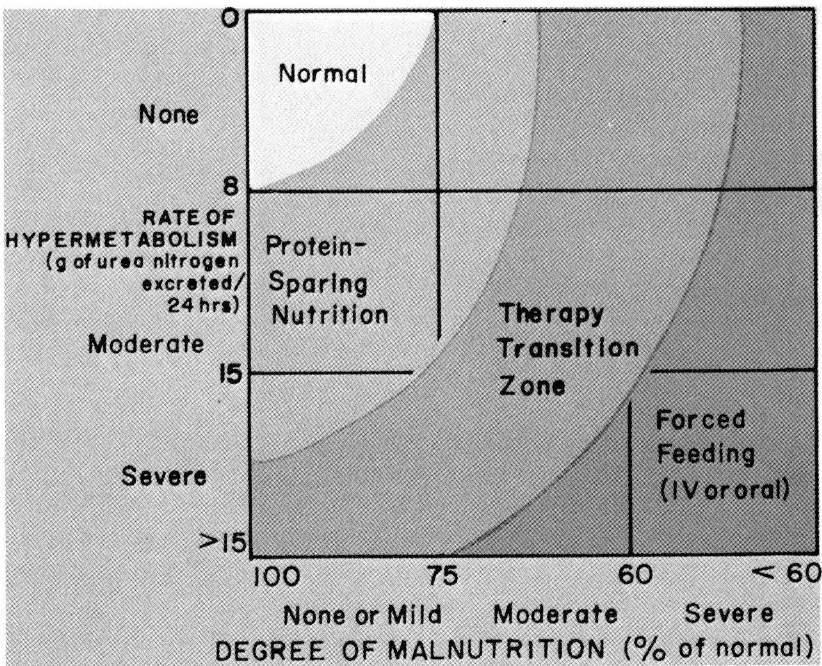

Figure 14-8. Clinical guide to nutritional needs. Nutritional needs are governed by the rate of hypermetabolism and the degree of malnutrition. When both are severe, only forced feeding, as with hyperalimentation, will provide optimal sustenance. When either is mild or both are moderate, protein-sparing nutrition with infused amino acid probably suffices. A fairly wide transitional zone will call for a clinical decision. Adapted from Dudrick, S.J., 1976.

nutrition, which require hyperalimentation, and which are in the transition zone where the appropriate nutritional prescription will require clinical judgment.

PATIENT EVALUATION AND SELECTION OF THERAPY

The enteric route is always the preferred nutritional route when it can be used; however, it is not always possible to aliment a patient adequately by mouth or by gavage tube. If oral and enteral feeding are not possible, either protein-sparing, TPN, or IVH shuld be employed as indicated. Patients requiring nutritional support can be classified into four general categories, the first three of which are considered nutritionally sound: (1) nonhypermetabolic, (2) slight to moderate deficit and/or slightly hypermetabolic, (3) hypermetabolic, and (4) severe nutritional deficits or protein-calorie malnutrition.

Nonhypermetabolic

The first group of patients requiring nutritional support are those who are nutritionally sound and are nonhypermetabolic, i.e., those whose normal metabolic rate is little changed, but whose disease state or surgery is expected to result in protein deficits if preventive therapy is not instituted. Based on the anergic/metabolic profile, these patients are either nutritionally adequate or show only a mild to moderate deficit. This group may include stroke, cancer/chemotherapy, and some surgical patients, or any other patient who is not undergoing a high degree of stress or infection.

The goal of therapy for these patients is the maintenance of the current nutritional level; therefore, a nitrogen balance from 0 to −2 is acceptable. These goals can usually be achieved by protein-sparing nutrition in patients with abundant fat stores and without renal or hepatic diseases. If the nitrogen balance significantly exceeds −2 or the visceral protein markers indicate a downward trend, the peripheral administration of additional nonprotein calories in the form of fat and/or carbohydrates may be appropriate.

Slight to Moderate Deficit and/or Slightly Hypermetabolic

The second category includes those patients who are nutritionally sound or show mild to moderate deficits and/or a nitrogen balance of −2 to −5. The metabolic rate of these patients will show a minor increase over the normal rate of an unstressed individual. In many cases, these patients may have been originally placed on protein-sparing nutrition, but a nitrogen balance in the −2 to −5 range indicated a declining patient trend toward the development of deficits. These patients require more calories than can be supplied by protein-sparing nutrition, but do not require the levels supplied by IVH or central TPN.

The goals of therapy are the maintenance of the currently acceptable nutritional level and the achievement of a nitrogen balance in the 0 to −2 range. Peripheral TPN should be instituted to meet these therapeutic goals.

Peripheral TPN can supply approximately 1400 to 2000 kcal per day to repair minor deficits and prevent the development of severe nutritional deficits.

Hypermetabolic

The third category of patients requiring intensive nutritional support includes those patients who are nutritionally sound but are hypermetabolic. These patients show an adequate nutritional level or only a mild to moderate deficit. However, by definition of a hypermetabolic state, nutritional and metabolic needs will be at levels that are so great they cannot be met by hypocaloric (protein) feeding. Consider that these demands are often double those of a healthy person and that caloric needs may reach 5000 to 6000 kcal and 24 to 36 g of nitrogen per day. Clearly, if these exceptionally large quantities of calories and protein are not supplied, a severe deficit will rapidly develop. These hypermetabolic states include most victims of major burns, trauma, and infection.

The goals of therapy for hypermetabolic patients are the maintenance of the currently adequate nutritional level and the achievement of a 0 nitrogen balance. The needs of these patients and the goals of therapy can be met only with hyperalimentation. Zero nitrogen balance under these circumstances indicates that adequate nonprotein calories and protein are being provided for repair of injury and the preservation of existing protein compartments. The status of the protein compartments affects the patient's ability to withstand stress. The hypermetabolic patient is in a state of severe stress and greatly increased nutritional needs.

Severely Malnourished

The fourth category is the severely malnourished patient. This state is delineated by a weight loss, anthropometric measurements, laboratory values, and responses to a battery of challenge antigens. The therapeutic goals in the severely malnourished are the repair of protein deficits and movement from the high-risk to the lower-risk category. This is paralleled by the achievement of at least a +4 to +6 positive nitrogen balance. The only therapeutic alternative that can repair those deficits and supply enough nitrogen to achieve a +4 to +6 positive nitrogen balance is intravenous hyperalimentation. The classification of the types of malnutrition are kwashiorkor, marasmus, or kwashiorkor-marasmus mix.

ADULT KWASHIORKOR-LIKE STATE (ICDA 267.0)

Kwashiorkor is a protein deficit without a significant calorie deficit, and is caused by a protein-deficient diet, such as one in which an overabundance of calories is delivered in the form of carbohydrates. Because carbohydrates elevate serum insulin, the somatic and fat compartments are favored at the expense of the visceral protein compartment. Kwashiorkor is characterized, therefore, by a depletion of visceral protein stores, but a maintenance of adequate reserves of fat and somatic mass as assessed by anthropometric measurements. The deficiency of the visceral protein compartment is manifested by lower levels of serum albumin, transferrin or total iron-binding capacity, and lymphocyte count. Anergy is frequent in severe kwashiorkor and particularly prone to develop in patients who were obese prior to illness and subsequently maintained on a 5% dextrose and electrolyte solution for prolonged periods of time.

ADULT MARASMUS OR CHRONIC INANITION (ICDA 268.0)

Marasmus is a prolonged and gradual wasting of muscle mass and subcutaneous fat due to an inadequate intake of both protein and calories. These substrates are transferred to the visceral protein compartment; therefore, serum albumin and other visceral proteins will remain normal and anthropometric measurements will decrease. Anergy may also be found with severe marasmus. Marasmus, observed in simple and uncomplicated starvation, is most frequently seen in postgastrectomy dumping syndromes and in carcinoma of the mouth and esophagus.

MARASMIC "KWASHIORKOR-LIKE" MIXTURE (ICDA 269.9)

This is a life-threatening form of malnutrition. The body mobilizes and exhausts its reserves of fat and lean somatic mass and then cannibalizes visceral proteins. The anthropometric measurements and levels of serum albumin, transferrin, and lymphocyte counts are lower. Immune competence is frequently impaired. This anergic state frequently results from placing a marasmic patient on 5% dextrose or from severe and life-threatening stress or infection.

The decision process of the need for nutritional support that can best meet the requirements of the patient's level of impairment and degree of metabolism is outlined in Figure 14-9.

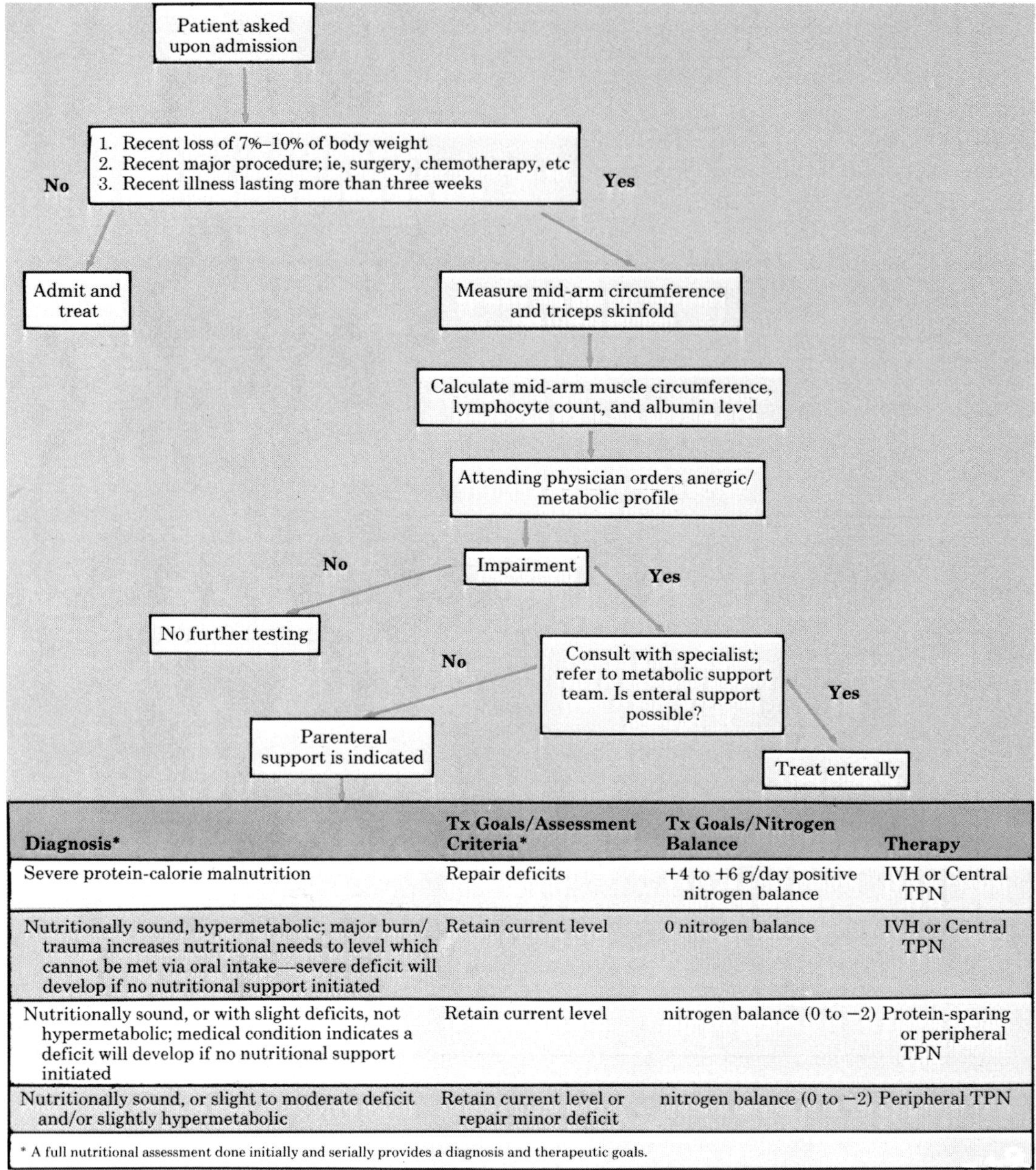

Diagnosis*	Tx Goals/Assessment Criteria*	Tx Goals/Nitrogen Balance	Therapy
Severe protein-calorie malnutrition	Repair deficits	+4 to +6 g/day positive nitrogen balance	IVH or Central TPN
Nutritionally sound, hypermetabolic; major burn/ trauma increases nutritional needs to level which cannot be met via oral intake—severe deficit will develop if no nutritional support initiated	Retain current level	0 nitrogen balance	IVH or Central TPN
Nutritionally sound, or with slight deficits, not hypermetabolic; medical condition indicates a deficit will develop if no nutritional support initiated	Retain current level	nitrogen balance (0 to −2)	Protein-sparing or peripheral TPN
Nutritionally sound, or slight to moderate deficit and/or slightly hypermetabolic	Retain current level or repair minor deficit	nitrogen balance (0 to −2)	Peripheral TPN

* A full nutritional assessment done initially and serially provides a diagnosis and therapeutic goals.

Figure 14-9. Decision tree for metabolic support.

Certain basic conclusions may be drawn from this discussion of types of nutritional support and patient categories. If the patient is nutritionally sound and not hypermetabolic, institute protein-sparing nutrition. If, however, the patient is hypermetabolic or severely malnourished, IVH or central TPN should be employed.

Between these two categories exists a spectrum of patients who require TPN through the peripheral vein.

The decision tree emphasizes that the most important consideration is the patient's current status and metabolic rate; the mode of therapy is selected to achieve specific therapeutic goals.

The major nutritional goal of hyperalimentation is the preservation or restoration of somatic and visceral protein compartments; i.e., muscle mass and function with maintenance or repair of visceral proteins as manifested by a normal albumin, transferrin, and lymphocyte count and, most significantly, cell-mediated immunity. This goal is accomplished by the administration via a central vein of both protein and nonprotein calories in water to which vitamins and appropriate amounts of intra- and extracellular electrolytes, including sodium, chloride, potassium, magnesium, calcium, phosphate, zinc, and copper, are added.

Amino Acids

Nitrogen requirements are met by crystalline amino acid solutions, which are available commercially. In order to achieve positive nitrogen balance in the stressed patient, i.e., protein synthesis in excess of breakdown, amounts of amino acids greater than are required by the normal unstressed person should be supplied. The requirement in the stressed patient may increase to four times greater than normal, e.g., in the burn patient.[36] Approximately 10.5 g of nitrogen per day must be supplied for equilibrium maintenance; however, the presence of disease or trauma may create a nitrogen requirement approaching 20 g to achieve protein synthesis in excess of breakdown. It may not be possible to infuse desirable amounts of amino acids because of azotemia or hepatic failure.

It is important that an optimal ratio of protein to nonprotein calories be achieved and maintained so that nonprotein calories are metabolized for energy and the protein calories can be used by the body to repair protein deficits. A ratio of 100 to 250 kcal of nonprotein calories per gram of nitrogen is routinely used in solutions of this sort.

The infusion of amino acids is crucial to the reversal of both somatic and visceral protein depletion—the major goal of nutritional therapy. Nitrogen is required for the repletion or maintenance of the somatic and visceral protein compartments.

Carbohydrates

Caloric requirements may be met by either carbohydrate supplied by glucose or by fat and glucose. Large amounts of nonprotein calories are required to spare the utilization of nitrogen for protein synthesis. To provide the energy needs of the uncomplicated, nonstressed patient at rest, 30 kcal/kg of body weight per day are necessary; however, caloric requirements may double or triple in the presence of extreme stress, sepsis, trauma, or burns.[37]

The most commonly used source of nonprotein calories in IVH solutions is glucose. It is readily available as a source of energy (approx 3.4 kcal/g), can be obtained in pure form, and is relatively inexpensive. Glucose solutions, available in concentrations of 5 to 70%, must be administered in concentrated form if used as the sole source of calories.[31]

Certain body tissues, including the brain, erythrocytes, bone marrow, peripheral nerves, and adrenal medulla, utilize glucose as a source of energy. In addition, fibroblasts and phagocytes essential to wound healing use glucose as the principal energy source.[38]

Carbohydrates supply the calories required to allow nitrogen to be used for tissue repair and for the reversal of the depletion of the somatic and visceral protein compartments; however, fats may also be used as a principal or secondary source of nonprotein calories.

Fat Emulsions

Since 1976, the Food and Drug Administration has permitted U.S. physicians to use lipid emulsions to supplement amino acids and glucose in patients who require maximal intravenous calories. Lipid emulsions have a number of applications in intravenous nutritional therapy: they are isotonic and do not damage venous endothelium; they avoid fatty liver and liver dysfunction, as seen when IVH is employed; they provide essential fatty acids; they do not require insulin to promote nitrogen utilization, and hence, no hyperinsulinemia or rebound hypoglycemia occurs, making the technical management of infusions easier. Exogenous insulin, which is often required in septic patients and those with adult-onset diabetes when IVH is administered, is rarely needed when lipid is used as a source of calories.

Fat emulsions have been tried as a source of calories since the 1940's. These initial emulsions were found to be toxic and were not used in the United States. Recently, through improved understanding and technology, safe emulsions became available. A safe emulsion is composed of a triglyceride with a fatty acid pattern compatible with the human body, a phospholipid that is not toxic, and a metabolizable agent (glycerol) to maintain osmotic pressure. In addition, the particle size is comparable with that of chylomicrons, and the lipid is not taken up by the reticuloendothelial system, does not block immune response,[39] and is cleared by the enzyme lipoprotein lipase.

In the adult, the clearance rate depends on the degree of malnutrition and is greatest in malnourished and hypercatabolic patients. Results of clearance studies indicate that 2g/kg per day are easily utilized, and the rate may increase to 4g/kg per day in malnourished and catabolic patients.[39] It is recommended that fat emulsion not be used as a complete source of calories. Investigators agree that lipid emulsion should be administered with dextrose and amino acids.[40]

The type of patient for whom the administration of fat emulsions is beneficial and the percentage of total solution composition that should consist of fat emulsions are controversial. Jeejeebhoy and his colleagues[9] demonstrated the protein-sparing effect of fat. Nitrogen conservation, particularly in patients with gastrointestinal diseases and in septic animals, is comparable with that of glucose. This study demonstrated that "lipid and glucose-lipid systems promote weight gain, fistula healing and an increase in serum protein levels." These workers further concluded that fat emulsions may be valuable in burned or injured patients who are unable to secrete adequate insulin in the presence of glucose and have glucose/insulin ratios in the so-called "catabolic range."

Beisbarth[41] concludes that "IV fat exerts a nitrogen-sparing effect in adults in certain hypercatabolic states provoked by severe stress (e.g., severe burns) and in children."

Long,[42] however, reported that severely traumatized or burned patients should receive 80% of nonprotein calories in the form of carbohydrates; fats should be used only as a source of additional calories to meet additional energy requirements to promote weight gain or to provide a source of essential fatty acids. He further concluded that fat emulsions do not appear to have a protein-sparing effect on this group of patients.

Blanchard and Gillespie[43] also have stated that fat emulsions should be used only for patients receiving short-term parenteral nutrition and not for patients in extreme catabolic states.

There is general agreement, however, that for certain high-risk patients for whom central venous catheterization offers too great a probability of severe complications, the use of fat emulsions provides a means of providing sufficient nonprotein calories peripherally. These high-risk categories include persistent bacterial septicemia, refractory hyperosmolar states, and candidiasis.[44] Furthermore, it is generally agreed that fat emulsions may be necessary to prevent the development of fatty liver and essential fatty acid deficiencies, thereby maintaining tissue synthesis.[9]

The infusion of fat emulsions as a major source of calories results in a fall of circulating pyruvate and lactate, a rise in free fatty acids and ketones, and a fall in insulin levels and the respiratory quotient. Increased insulin secretion is not required for the utilization of fat. Hence, lipids are utilized well in states in which insulin output is low.

It is commonly believed that fats may impair liver function. However, liver function abnormalities occur in the absence of fat, and patients with abnormal liver function improve when given lipid.[45]

TABLE 14-6. Examples of Nutritional Support Infusions*

	Quantities/Liter				Quantities/Day (3 liters/day)				
Therapy	Nitrogen (g)	Nitrogen (kcal)	CHO (kcal)	Fat (kcal/ 500 ml)	Nitrogen (g)	Nitrogen (kcal)	CHO (kcal)	Total Fat (kcal)	Total kcal
Protein	5.5	140	—	—	16.5	420	—	—	420
Sparing	5.5	140	170	550	16.5	420	510	550	1480
Peripheral	5.5	140	170	550	16.5	420	510	1100	2030
TPN	5.5	140	425	550	16.5	420	1275	1650	3345
Central	7.8	199	425	550	23.4	597	1275	1650	3522
TPN	5.5	140	850	—	16.5	420	2550	—	2970
IVH	7.8	199	850	—	23.4	597	2550	—	3147

* All solutions contain appropriate vitamins, minerals, and electrolyte additives.
The caloric contribution of amino acids is traditionally excluded from the total calories provided.

Table 14-6 indicates the amounts of nitrogen, carbohydrates, and fat generally administered for the various therapeutic approaches.

"Total parenteral nutrition has been a reality in this country for less than 10 years, but already thousands of patients are in its debt, many for their lives."[46] We can conclude that IVH does have a place in the total therapeutic program of thousands, if not millions, of hospitalized patients. If the nutritional needs of these patients are ignored, their chances of recovery and survival will be significantly reduced. Nutritional support cannot be considered simply as an occasional adjunct to other therapies, but rather as an integral part of the total therapeutic program.

BIBLIOGRAPHY

1. Abbott, W.M.: Indications for Parenteral Nutrition, *In* Total Parenteral Nutrition. J.E. Fischer, ed. Boston, Little, Brown and Co., 1976, p. 12.
2. Blackburn, G.L., et al.: Manual for nutritional/metabolic assessment of the hospitalized patient. Presented at the 62nd Annual Clinical Congress of the American College of Surgeons, Chicago, Oct. 11–15, 1976.
3. Blackburn, G.L., Maini, B.S., and Pierce, E.C.: Nutrition in the critically ill patient. Anesthesiology, *47:*0104, 1977.
4. Abbott Laboratories: Nutritional Assessment & Intravenous Support. The Use of Amino Acids for Protein-Sparing Nutrition (Physician's Monograph). Abbott Laboratories, North Chicago, IL, July 1977.
5. Jeejeebhoy, K.N., et al.: Metabolic studies in total parenteral nutrition with lipid in man: Comparison with glucose. J. Clin. Invest., *57:*125, 1976.
6. Gazziniga, A.B., Bartlett, R.H., and Shobe, J.B.: Nitrogen balance in patients receiving either fat or carbohydrate for total intravenous nutrition. Ann. Surg., *182:*163, 1975.
7. Wannemacher, R.W., Jr., et al.: Protein-sparing therapy during pneumococcal sepsis in the rhesus monkey. JPEN, *2:*507, 1978.
8. Jeejeebhoy, K.N.: Total parenteral nutrition. Review article. Ann. R. Coll. Phys. Surg. Can., Oct. 1976, pp. 287-300.
9. Jeejeebhoy, K.N., et al.: Lipid in Parenteral Nutrition: Studies of Clinical and Metabolic Features, *In* Fat Emulsions in Parenteral Nutrition. Chicago, American Medical Association, 1976.
10. Holroyde, C.P., et al.: Metabolic response to total parenteral nutrition. Cancer Res. *37:*3109, 1977.
11. Meakins, J.L., et al.: Delayed hypersensitivity: Indicator of acquired future of host defenses in sepsis and trauma. Ann. Surg., *186:*241, 1977.
12. Pietsch, J.B., Meakins, J.L., and MacLean, L.D.: The delayed hypersensitivity response: Application in clinical surgery. Surgery, *82:*349, 1977.
13. Harvey, K.B., et al.: Hospital morbidity: Mortality risk factors using nutritional assessment. Clin. Res., Apr., 1978.
14. Willcutts, H.D.: Nutritional assessment of 1000 surgical patients in an affluent suburban community hospital. Presented at the Second Annual Clinical Congress of the American Society of Parenteral and Enteral Nutrition, Houston, Feb. 1-4, 1978.
15. Zohrab, W.J., McHattie, J.D., and Jeejeebhoy, K.N.: Total parenteral alimentation, with lipid. Gastroenterology, *64:*583, 1973.
16. MacFadyen, B.V., Jr., and Dudrick, S.J.: Total parenteral nutrition of the critically ill patient. Dietetic Curr., *5:*1, 1978.
17. Fleming, C.R., et al.: Subject review: Total parenteral nutrition. Mayo Clin. Proc., *51:*187, 1976.
18. Dudrick, S.J., Copeland, E.M., III, and MacFadyen, B.V., Jr.: Long-term parenteral nutrition: Its current status. Hosp. Pract., *10:*47, 1975.
19. Greenberg, G.R., Haber, G.B., and Jeejeebhoy, K.N.: Total parenteral nutrition (TPN) and bowel rest in the management of Crohn's disease (abstr). Gut, *17:*828, 1976.

20. Dudrick, S.J., Ruberg, R.L.: Principles and practice of total parenteral nutrition. Curr. Clin. Concept, *61:*901, 1971.
21. Wilmore, D.W., and Pruitt, B.A.: Parenteral Nutrition in Burn Patients, *In* Total Parenteral Nutrition. J.E. Fischer, ed. Boston, Little, Brown and Co., 1976.
22. Copeland, E.M., et al.: Intravenous Hyperalimentation and Cancer. University of Texas Medical School at Houston.
23. Schwartz, G.F., et al.: Combined parenteral hyperalimentation and chemotherapy in the treatment of disseminated solid tumors. Am. J. Surg., *121:*169, 1971.
24. Copeland, E.M., MacFadyen, B.V., Jr., and Dudrick, S.J.: Intravenous hyperalimentation in cancer patients. J. Surg. Res., *16:*241, 1974.
25. Heird, W.C.: Columbia University College of Physicians and Surgeons and the Babies Hospital, Columbia-Presbyterian Medical Center, New York, personal communication, 1978.
26. Muttart, C.R.: Role of pediatric nurse in total parenteral nutrition. Presented at the Second Annual Clinical Congress of the American Society of Parenteral and Enteral Nutrition, Feb. 2–4, 1978.
27. Lebenthal, E., Antonowics, I., and Shwachman, H.: The interrelationship of enterokinase and trypsin activities in intractable diarrhea of infancy, celiac disease, and intravenous alimentation. Pediatrics, *56:*585, 1975.
28. Avery, G.B., et al.: Intractable diarrhea in early infancy. Pediatrics, *41:*712, 1978.
29. Greene, H.L., McCabe, D., and Merenstein, G.B.: Protracted diarrhea and malnutrition in infancy: Changes in intestinal enzymes after intravenous nutrition or oral alimentation diets. J. Pediat., *87:*695, 1975.
30. Blackburn, G.L.: Factors Influencing Preservation of Body Cell Mass Using Hypocaloric Feeding of Isotonic Amino Acid, *In* Clinical Nutrition Update. Chicago, American Medical Association, 1977.
31. Meng, H.C.: Parenteral nutrition: Principles, nutrient requirements, and techniques. Geriatrics, *30:*97, 1974.
32. Rudman, D., et al.: Elemental balances during hyperalimentation of underweight adult subjects. J. Clin. Invest., *55:*94, 1974.
33. Blackburn, G.L., and Flatt, J.P.: Metabolic response to illness: Protein-sparing therapy. Comp. Ther., *1:*23, 1974.
34. Butterworth, C.E., and Blackburn, G.L.: Hospital malnutrition and how to assess the nutritional status of a patient. Nutr. Today, *10:*8, 1975.
35. Kaminski, M.V., Jr.: Hyperalimentation: Who, what, and why. Surg. Team, *5:*23, 1976.
36. Long, J.M., III: Hyperalimentation: Theory behind the technic. Am. J. IV Ther., *3:*41, 1976.
37. Law, D.H.: Current concepts in nutrition: Total parenteral nutrition. N. Engl. J. Med., *297:*1105, 1977.
38. Harper, H.A., and Sheldon, G.F.: Metabolic and Nutritional Considerations in Surgery, *In* Current Surgical Diagnosis and Treatment. J.E. Dunphy, and L.W. Way. Los Altos, CA, Lange Medical Publications, 1975.
39. Hallberg, D., et al.: Studies on the elimination of exogenous lipids from the bloodstream. The kinetics of elimination of a fat emulsion and of chylomicrons in the dog after single injection. Acta Physiol. Scand., *65:*153, 1965.
40. Elsberry, V.A., et al.: The lipid phase in TPN. Am. J. IV Ther., *4:*22, 1977.
41. Beisbarth, H.: Influence of Stress on Intravenous Fat Requirements, *In* Fat Emulsions in Parenteral Nutrition. Chicago, American Medical Association, 1976.
42. Long, J.M., III: Use of Intravenous Fat Emulsion after Trauma and Burns, *In* Fat Emulsions in Parenteral Nutrition. Chicago, American Medical Association, 1976.
43. Blanchard, R.J., and Gillespie, D.J.: Some Comparisons Between Fat Emulsion and Glucose for Parenteral Nutrition in Adults at the Winnipeg Health Sciences Centre, *In* Fat Emulsions in Parenteral Nutrition. Chicago, American Medical Association, 1976.
44. Thompson, W.R.: Peripheral Venous TPN in the Treatment of Critically Ill Surgical Patients, *In* Fat Emulsions in Parenteral Nutrition. Chicago, American Medical Association, 1976.
45. Jeejeebhoy, K.N., et al.: Total parenteral nutrition at home for 23 months, without complications, and with good rehabilitation. A study of technical and metabolic features. Gastroenterology, *65:*811, 1973.
46. Fischer, J.E., ed.: Total Parenteral Nutrition. Boston, Little, Brown and Co., 1976, p xi.

Chapter 15

Calories and Parenteral Nutrition

Robert A. Quercia, M.S., R.Ph.
Supervisor of Drug Information Service
Hartford Hospital
Hartford, Connecticut and
Assistant Clinical Professor
University of Connecticut
School of Pharmacy
Storrs, Connecticut

Energy plays a vital role in our concepts of nutritional therapy. It is defined as the capacity to do work, and the calorie (kilocalorie) is the unit of energy most commonly used in human nutrition. One kilocalorie is the amount of heat necessary to raise one kilogram of water from 15°C to 16°C.[1] The available energy in nutrition is used for muscular work, brain and nerve activity, maintenance of body temperature, and synthesis of tissue.

The human body is able to convert carbohydrates, fats, and proteins to glucose, fatty acids, and amino acids before they reach the cell. Within the cell, these nutrients are oxidized through a number of pathways (Figure 15-1) to produce energy that is used to form adenosine triphosphate (ATP). ATP contains high-energy phosphate bonds, which are very labile and can be released instantly, as needed, for muscle contraction, synthesis of body tissue, and active transport. Thus, ATP formation is the mechanism the body has devised for capturing, storing, and releasing energy as it is needed in the human biochemical system.

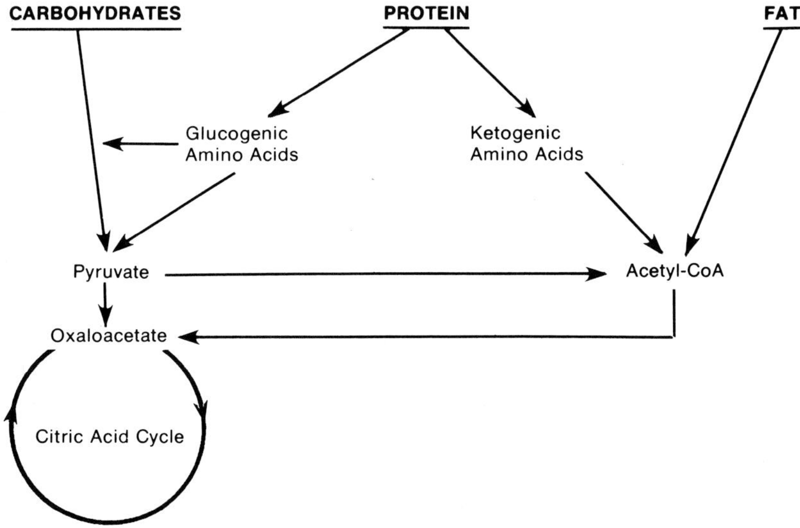

Figure 15-1. Metabolic energy-producing pathways of carbohydrate, fat, and protein.

MEASUREMENT OF ENERGY EXPENDITURE

The measurement of energy expenditure plays an important role in determining the caloric requirements of the hospitalized patient, since energy metabolism is altered in the injured or diseased patient. Heat production in the human body is directly related to the combustion of carbohydrates, fat, and proteins. Energy that does not appear as work is dissipated as heat. The measurement of the dissipated-heat loss can be used as a method of determining energy expenditure. Calorimetry can be used to measure heat loss directly or indirectly. In the direct method, the individual is placed in a specially constructed chamber, and the heat is measured by physical techniques. The indirect method uses oxygen consumption, carbon dioxide production, and nitrogen excretion as a measure of heat production.[2,3] The indirect method may be applied when the body is lying at rest or is engaged in various activities. Direct calorimetry is costly and not practical in the clinical setting; the indirect method is less expensive and clinically more feasible.

Energy Requirements

In the hospital setting, energy requirements for patients suffering from disease or injury are increased and are often expressed as a percentage above the measured or estimated Basal Energy Expenditure (BEE) or over the Resting Metabolic Expenditure (RME). The increase in caloric requirement varies considerably from one patient to another and depends on a number of factors, including:

A. Either the Basal Energy Expenditure or the Resting Metabolic Expenditure;
B. Physical activity;
C. Specific Dynamic Action (SDA) of food;
D. Degree of hypermetabolism

Basal Energy Expenditure is an important part of the energy requirement for any person, since it represents the life critical requirement for the nonactive person. The BEE is defined as the amount of energy needed to perform necessary physiologic work at rest, in the postabsorptive state (12 to 14 hours after the last meal), in a thermoneutral environment. The RME differs from the BEE in that it is the energy expenditure at rest, under normal environmental conditions; it is approximately 10 to 15% over the BEE.[4] The basal energy expenditure and the resting metabolic expenditure can be measured by direct or indirect calorimetry. Indirect calorimetry is probably the most accurate, reliable, and practical method of assessing the optimal caloric requirements of the critically ill patient. The equipment required is usually available in most modern hospitals with a cardiopulmonary laboratory.[5] Indirect calorimetry takes into consideration all the factors of the patient's illness, including temperature, sepsis, respiratory rate, and other catabolic processes.

Physical activity for most hospitalized patients is limited, but work by Long and Blakemore[2] demonstrated through indirect calorimetry that most hospitalized patients need approximately 20% more calories above their resting energy needs for their limited physical activity. Specific Dynamic Action of food refers to the increase over the RME that results from excess heat production while eating. The SDA of protein is approximately six times greater than that of carbohydrates or fat. This additional energy expenditure from the specific dynamic action of food, which can vary from 6 to 15% of the total food calories, must be accounted for when calculating the total caloric requirements of the hospitalized patient.[6] Thus, it becomes apparent that to provide adequate protein deposition for the hospitalized patient on TPN, suffering from disease, injury, or surgical trauma, calories in excess of the RME are essential. Kinney has recommended an intravenous caloric intake that is 50% above the resting metabolic expenditure, in order to achieve positive nitrogen balance (Table 15-1).

Increased energy requirements for severe-burn patients can be explained, in

TABLE 15-1. Resting Metabolic Expenditure*

Conditions	Actual RME[1]	Calculated Daily Caloric Intake[1] RME + 50%
Postoperative	1800	2700
Multiple fractures	2160	3240
Major sepsis	2520	3780
Major burn	3240	4860

* For an average 70 kg male surgical patient.

part, by the loss of skin covering, which allows for large fluid losses from the body surface. Every ml of water that leaves the body's surface at 37° C requires half a calorie for the latent heat of vaporization. It is not unusual for a severe-burn patient to lose 4 L of fluid per day, which is equivalent to approximately 2000 kcal needed as a result of water loss alone.[2] When this is added to the patient's other caloric requirements, he may need 4000 kcal per day just to prevent a severe loss of weight.

In those clinical settings where indirect calorimetry is not possible, the BEE can be calculated from the Harris-Benedict Formula, which uses age, sex, height, and weight.[7]

For Males:

$$BEE = 66.473 + (13.752 \times W) + (5.003 \times H) - (6.755 \times A)$$

For Females:

$$BEE = 655.096 + (9.563 \times W) + (1.849 \times H) - (4.675 \times A);$$

W = Weight (in kg);
H = Height (in cm);
A = Age (in yrs).

Rutten et al.[8] have demonstrated that, in mild to moderate stress, with delivery of TPN at a daily caloric intake from 1.75 to 2.0, the calculated BEE produces positive nitrogen-balance. In the severe hypercatabolic patient (e.g., major burn, severe sepsis, major trauma), calories in excess of 2.0 calculated BEE are required.[9,10]

It becomes important, when calculating caloric requirements with the BEE formula, to be able to assess the degree of the patient's hypermetabolism. The rate of hypermetabolism can be estimated by obtaining a 24-hour urine urea-nitrogen excretion while the patient is on a protein-free diet. The degree of hypermetabolism can then be estimated by comparing the quantity of urine urea excreted to already established relationships of urea-nitrogen excretion and degree of net catabolism (Table 15-2).

TABLE 15-2. Classification of Hypermetabolism

Degree of Net Catabolism	Urea Nitrogen Excreted/ 24 hrs[8]	% Increase of RME Over BEE[8]
1° (Normal)	<5 g	None
2° (Mild)	5-10 g	0-20
3° (Moderate)	10-15 g	20-50
4° (Severe)	>15 g	>50

When calorimetric or calculated BEE methods cannot be used to determine caloric requirements for TPN patients, the more empiric method of using kcal/kg nomogram can be followed (Table 15-3).

TABLE 15-3. Calorie Requirements for Positive Nitrogen Balance

Condition	Calorie Requirement[4]
Minor abdominal surgery	40 kcal/kg
Major trauma	55 kcal/kg

Regardless of the method used to determine caloric requirements (Figure 15-2), accurate nitrogen-balance monitoring is essential in order to provide for optimal use of infused amino acids. A nitrogen-balance determination should be performed at least weekly, and more often if the patient is severely hypermetabolic or if it appears that the patient's hypermetabolic status is rapidly changing.

The infusion of the measured or calculated nonprotein caloric requirements is es-

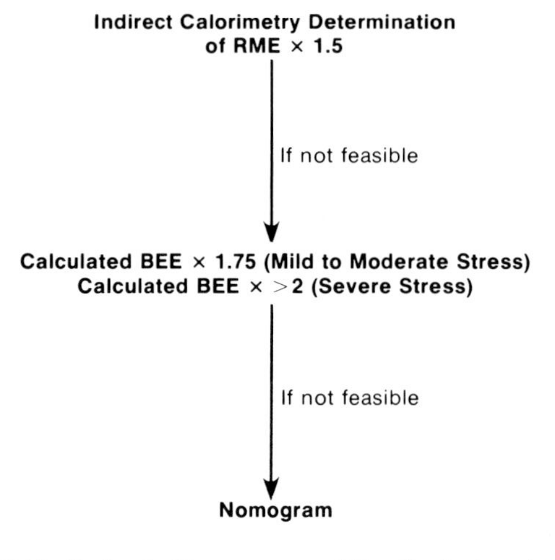

Figure 15-2. Methods of determining calorie requirements for positive nitrogen balance.

sential for patients who are hypermetabolic (e.g., burn, trauma, sepsis, etc.), even though the average-size adult has approximately 25,000 protein calories.[11] The reason is that all this protein is part of vital structural or functional compounds in the body and must be protected. The delivery of these nonprotein calories by total parenteral nutrition (TPN) in a fixed ratio is essential for the efficient use of both calories and amino acids in protein synthesis. The nitrogen-to-nonprotein caloric ratio (N/kcal) for TPN has not been specifically determined, but with disease, injury, and trauma, the optimal N/kcal ratio has been reported to range from 1:150 to 1:200.[12,13] Most commercially available parenteral nutrition solutions have N/kcal ratios around 1:150; thus tying the nitrogen intake to the caloric intake. The use of indirect calorimetry and BEE formulas, as described above for calculating energy requirements may not be appropriate for patients with acute renal failure, since clinically it may not be feasible to deliver the total estimated energy requirements. Patients with acute renal failure also require high nitrogen-to-nonprotein calorie ratios (e.g., 1:800) when being supported by parenteral nutrition.

CALORIE SOURCES

Although several sources of the nonprotein calories needed to meet the metabolic demands of the hospitalized patient on parenteral nutrition are available, some controversy exists about which source is most satisfactory in TPN. The available sources of calories that have the potential of meeting the large energy demands are shown in Table 15-4.

TABLE 15-4. Source of Calories

Substrate	Kcal/g[14]
Glucose*	4.0
Fructose	4.0
Ethanol	7.0
Sorbitol	4.0
Xylitol	4.0
Fat	9.1

* Glucose monohydrate provides 3.4 kcal/g.

Glucose

Glucose is one of the more common monosaccharides, with the empiric formula $C_6H_{12}O_6$. It is also known as grape sugar or dextrose. This substrate is a valuable calorie source in the provision of parenteral nutrition, because it can be metabolized by all tissues of the body.[15] Glucose provides 3.4 kcal/g in solution and can be used by most patients at a maximum rate of 0.5 g/kg per hour.[16] Some significant differences exist in the mechanisms by which glucose is metabolized by these various tissues. The central nervous system and erythrocytes rely completely on glucose for their energy requirements. It appears that the transport of glucose into the brain and erythrocytes takes place by a facilitated carrier, but it does not depend on the actions of insulin. Under extreme conditions, such as starvation, the brain will use ketone bodies as a source of energy, but prolonged hypoglcemia can result in brain-cell death. The liver is also freely permeable to glucose, but it requires insulin to store glucose in the form of glycogen. In those tissues that can use other sources of energy besides glucose (e.g., muscle, adipose tissue), insulin is necessary for the transport of glucose across the cell membrane, except for glucose uptake during muscular work. The quantity of glucose taken up during muscular work, however, is much smaller than the quantity of glucose taken up during maximal stimulation by insulin. In addition, glucose taken up during muscular work is primarily converted to lactate and CO_2, while most of the glucose taken up during insulin stimulation is converted to glycogen. Muscle is the most important tissue in glucose combustion, while adipose tissue is responsbile for most glucose storage (in the form of triglycerides). The purpose of the impermeability of the muscle and adipose-tissue membrane to glucose is to conserve glucose for those tissues that use it as their only substrate (e.g., brain and erythrocytes).[17]

Fructose

Fructose is also a monosaccharide that can be used as a calorie source in parenteral nutrition. It has been suggested that fructose is a good substitute for glucose because it is apparently independent of insulin.[18] It is probably true that, for hepatic uptake, phosphorylation, and conversion to glucose, fructose is insulin-independent, but its use by tissue does not appear to be insulin-independent. Several studies in animals have indicated that fructose is hepatically metabolized to glucose, and that all further reactions are insulin-dependent. Similar studies in man have led to the same conclusions.[17]

There are also some adverse effects of fructose, including lactic acidosis, hepatocellular toxicity, hepatic depletion of phosphorus and adenine nucleotides, and hyperuricemia.[10]

Sorbitol

Sorbitol is a polyalcohol that was thought to be a good substitute for glucose. It was claimed to be less irritating to veins in high concentrations and to have a metabolism independent of insulin. There is no question that sorbitol can be used as a source of energy, but the first step in its metabolism is hepatic conversion to fructose by sorbitol dehydrogenase. Subsequently, it is metabolized by the liver as fructose, of which it has all the disadvantages. It seems not to offer any advantage over fructose and definitely none over glucose.[17,18] It appears to have little or no role as a calorie source in total parenteral nutrition.

Xylitol

Xylitol is also a polyalcohol. It has been considered a potential calorie source in parenteral-nutrition programs. The initial hepatic conversion of xylitol to xylulose and then to glucose is insulin-dependent, but the subsequent metabolism of glucose is insulin-independent. Thus, as with fructose, it is only the first few metabolic steps of hepatic metabolism that are insulin-dependent. Serious adverse reactions have been reported with the use of xylitol as a calorie source. They include metabolic acidosis, osmotic diuresis, renal tubule deposits of calcium oxalate crystals, altered cerebral function (i.e., nausea, confusion, disorientation and stupor, loss of consciousness), elevated total serum bilirubin, elevated SGOT, hyperuricemia, metabolic acidosis, and oliguric renal failure.[20] Thus, as with fructose and sorbitol, xylitol offers no advantage over glucose, and the adverse reactions associated with its use should preclude it as a substitute for glucose.

Ethanol

Ethanol is a primary alcohol that can provide 7 kcal/g. Its nitrogen-sparing effect has long been known, and it has been used in parenteral nutrition at a rate of 1.5 g/kg of body weight per 24 hours in alcoholic concentrations not exceeding 4%. However, ethanol and amino acids alone are not sufficient to maintain nitrogen-balance, and some carbohydrate is necessary for adequate anabolic response.[21] The use of ethanol is also associated with a number of undesirable properties that include potential intoxication following infusion of large volumes, impairment of respiratory function, hepatotoxicity, CNS depression, irritation of bowel mucosa, and its contraindication in cirrhosis and pancreatitis.[18] Thus, the use of ethanol as a calorie source in TPN is metabolically unwise and offers no advantage over glucose.

In comparing the caloric value of the carbohydrates and alcohol in TPN, it appears that glucose is the substrate of choice in modern parenteral nutrition. Just a few of the reasons for this are as follows:

1. Glucose is capable of being completely utilized by all organs.
2. It has a strong anabolic effect when endogenous or exogenous insulin is present.
3. It has no serious adverse effects, except, probably, hyperglycemia, which can be determined relatively simply at any time.
4. It is comparatively inexpensive and readily available.

Fat

Fat possesses the highest calorie value of all available nutrients. It supplies about 9.1 kcal/g and is the major reserve fuel of the body. Fat has a definite protein-sparing effect, and several metabolic studies have shown that soybean oil is comparable to glucose in promoting positive nitrogen-balance.[22,23]

The only parenteral form of fat available in the United States as a calorie source is 10% soybean oil emulsion (Intralipid). It contains 10% soybean oil emulsified with 1.2% eggyolk phospholipids and 2.25% glycerin to make the emulsion isotonic.

The fatty acid composition of Intralipid is described in Table 15-5. The emulsion provides 1.1 cal/ml and has an osmolarity of 280 mOsm/L. Since the lipid particles are comparable in size to natural chylomicrons, they are distributed and metabolized in a similar manner.[24]

It is recommended that when the soybean oil emulsion is used as a source of calories in

TABLE 15-5. Fatty Acid Composition of Intralipid

Fatty Acids	Percent
Linoleic	54.0
Oleic	26.0
Palmitic	9.0
Linolenic	8.0
Stearic	2.5

TPN, no more than 60% of the total calories be supplied as fat calories and that the remaining calories be supplied by glucose and amino acids. Carbohydrate calories are required to satisfy the glucose requirements of the brain and to prevent gluconeogenesis as a result of inadequate glucose supply. Regardless of what the caloric requirements are for any given patient, the amount provided in fat should not exceed 2.5 g/kg of body weight per day. The pediatric patient should not receive more than 4 g/kg of body weight per day.[24]

This method of TPN can be accomplished by administering Intralipid and a solution of 5% dextrose and 4.25% crystalline amino acids with electrolytes and vitamins. The Intralipid and the solution of amino acid and dextrose are given simultaneously through separate lines that come together just before entering a peripheral vein.

In comparing glucose and lipid as a source of calories, one can look at an average 3-L TPN regimen for both the glucose system and lipid system. Table 15-6 clearly shows that with the glucose system, in which 83% of the calories are supplied by glucose, the patient receives 77% more nonprotein calories and 50% more nitrogen than with the lipid system, in which 60% of the calories are supplied by lipid. When glucose is used as the only source of nonprotein calories in a TPN regimen, not only is a significantly greater number of calories delivered, but it is done at a substantial price savings (34%) to the patient. It is interesting to note that Intralipid is often considered the concentrated source of calories, but it has to be

TABLE 15-6. Comparison of Lipid System and Glucose System

System	Total Volume of TPN	Total Non-protein Calories	Total g Nitrogen	Total Daily Cost* to Patient	Cost/Cal
Glucose (4.25% amino acids 25% dextrose)	3 Liters	2550	18.75	$97.00	$0.038
Lipid (2 Liters-4.25% amino acids, 5% dextrose, 1 Liter Intralipid)	3 Liters	1440	12.50	$148.00	$0.10

* Patient cost at Hartford Hospital.

remembered that it is only a 10% fat emulsion and provides 1.1 kcal/ml in comparison to 0.85 kcal/ml from a 25% glucose solution. When a liter of Intralipid is administered with 2L of 5% dextrose (see Table 15-6), only 0.48 kcal/ml is delivered. In addition, the lipid system becomes impractical when more than 2000 nonprotein calories need to be provided peripherally (because of problems with phlebitis and meeting the dosage requirements of fat).

In summary, when fat is used as the major source of calories in TPN, it has the advantage of peripheral administration, but it delivers only a limited number of calories and nitrogen at a high cost to the patient. In contrast, when glucose is used as the only nonprotein source of calories in TPN, there is essentially no problem in delivering as many calories and grams of nitrogen as the patient requires for an anabolic response. The administration of 25% glucose does necessitate the use of a central venous line, but in most modern hospitals this should not present a major problem. In our institution, we usually recommend glucose as the source of calories in TPN, with Intralipid used primarily as a source of essential fatty acids for long term TPN patients.

SUMMARY

The task of parenteral nutrition is to insure the continuing existence and functional capability of body proteins. Energy, in the form of nonprotein calories, is required to synthesize proteins from amino acids, so it becomes important, for efficient protein synthesis, to determine as accurately as possible the specific caloric requirements of individual patients on TPN. We also have an obligation to provide the caloric requirements with the safest and most economical substrate. In our present state of knowledge, glucose seems to be the preferable substrate for nonprotein calories.

BIBLIOGRAPHY

1. Kinney, J.M.: Energy Requirements of the Surgery Patient, *In* Manual of Surgical Nutrition. W.F. Ballinger, et al., eds. Philadelphia, W.B. Saunders, 1975.
2. Long, C.G., and Blakemore, W.S.: Energy and protein requirements in the hospitalized patient. JPEN, *3:*69, 1979.
3. Gump, F.E., and Kinney, J.M.: Oxygen consumption and caloric expenditure in surgical patients. Surg. Gynecol. Obstet., *137:*499, 1973.
4. Tilstone, W.J.: Energy Requirements: Balance Concepts, *In* Parenteral Nutrition in Acute Metabolic Illness. H.A. Lee, ed. London, Academic Press, 1974.
5. Gazziniga, A.B., et al.: Indirect calorimetry as a guide to caloric replacement during total parenteral nutrition. Am. J. Surg., *136:*128, 1975.
6. Krause, M.V., and Hunscher, M.A.: Energy, *In* Food, Nutrition, and Diet Therapy. Philadelphia, W.B. Saunders, 1972.
7. Harris, H., and Benedict, B.: A biometric study of basal metabolism in man. Publication #279 of the Carnegie Institute, Washington, D.C., 1979.
8. Rutten, P., et al.: Determination of optimal hyperalimentation infusion rate. J. Surg. Res., *18:*477, 1975.
9. Blackburn, G.L., and Bistrian, B.R.: Nutritional care of the injured and/or septic patient. Surg. Clin. North Am., *56:*1206, 1976.
10. Wilmore, D.W., et al.: Catecholamines: mediator of the hypermetabolic responses to thermal injury. Ann. Surg., *180:*653, 1974.
11. Kaminski, M.V.: Hyperalimentation switching off

catabolism. Am. J. IV Ther., *Feb./March:*34, 1976.
12. Long, J.M.: Practical aspects of parenteral nutrition. Hospital Physician, *May:*36, 1974.
13. Spiro, H.M., et al.: Parenteral nutrition: total or partial; central or peripheral. Current Prescribing, *5:*33, 1979.
14. Bassler, K.H.: Metabolism of the Nutrient Substances Used for Parenteral Nutrition, *In* Parenteral Nutrition. F.W. Ahnefeld, et al., eds. Berlin, Springer-Verlag, 1976.
15. Goschke, N.A., et al.: Advantages and Disadvantages of Parenteral Hyperalimentation, *In* Parenteral Nutrition. F.W. Ahnefeld, et al., eds. Berlin, Springer-Verlag, 1976.
16. Hull, R.L.: Physiochemical considerations in intravenous hyperalimentation. Am. J. Hosp. Pharm., *31:*236, 1974.
17. Froesch, E.R.: The Metabolism of Glucose, Its Endocrine Control and Comparative Aspects with Fructose, Sorbitol, and Xylitol Metabolism, *In* Parenteral Nutrition in Acute Metabolic Illness. H.A. Lee, ed. London, Academic Press, 1974.
18. Wretland, A., and Schumer, W.: Carbohydrates and Fats, *In* Total Parenteral Nutrition. P.L. White and M.E. Nagy, eds. Acton, MA, Publishing Sciences Group, 1974.
19. Woods, H.F., and Alberti, K.G.M.M.: Dangers of intravenous fructose. Lancet, *2:*1354, 1972.
20. Thomas, D.W., Edwards, J.B., and Edwards, R.G.: Examination of xylitol. N. Engl. J. Med., *283:*437, 1970.
21. Lee, H.A.: The Alcohols—Ethanol, Sorbitol, Xylitol, *In* Parenteral Nutrition in Acute Metabolic Illness. H.A. Lee, ed. London, Academic Press, 1974.
22. Jeejeebhoy, K.N., et al.: Metabolic studies in total parenteral nutrition with lipid in man. J. Clin. Invest., *57:*125, 1976.
23. Hanson, L.M., Hardic, W.R., and Hildalgo, J.: Fat emulsion for intravenous administration: clinical experience with Intralipid 10%. Ann. Surg., *184:* 80, 1976.
24. Anon: Intralipid 10% IV fat emulsion: a major advance in IV lipid nutrition. Berkeley, CA, Cutter Laboratories, Inc., 1978.

Chapter 16

Total Parenteral Nutrition in Pediatrics

William R. Crom, Pharm.D.
Clinical Division of Pharmacy

Larry F. Barker, M.S., R.Ph.
Director of Pharmacy
St. Jude Children's Research Hospital
Memphis, Tennessee

Total parenteral nutrition (TPN) has become a widely used form of therapy, despite its relatively recent development. The first reported case of successful TPN was published by Helfrick and Abelson[1] in 1944. Using alternate infusions of a mixture of 50% glucose-10% casein hydrolysate and electrolytes, followed by a "do-it-yourself" homogenized olive oil-lecithin emulsion, these investigators were able to infuse 130 calories in 150 ml/per day via the ankle veins of a 5-month-old boy. Despite repeated thrombophlebitis, TPN was administered for 5 days. The child, who had been near death at the initiation of TPN, survived.

This success was not repeated until 1968, when Wilmore and Dudrick[2] treated a female infant with a short gut. Following surgery, her weight decreased steadily from 5 pounds 2 ounces at birth to 4 pounds at 19 days. She was then put on a 25% glucose-fibrin hydrolysate solution, administered via a catheter in her superior vena cava. She steadily gained weight to 18.5 pounds over 22 months of TPN.

In the decade since that first attempt to administer hypertonic TPN solution via a central venous catheter, TPN has become a valuable and sometimes lifesaving form of nutritional support. Today, a variety of commerical products are available for preparation of TPN solutions, and research and clinical experience have identified—and in some cases solved—the problems associated with this form of therapy.

CLINICAL USES

Many patients may become candidates for TPN. In pediatric practice, patients with surgical disease of the gastrointestinal tract, especially newborn infants, form one important group. Other patients in whom TPN is used are those with chronic intestinal obstruction resulting from adhesions or peritoneal sepsis, bowel fistulas, chronic severe diarrhea, extensive body burns, and abdominal tumors treated by surgery, irradiation, and chemotherapy. Low-birth-weight infants have also been treated with TPN, although the efficacy and safety of TPN in this group of patients has not been conclusively demonstrated.[3] Among older children and adults, those who have surgery or trauma to the GI tract, chronic disease of the GI tract (ulcerative colitis, Crohn's disease), or cancer of the abdomen or GI tract often benefit from TPN.

Some patients with severely impaired GI function have received long-term TPN at home. With the example of home hemodialysis, or "artificial kidney," for renal-failure patients, home TPN has been described as the "concept of artificial gut." This therapy requires that the patient remain in a relatively stable clinical state and have a suitable home environment with supportive family members who are able to prepare and administer the TPN solutions.

Malnutrition is often a problem in patients with renal failure or hepatic failure. Such patients also benefit from TPN, but they have special requirements that necessitate a somewhat different approach. (Nutritional therapy in these disease states will not be discussed in greater detail here, but a new amino-acid solution [Nephramine] has been marketed specifically for use in patients with renal failure. A corresponding amino-acid solution for patients with hepatic failure is currently in clinical trials.)

NUTRITIONAL REQUIREMENTS

The general nutritive requirements for TPN are amino acids, calories, electrolytes and minerals, vitamins, essential fatty acids, and trace minerals. The available sources for meeting these requirements have dramatically increased in number and improved in quality over the past decade. Amino acids may be administered as either casein hydrolysates or as crystalline amino acids (CAA) mixtures. The CAA solutions are rapidly becoming the preferred source, due to less lot-to-lot variation in the composition of the CAA mixtures. Additionally, only about 50% of the total nitrogen content of protein hydrolysates consists of amino acids. The remainder consists of di-, tri-, or even larger polypeptides, the precise metabolic fate of which is unknown. Nearly 100% of the nitrogen content of CAA solutions is available as free amino acids.

Calories are usually administered as a glucose solution, although fat emulsions are increasingly being used as a calorie source. When administered as hydrous glucose, a gram of glucose provides 3.4 calories, so a 25% glucose solution has about 0.85 kcal/ml. A 10% fat emulsion has about 1.1 kcal/ml, of which 0.9 calories are provided by lipid. One advantage of lipid fat emulsions as a calorie source is isotonicity. A 25% glucose solution has an osmolarity of about 1800 mOsm/L, and it can be administered only by a central-vein catheter. A 10% fat emulsion has an osmolarity of about 300 mOsm/L, and it can be administered via a peripheral vein. Thus, fat emulsions are an additional important caloric source in TPN.

Electrolytes (such as potassium, sodium, and chloride) and minerals (such as calcium, magnesium, and phosphorus) are available as a variety of salts for parenteral use. Fat and water-soluble vitamins are available as a mixture in fixed concentrations for parenteral use (MVI), but this product does not contain vitamins K, B_{12}, or folic acid. These may be administered intramuscularly at regular intervals or may be added to the TPN solutions in excess amounts (since not all of the vitamins will necessarily be utilized, because of compatibility problems).

Essential fatty acids are administered in sufficiently large amounts when fat emulsions are used as a calorie source. Alternatively, prevention of essential-fatty-acid deficiency has been achieved by daily cutaneous application of sunflower-seed oil.

Body stores of such trace minerals as zinc, copper, iodine, chromium, manganese, and iron may become deficient after several weeks of TPN. Only recently have trace mineral products for parenteral use become commercially available, and in the past many institutions extemporaneously prepared sterile solutions of trace minerals for addition to TPN solutions. Periodic blood or plasma transfusions have been suggested as another means of meeting these requirements. Iron is usually administered intramuscularly on a weekly basis, when required.

Protein and calorie requirements vary according to age, weight, and clinical condition. In general, protein and calories should be provided in a ratio of 150 nonprotein calories per gram of nitrogen. The nitrogen content of protein varies, but it is usually one gram per 6.0 to 6.25 grams of protein. Thus a balance of 24 to 25 nonprotein calories per gram of protein is considered the optimum

TABLE 16-1. Protein Requirements

	Infants and Young Children[6]	Adults[7]
Normal	2.4 g/kg/day	1.0-1.5 g/kg/day
Post-surgery	2.5-3.0 g/kg/day	1.3-1.5 g/kg/day
Infection	2.5-3.5 g/kg/day	1.5-1.8 g/kg/day
Severe sepsis	3.0-3.5 g/kg/day	1.7-2.2 g/kg/day
Burns (30-100% body-surface area)	3.5-4.0 g/kg/day	1.8-2.7 g/kg/day

for utilization of amino acids in anabolic processes. Any caloric contribution of the protein content of TPN solutions is disregarded, since the goal of TPN is to produce a positive nitrogen balance and anabolism, and the protein in TPN is not intended for use by the body as a caloric source.

The usual daily requirements for infants, children, and adults of protein, calories, electrolytes and minerals, and trace elements are summarized in Tables 16-1 through 16-4. These figures provide only a general guideline for a starting point in TPN, and each patient must be carefully monitored to assess individual needs and tolerances, with the dosage of each ingredient adjusted accordingly.

TABLE 16-2. Calorie Requirements

Age	kcal/kg/day
0-6 mos.	120
6-12 mos.	100
Over 12 mos.	1000 + (100 × age in years)
Adult	2500+

COMPLICATIONS

As might be anticipated, administration of large amounts of nutrients parenterally may lead to a variety of metabolic complications. Because of the large quantities of glucose being administered carbohydrate metabolism is markedly altered. Hyperglycemia and glycosuria, with osmotic diuresis and secondary changes in water and electrolyte metabolism, are constant threats, especially during the early stages of TPN. This adverse effect can be minimized by slowly increasing the rate of glucose administration to the desired number of calories, over a period of 3 to 5 days, thus allowing the body to adjust endogenous insulin production. Hyperglycemia and glycosuria can be corrected by slowing the rate of infusion, decreasing the concentration of glucose in the TPN solution, or adding exogenous regular insulin to the TPN solution. Hypoglycemia may occur when TPN with a high glucose concentration is abruptly stopped. This is a rebound effect, caused by circulating levels of endogenous insulin that have been induced by the high glucose load. This may be avoided by slowly decreasing the rate of

TABLE 16-3. Electrolyte and Mineral Requirements[5]

	Infants and Young Children	Adults
Sodium	3-5 mEq/kg/day	60 + mEq/day
Potassium	3-5 mEq/kg/day	60 + mEq/day
Chloride	Same as sodium	Same as sodium
Calcium	0.1 mEq/kg/day	10-20 mEq/day
Phosphorus	0.65-1.3 mMoles/day	10-15 mMoles/day
Magnesium	0.3-0.5 mEq/kg/day	10-30 mEq/day

TABLE 16-4. Trace Mineral Requirements[5,8]

	Infants and Young Children	Adults
Zinc	100 μg/kg/day*	2.5-4.0 mg/day
Copper	20 μg/kg/day	0.5-1.5 mg/day
Iron	1 mg/kg/day	1-2 mg/day
Manganese	2-10 μg/kg/day	0.15-0.8 μg/day
Iodide	3-5 μg/kg/day	1-2 mg/day
Fluoride	1 μg/kg/day	1-2 mg/day
Chromium	0.14-0.2 μg/kg/day	10-15 μg/day

* The zinc dosage for premature infants (weight less than 1500 g) up to 3 kg of body weight is 300 μg/kg/day. For children over 5 years of age, the adult zinc dosage applies, up to a maximum dosage of 4 mg/day.

TPN administration before stopping TPN. If the infusion is suddenly terminated, then 10% dextrose solution in water should be administered by either the central line or a peripheral vein for a few hours to prevent rebound hypoglycemia. This will allow insulin production to decrease to more usual levels.

There are also problems related to amino acid metabolism. Hyperammonemia has been reported,[3] generally in infants less than 6 months of age. Initially, this was thought to be a result of excessive amounts of preformed ammonia in protein hydrolysates or due to hepatic immaturity. However, it has also occurred during therapy with FreAmine, a CAA solution. This condition responds readily to arginine infusions and may be due to a relative deficiency of arginine in FreAmine. It is a rare complication with newer CAA solutions. Prerenal azotemia may occur as a result of excessive protein infusion or inappropriate ratio of calories (nonprotein) to protein.

Imbalances of electrolytes and minerals may also occur. Deficiencies of phosphorus may lead to decreased levels of erythrocyte 2,3-DPG and to increased affinity of hemoglobin for oxygen. This may further compromise oxygenation of tissues in a patient who has a respiratory disease or anemia. This can be avoided by monitoring serum phosphorus levels and adjusting the phosphorus content of the TPN solution accordingly.

Hypo- or hypercalcemia may be seen in patients receiving TPN. Hypocalcemia may result from inadequate calcium administration or as a reciprocal response to phosphorus repletion without simultaneous calcium infusion. Hypercalcemia may result from excessive calcium administration. Malnourished patients may also have low albumin levels, and the ratio of free to protein-bound calcium may be altered.

Deficiencies or excesses of sodium, chloride, potassium, and magnesium may occur as the result of too much or too little of these minerals in TPN solutions. This can be avoided or corrected by close monitoring of serum levels and adjustment of the amount of each in TPN solutions. It is important to keep in mind that hypokalemia and hypomagnesemia are likely to occur when anabolism and new tissue growth are taking place, since both are intracellular cations and requirements for both will be correspondingly high during periods of new cell formation. Although uncommon, hypomagnesemia has been reported to cause seizures in patients receiving TPN.

Essential fatty acid deficiencies may result after long periods of lipid-free TPN. This is less common now, with the routine use of intravenous fat emulsions. This deficiency is manifested as a generalized skin rash—a dry, scaly, usually erythematous skin eruption. Diffuse hair loss is frequently seen, especially in infants. Wound healing may be impaired.

Body stores of copper and zinc may become deficient if these trace minerals are not added to TPN solutions.[4] Copper deficiency may be manifested by anemia, neutropenia, hypoproteinemia, osteoporosis, deep pigmentation of skin and hair, hypotonia, and psychomotor retardation. Zinc deficiency may produce psoriasiform dermatitis, hair loss, inflammatory paronychia-like lesions, growth retardation, and diarrhea. Neither deficiency may be observed until the patient has received several weeks of TPN therapy. Although other trace minerals are often added to TPN solutions, deficiencies of these minerals have not been well described.

Vitamin deficiencies may be avoided by daily addition of vitamins to TPN solutions. Vitamin K deficiencies may result in abnormal blood coagulation (elevated prothrombin time).

Disorders of hepatic function and structure may be seen.[3] There are consistent, modest rises in serum transaminases, lactic dehydrogenase, and bilirubin concentrations when TPN is initiated. Hepatomegaly is sometimes seen as well. This may be related to excess deposition of glycogen or fat in the liver. The condition is usually transient, despite continuation of TPN.

Metabolic acidosis has occasionally been a problem, especially in infants. Although the administration of large quantities of amino acids might be expected to produce this condition, the actual amount of titratable acidity in the amino acid solutions is insufficient to account for the degree of acidosis seen. The cause has been identified as a "cation gap" in the CAA mixtures.[3] Both arginine and lysine are present in some products as hydrochloride salts, which generate hydrochloric acid on metabolism. The acidosis can be corrected (or avoided) by determining the chloride content of the protein source being used and then adding a corresponding amount of sodium or potassium as the acetate salt, instead of the chloride salt. Ideally, the total chloride content of a TPN solution should match the sodium content. The balance of the cations in the TPN solution may be added as other salts (phosphate, acetate, gluconate, and the like). Acetate is a metabolizable salt and a bicarbonate source.

The most significant nonmetabolic complication of TPN is sepsis. Although the hypertonicity of TPN solutions inhibits bacterial growth, they provide a good medium for fungal growth, especially Candida species. The most effective control of this complication is adherence to strict aseptic principles during catheter insertion, catheter care, and mixing of TPN solutions. Central-vein catheters should not be used for other purposes, such as infusion of other drugs, obtaining blood samples, or taking central-venous-pressure readings. Fungal infections usually resolve after removal of the central-vein catheter, but, occcasionaly, immunosuppressed patients, such as those receiving cancer chemotherapy, may require systemic therapy with amphotericin B. There does not appear to be any evidence supporting the suggestion that amphotericin, pushed periodically through the catheter, may reduce sepsis from Candida, and the adverse effects of this drug outweigh any potential benefit of this technique.

Thrombosis and catheter displacement occur occasionally. Malposition and perforation are avoidable with good technique.

SUMMARY

Total parenteral nutrition is most successful in those institutions that use an interdisciplinary team with specific responsibility for care of the patient receiving TPN. The essential members of this team are a physician, nurse, and pharmacist. Responsive microbiologic and chemistry laboratory support is also of paramount importance. The metabolic and septic complications of TPN are largely avoidable when it is administered by a well-trained and dedicated team. It is likely that as further definition of the risks and indications and refinements of technique are made, TPN will become even more widely used and important in pediatric practice.

BIBLIOGRAPHY

1. Helfrick, F.W., and Abelson, N.M.: Intravenous feeding of a complete diet in a child: report of a case. J. Pediatr. *25:*400, 1944.
2. Wilmore, D.W., and Dudrick, S.V.: Growth and development of an infant receiving all nutrients exclusively by vein. JAMA, *203:*860, 1968.
3. Heird, W.C., and Winters, R.W.: Parenteral Nutrition: Pediatrics, *In* Nutritional Support of Medical Practice. H.A. Schneider, C.E. Anderson, and D.B. Coursin, eds. Hagerstown, MD, Harper and Row, 1977.
4. Briggaman, R.A., and Crounse, R.G.: Skin, *In* Nutritional Support of Medical Practice. H.A. Schneider, C.E. Anderson, and D.B. Coursin, eds. Hagerstown, MD, Harper and Row, 1977.
5. Shils, M.C.: Guidelines for total parenteral nutrition. JAMA, *220:*1721, 1972.
6. Dudrick, S.J., Copeland, E.M., and MacFadyen, B.V.: Long-term parenteral nutrition: its current status. Hosp. Pract., *10:*47, 1975.
7. Blackburn, G.L., and Bistrian, B.R.: Curative Nutrition: Protein-Calorie Management, *In* Nutritional Support of Medical Practice. H.A. Schneider, C.E. Anderson, and D.B. Coursin, eds. Hagerstown, MD, Harper and Row, 1977.
8. AMA Department of Foods and Nutrition: Guidelines for essential trace element preparations for parenteral use; a statement by an expert panel. JAMA, *241:*2051, 1979.

Chapter 17

Central Versus Peripheral Nutrition: The Controversy

Brack A. Bivins, M.D.
College of Medicine

Robert P. Rapp, Pharm.D.
College of Pharmacy
Department of Surgery
University of Kentucky Medical Center
Lexington, Kentucky

Clinical nutrition is a rapidly growing area for scientific inquiry and clinical practice. More than 35,000 articles were published on nutrition-related topics worldwide during the 5-year period 1975 to 1978.[1] This information explosion makes it difficult to select either a starting point for study or a conclusion for practical application. The current controversy concerning the validity of peripheral parenteral nutrition versus central parenteral nutrition reflects many unknowns of the clinical applications of nutrition science.

"Nutrition" may be defined as the act or process of nourishing. "Nourish" means to promote growth. Utilizing these two definitions then, "parenteral nutrition" must be the administration of nutrients by the intravascular route to promote growth. Basically, two parenteral nutrition systems are available at the present time—central and peripheral (see Table 17-1). The central nutrition scheme can be divided into two types: the first is the glucose and amino acid system pioneered in this country by Dudrick and his associates[2–5]; the second is the lipid system developed in Europe.[6–9] These two systems differ only in the role of intravenous fat in total parenteral nutrition, since both systems require central venous administration of hypertonic glucose and amino acids, and both systems are designed to promote growth of tissue. The European lipid system uses fat more liberally as a calo-

TABLE 17-1. Central and Peripheral Nutrition Systems

	Central		Peripheral
	Glucose System	Lipid System	Amino Acid System
Administration	Central	Central (Peripheral**)	Peripheral
Objective	Synthesis	Synthesis	Stasis
Nutrients			
Glucose	Yes	Yes	No
Lipid	(Yes*)	Yes	No
Amino acids	Yes	Yes	Yes

* Lipid given as source of essential fatty-acids rather than as a caloric source.
** Peripheral use limited by the development of infusion phlebitis.

ric source than is usually the case in the United States, where lipid is most often used as a dietary supplement to prevent essential-fatty-acid deficiency. The peripheral nutrition scheme, as outlined by Blackburn and his associates, is designed to spare endogenous protein by promoting intravenous amino acids as an energy source.[10–14] Since hypertonic glucose is not required, the solutions may be given by peripheral vein. The objective of the peripheral amino-acid system is to prevent deterioration (i.e., achieve stasis) rather than to promote growth.

The controversial aspects of the two systems revolve around two questions. The first is the metabolic question of whether or not carbohydrate is required to achieve protein sparing. The second is the clinical question of what should be the objective of nutrition therapy. To attempt to answer these two questions requires an overview of the clinical significance of malnutrition, the essentials of starvation metabolism, and the effects of parenteral nutrition.

MALNUTRITION

Malnutrition, defined as faulty or inadequate nutrition, encompasses the morbidly obese, the cola and french fries fast-food culture, the protein-calorie malnourished third-world populations, and the critically ill catabolic patients seen in our hospitals. The clinical problem of malnutrition is seen in the latter group who, as defined by Dudrick "cannot eat, should not eat, will not eat, or cannot eat enough."[5]

The extent of malnutrition can be calculated in a variety of ways.[15] One traditional technique is to express malnutrition as a function of weight loss, body appearance, and strength. Slightly more sophisticated are the anthropomorphic measurements, including the skin-fold thickness and arm-muscle circumference. The creatinine-height index is a reflection of body muscle mass. Severe protein-calorie malnutrition is marked by decreases in serum albumin, transferrin, and total iron-binding capacity. Starvation may be associated with anergy to common skin-test antigens, such as mumps. Nutritional repletion restores the delayed hypersensitivity reaction. Nitrogen-balance studies relate the intake of protein to the excretion of the protein-catabolic product urea. Protein utilization may also be determined.

When these nutritional assessment techniques are applied to hospitalized patients, 40 to 70% can be shown to be malnourished to some extent.[16–19] Severe malnutrition is generally accepted as an indication for nutritional support, but unfortunately, the clinical significance of mild and moderate degrees of malnutrition is not known. Clinically, the severely malnourished patient is weak, tired, irritable, and depressed.[20] The patient is anemic and may have leukopenia, and of course, there is evidence of weight loss.[20]

The severely malnourished patient may evidence poor healing of soft tissue and bone, diminished ability to combat infection, and decreased ability to withstand operative stress. Studley in 1936 found that patients who had lost greater than 20% of their ideal weight preoperatively had a tenfold greater operative mortality than did patients with less than a 20% weight loss.[21] One reason for this increased mortality was outlined by Daly in 1972, when he demonstrated that colonic tissue in malnourished rats had a lower tinsel strength and poorer healing ability than the colon of normal rats.[22] Alexander has extended these studies to include the immune system in human patients.[23] Burn patients who were supported nutritionally had both a lower sepsis rate and a lower death rate than did patients who were not on nutritional support.

Adequacy of nutritional support varies with the clinical situation. The average 70 kg male requires approximately 1800 kcal per day to maintain ideal weight. A 70 kg male who has undergone an uncomplicated operative procedure also requires 1800 kcal per day, but if this is to be provided parenterally, then approximately 2700 kcal must be given to get 1800 kcal utilized (due to the less effective use of parenteral calories.[24,25] A severely injured patient may increase his basal metabolic rate by 80%, so that 3200 calories may be required for nutritional balance. When the poor utilization of parenteral calories is considered, then the severely injured may require 5000 or more calories just for maintenance.

STARVATION METABOLISM

The human body stores the majority of excess calories as fat (9.4 kcal/g); a smaller number of calories are stored as protein (5.6 kcal/g); and only a small fraction of total body calories are carbohydrate (hydrated carbohydrate, 3.4 kcal/g). The sequence of starvation metabolism has been outlined in a series of articles by Cahill.[26–28] Circulating carbohydrate is adequate for fuel for only a short period of time. Within 24 hours, a 75 kg male will begin breaking down approximately 75 g of protein per day and approximately 60 g of fat per day. The protein is fragmented into amino acids which enter the gluconeogenic system. The fat stores are mobilized as triglycerides, which are broken down into glycerol and free fatty acids, which then form ketones used by peripheral muscle.

If starvation is continued over a 5- to 6-week period, further metabolic adaptation occurs. Protein utilization as a calorie source decreases from 75 g per day to 20 g per day. The utilization of triglycerides increases. Ketones are used as the predominant calorie source.

The adaptive phases of starvation can be summarized as follows: (1) in early starvation, fat and protein serve as caloric sources while glycogen is recycled; (2) in late or prolonged starvation, fat predominates as the calorie source, so less protein is utilized and available glucose is recycled.

Utilizing this scheme as an outline for the effects of starvation, it appears that fat, protein, and carbohydrate may be administered as energy sources. In fact, each of these can be and have been used for parenteral nutrition. Gamble demonstrated the protein-sparing effects of glucose in the 1920s; Elman used parenteral amino acids as a calorie source in the 1930s; and in the 1960s, fat was effectively used as a parenteral source of calories.[29–34] The problem encountered with each of these nutritional schemes was how to supply an adequate number of calories. Coupled with that is the observation that the number of nonprotein calories seemed to be critical if long-term support with a positive nitrogen balance was to be achieved.[6,9]

CENTRAL TPN

The Hypertonic Glucose and Amino Acid System

The use of hypertonic glucose resolved the problem of adequate nonprotein calories. The destruction of veins by the hypertonic solution initially limited the duration of glucose-based nutrition. Dudrick, Wilmore, Vars, and Rhoads applied the central-venous cannulation technique, developed by Aubianiac in 1952, to total parenteral nutrition.[2,3,35] Cannulation of the subclavian vein provided a high-flow site for administration of the hypertonic solution. The central-venous catheter could be left in place for days, weeks, or in some cases, months, so that total parenteral nutrition with adequate calories and other nutrients for growth became a reality.

The initial solutions contained 20% glucose, added amino acids from protein hydrolysate, electrolytes, vitamins, and trace minerals.[2–5] The ratio of calories commonly used is 120 to 220 carbohydrate calories per gram of nitrogen in the final mixture. Parenteral fat becomes a necessity when total parenteral nutrition continues beyond 2 to 3 weeks to prevent the development of essential fatty-acid deficiency.[32,33,36]

This system has proven its utility for a variety of difficult clinical situations. It can be used as supportive therapy for the surgical patient, for restoration of weight and positive nitrogen-balance preoperatively, or as nutritional support postoperatively to allow time for gastrointestinal recovery.[4,5,38] The patient with anorexia nervosa can be treated with total parenteral nutrition.[5] Intravenous nutrition may be used as adjunct to cancer chemotherapy.[39,40] Centrally administered nutrition may serve as a primary therapy for patients with enterocutaneous fistulas or Crohn's disease.[4,5,38,41]

The central system of total parenteral nutrition can be hazardous. Metabolic complications are associated with the administration of glucose and amino acids.[42] The glucose-related complications include hyperglycemia, coma, and reactive hypoglycemia. Aminoacidemia, hyperchloremic alkalosis, and hypophosphatemia may complicate amino acid administration. Deficiency states of trace minerals and essential fatty acids may, also, develop. The technical complications associated with placement of the central venous catheter may be expected in 36% of patients.[43–45]

The Lipid System

The lipid system of total parenteral nutrition differs little in concept from the glucose system. In the lipid system, parenteral fat is utilized for a substantial portion of the nonprotein calories.[6–9,37] Originally, it was hoped that the combination of fat, low-concentration glucose, amino acids, electrolytes, vitamins, and minerals would be adequate for nutritional support, and that this could be administered through a peripheral vein (since parenteral fat is isoosmotic in concentrations up to 30%). Unfortunately, peripheral use of this solution is limited by infusion thrombophlebitis, so that within a few days of therapy, a central venous catheter must be placed.[6,37]

PERIPHERAL PROTEIN-SPARING

The peripheral system for parenteral nutrition relies on infused amino acids with no nonprotein calorie source added.[10–14] The basis for this scheme is adaptive starvation, whereby ketones become the primary energy source and protein is spared.[12–14,26–28] Infused amino acids are then used as an energy source. Blackburn, one of the principal proponents of amino-acid infusion, suggests that there is a metabolic fuel-regulatory system that is influenced by input of glucose or amino acids.[10] Addition of glucose increases insulin production and decreases the mobilization and utilization of free fatty acids and amino acids. In contrast, the addition of amino acids suppresses insulin production, so that gluconeogenesis is preserved and free fatty-acid mobilization is increased.

This system conflicts with at least two areas of standard teaching. First, it has been believed that certain body tissues, especially the central nervous system, could use only glucose as an energy substrate. If that were so, adaptive starvation with the use of ketones as a primary energy source would not apply to all tissues, and there would be a continuing need for glucose whether given parenterally or derived through gluconeogenesis from the catabolism of muscle protein. More recent studies have demonstrated that ketones can be used as energy substrates in the so-called "glucose-dependent" tissues such as red blood cells and neural tissue.[46,47]

The second major area of conflict lies with the concept of protein sparing. It has been believed since the early work by Gamble that, without a glucose source, endogenous protein would be catabolized. Work by Blackburn and others has demonstrated that protein catabolism can be suppressed by adaptive starvation and that protein sparing can be enhanced by the administration of amino acids.[10–14,45,48–50] Unfortunately, the result is not a consistently positive nitrogen balance and growth, but merely a slowing of the rate of protein breakdown.[51] The goal of the proponents of peripheral amino-acid administration, then, is not growth and synthesis but, rather, preservation of protein, or stasis.

Within the limited objective of reducing the rate of protein catabolism, there seem to be two uses for peripheral amino-acid administration. First, since this solution is not hypertonic, it may be administered through a peripheral vein. This allows nutritional support to be given to the patient whose degree of malnutrition is not sufficient to justify the technical hazards of deep venous cannulation and administration of hypertonic glucose and amino acids. This may be of some benefit in the reasonably well-nourished patient who is expected to be deprived of oral nutrition for a short period of time. A second use of the amino-acid system would be for those patients in whom glucose administration is undesirable and fatty-acid mobilization is highly desirable, as in weight-reduction therapy.

A potential area for application of the amino-acid system may be the severely stressed patient with a major burn, systemic sepsis, or multiple trauma. These patients mobilize endogenous fats and proteins very quickly, while insulin production is suppressed and hyperglycemia appears.[52–54] Further increases in glucose by administration of hypertonic glucose would not be expected to improve utilization in the face of insulin suppression and resistance. As substrate utilization in these patients is clarified, a specific amino-acid mixture or lipid emulsion may be identified as the optimal energy source during the acute period of stress.

SUMMARY

When central and peripheral total parenteral nutrition are compared, the key clinical difference seems to be synthesis (growth) with central nutrition, contrasted to stasis (preservation of protein) with peripheral nutrition. The technical difference is that central nutrition requires placement of a central venous catheter, with the attendant hazards, whereas peripheral nutrition is carried out through a peripheral vein. Central nutrition has been demonstrated to be an effective means of nutritional support for large numbers of patients, while the precise role of peripheral amino-acid administration has not yet been defined.

BIBLIOGRAPHY

1. Rombeau, J.L.: Editorial comment. J. Paren. and Ent. Nutr., *2:*246, 1978.
2. Dudrick, S.J., et al.: Long-term total parenteral nutrition with growth, development, and positive nitrogen balance. Surgery, *64:*134, 1968.
3. Dudrick, S.J., et al.: Can intravenous feeding as the sole means of nutrition support growth in the child and restore weight loss in an adult? An affirmative answer. Ann. Surg., *169:*974, 1969.
4. Dudrick, S.J., and Copeland, E.M.: Parenteral hyperalimentation, *In* Surgery Annal. L.M. Nyhus, ed. New York, Appleton-Century-Crofts, 1973.
5. Dudrick, S.J., and Ruberg, R.L.: Principles and practice of parenteral nutrition. Gastroenterol., *61:*901, 1971.
6. Wretlind, A.: Parenteral nutrition. Surg. Clin. North Am. *58:*155, 1978.
7. Hallberg, D., Schuberth, O., Wretlind, A.: Experimental and clinical studies with fat emulsion for intavenous nutrition. Nutr. Dieta., *8:*245, 1966.
8. Schuberth, O., and Wretlind, A.: Intravenous infusion of fat emulsions phosphatides and emulsifying agents. Acta Chir. Scand., *278*(Suppl.):1, 1961.
9. Wretlind, A.: Complete intravenous nutrition. Theoretical and experimental background. Nutr. Metab., *14*(Suppl):1, 1972.
10. Blackburn, G.L., and Reinhoff, H.Y., Jr.: Isotonic Crystalline Amino Acids for Protein Sparing, *In* Advances in Parenteral Nutrition. I.D.A. Johnston, ed. Lancaster, England, MTP Press, 1978.
11. Blackburn, G.L. et al.: Peripheral intravenous feeding with isotonic amino acid solutions. Am. J. Surg., *125:*447, 1973.
12. Blackburn, G.L., et al.: Protein sparing therapy during periods of starvation with sepsis or trauma. Ann. Surg., *177:*588, 1973.
13. Flatt, J.P., and Blackburn, G.L.: The metabolic fuel regulatory system: Implications for protein sparing therapy during caloric deprivation or disease. Am. J. Clin. Nutr. *27:*175, 1974.
14. Miller, J.D., et al.: Failure of postoperative infection to increase nitrogen excretion in patients maintained on peripheral amino acids. Am. J. Clin. Nutr., *30:*1523, 1977.
15. Kaminsky, M.V., and Jeejeebhoy, K.N.: Nutritional assessment—Diagnosis of malnutrition and selection of therapy. Am. J. IV Therapy Clin. Nutr., *6:*31, 1979.
16. Butterworth, C.E., and Blackburn, G.L.: Hospital malnutrition. Nutr. Today, *10:*8, 1975.
17. Bistrian, B.R., et al.: Prevalence of malnutrition in general medical patients. JAMA, *235:*1567, 1976.
18. Bistrian, B.R., et al.: Protein status of general surgical patients. JAMA, *230:*858, 1974.
19. Willcutts, H.D.: Nutritional assessment of 1000 surgical patients in an affluent suburban community hospital. J. Paren. and Ent. Nutr., *125:*125, 1977.
20. Levenson, S.M., Crowley, L.V., and Siefter, E.: Starvation, *In* Manual of Surgical Nutrition. W.F. Ballinger, et al., eds. Philadelphia, W.B. Saunders, 1975.

21. Studley, H.O.: Percentage of weight loss, a basic indicator of surgical risk. JAMA, *106:*458, 1936.
22. Daly, J.M., Vars, H.M., and Dudrick, S.J.: Effects of protein depletion on strength of chronic anastomoses. Surg. Gynec. Obstet., *134:*15, 1972.
23. Alexander, J.W.: Emergent concepts in the control of surgical infections. Surgery, *75:*934, 1974.
24. Kinney, J.N.: A consideration of energy exchange in human trauma. Bull. NY Acad. Med., *36:*617, 1960.
25. Kinney, J.N., et al.: Carbohydrate and nitrogen metabolism after injury. J. Clin. Path., *23*(Suppl) (R. Coll. Path.):65, 1970.
26. Cahill, G.F., Jr.: Starvation in man. New Engl. J. Med., *282:*668, 1970.
27. Cahill, G.F., Jr., et al.: Hormone—fuel inter-relationships during fasting. J. Clin. Invest., *45:*1751, 1966.
28. Cahill, G.F., Jr., and Owen, O.E.: Amino acid metabolism during prolonged starvation. J. Clin. Invest., *48:*584, 1969.
29. Gamble, J.L.: Physiologic information gained from studies on the life ration. Harvey Lecture, *42:*247, 1947.
30. Elman, R.: Time factors in utilization of a mixture of amino acids (Protein hydrolysate) and dextrose given intravenously. J. Clin. Nutr., *1:*287, 1953.
31. Elman, R., and Weiner, D.O.: Intravenous alimentation with special reference to protein (amino acid) metabolism. JAMA, *112:*796, 1939.
32. Lehr, H.B., et al.: The use of intravenous fat emulsions in surgical patients. JAMA, *181:*745, 1962.
33. Lehr, H.B., et al.: Clinical experiences with intravenous fat emulsions. Metab., *6*(2):666, 1957.
34. Hakansson, I.: Experience in long-term studies on nine intravenous fat emulsions in dogs. Nutr. Dieta., *10:*54, 1968.
35. Aubianiac, R.: L'injection intraveneuse sousclaviculaire: avantages et technique. Presse Med., *60:* 1456, 1952.
36. MacFadyen, B.V., et al.: Triglyceride and free fatty acid clearances in patients receiving complete parenteral nutrition using a 10% soybean oil emulsion. Surg. Gynec. Obstet., *137:*813, 1973.
37. Wilmore, D.W.: Role of Lipid as a Source of Nonprotein Calories, *In* Advances in Parenteral Nutrition. D.A. Johnston, ed. Lancaster, England, MTP Press, 1978.
38. Dudrick, S.J., and Duke, J.H., Jr.: Nutritional Complications in the Surgical Patient, *In* Management of Surgical Complications. C.P. Ards and J.D. Hardy, eds. Philadelphia, W.B. Saunders, 1975.
39. Copeland, E.M., and Dudrick, S.J.: Nutritional Aspects of Cancer, *In* Current Problems in Cancer. Vol. 1. R.C. Hicky, ed. Chicago, Yearbook Medical Publishers, 1976.
40. Copeland, E.M., et al.: Intravenous hyperalimentation as an adjunct to cancer chemotherapy. Am. J. Surg., *129:*167, 1975.
41. MacFadyen, B.V., Jr., Dudrick, S.J., and Ruberg, R.L.: The management of gastrointestinal fistulas with parenteral hyperalimentation. Surgery, *74:* 100, 1973.
42. Dudrick, S.J., et al.: Parenteral hyperalimentation: Metabolic problems and solutions. Ann. Surg., *176:*259, 1972.
43. Hauswald, K.R., Bivins, B.A., and Griffen, W.O., Jr.: Analysis of safety factors in percutaneous deep venous cannulation. Am. J. Surg., *127:*623, 1974.
44. Smith, B.E., et al.: Complications of subclavian vein catheterization. Arch. Surg., *20:*288, 1965.
45. Henzel, J.H., and Deweese, M.J.: Morbid and mortal complications associated with prolonged central venous cannulation. Am. J. Surg., *121:*600, 1971.
46. Owen, O.E., et al.: Brain metabolism during fasting. J. Clin. Invest., *16:*1589, 1967.
47. Marliss, E.B., and Nakhooda, A.F.: Ketosis and protein-sparing in man. Clin. Res., *22:*751A, 1974.
48. Greenberg, G.R., et al.: Protein sparing therapies in postoperative patients: Effective added hydrochloric glucose or lipid. New Engl. J. Med., *294:* 1411, 1976.
49. Freeman, J.B., et al.: Current status of protein sparing. Surg. Gynec. Obstet., *144:*843, 1977.
50. Hoover, H.C., et al.: Nitrogen sparing intravenous fluids in postoperative patients. New Engl. J. Med., *293:*172, 1975.
51. Wolfe, B.M., et al.: Substrate interaction in intravenous feeding: Comparative effects of carbohydrate and fat on amino acid utilization in fasting man. Ann. Surg., *186:*518, 1977.
52. Gump, F.E., et al.: The significance of altered gluconeogenesis in surgical catabolism. J. Trauma, *15:*704, 1975.
53. Clowes, G.H.A., et al.: Energy metabolism in sepsis. Ann. Surg., *179:*684, 1974.
54. O'Donnell, T.F., et al.: Proteolysis associated with a deficit of peripheral energy fuel substrates in septic man. Surgery, *80:*192, 1976.

Chapter 18

The Role of Trace Elements in Intravenous Nutrition

Raymond J. Muller, M.S., R.Ph.
Sr. TPN Clinical Pharmacist
Division of Pharmacy Services
and Clinical Nutrition Service
Memorial Sloan Kettering Cancer Center
New York, New York

Terry L. Pipp, Pharm.D.
Clinical Instructor
Division of Clinical Pharmacy
School of Pharmacy
University of California, San Francisco

Certain minerals present in tissue, although in only minute quantities, are essential nutrients.[1] Their presence has been long overlooked because of the failure to recognize their physiologic importance coupled with the inability to analyze them. Trace elements, trace minerals, micronutrient elements, or minor elements are general terms used for these nutrients. They perform vital functions necessary for the maintenance of life, growth and reproduction. In general, trace elements are involved with the catalysis of enzymes, stabilization and synthesis of protein, nerve conduction, muscle contraction, and nutrient transport.[2]

To be considered essential, a trace element must be present in all healthy tissue of the organism and in relatively constant concentration. Additionally, the omission of the element should produce similar structural and physiologic defects in different species. These defects must be prevented or reversed by the addition of the trace element.[3]

The elements currently recognized as fulfilling these requirements include chromium, cobalt, copper, fluoride, iodine, iron, manganese, molybdenum, nickel, selenium, silicon, tin, vanadium, and zinc. To date, human deficiency states have been described with cobalt, copper, iodine, iron, and zinc. Some evidence also exists that chromium and manganese are essential, but the exact requirements are controversial.[4] There has been a recent report of a selenium deficiency during long-term total parenteral nutrition.[5] However, the need for selenium administration still needs further investigation. Fluoride gives caries resistance to enamel of teeth but it possesses no other known biologic function in man. The other trace elements, molybdenum, nickel, silicon, tin, and vanadium, are essential in man but there is insufficient information regarding their functions or doses to recommend their use in intravenous nutrition at this time.[4]

Zinc deficiency states have been described in several patients.[6–12] Zinc deficiency has characteristic symptoms. Copper deficiency symptoms have been described in many patients receiving prolonged intravenous nutrition without supplementation.[13–16] Recently, chromium deficiency has been reported which presented as glucose imbalance.[17,18]

In increasing numbers, patients are being treated with intravenous nutrition. Also, the indications and benefits of parenteral nutrition are being recognized more frequently by the medical community, and patients are being maintained on parenteral nutrition for longer periods of time. In the early years of intravenous nutrition, protein hydrolysates were the only available amino acid source. These products contained substantial inherent quantities of trace minerals. This may have been the reason for the infrequent occurrence or observation of trace-element deficiency. The increased reports of trace-element deficiency seemed to, in part, coincide with the increased use of intravenous crystalline amino acid preparations which contain inadequate inherent amounts of trace elements. It is now clear that supplemental trace elements are required in parenteral nutrition solutions, especially in long-term patients.[4,19,20]

This chapter will discuss and review the roles of zinc, copper, chromium, manganese, and selenium because of the current interest in these elements and their use in parenteral nutrition.

FUNCTIONS OF TRACE ELEMENTS

Zinc is intimately involved with protein and lipid metabolism and is associated with the function of the immune system.[22] Copper has an essential role in collagen synthesis; chromium, in glucose metabolism; selenium, in the activity of glutathione peroxidase, a human red blood cell enzyme; and manganese, in the metabolism of bone structure.[23] A detailed discussion regarding the physiologic functions of these and other common trace elements is beyond the scope of this chapter, but can be found elsewhere.[1–4,19–21,23] However, the physiologic functions of trace elements are summarized in Table 18-1.

ABSORPTION AND METABOLISM OF TRACE ELEMENTS

Absorption of all the metals occurs at the intestinal mucosa of the small intestine. Most trace elements are secreted through the gut, however. Bile is the major pathway for the excretion of some metals, notably copper and manganese. Zinc and chromium are excreted primarily by the kidneys. Urinary excretion for most trace elements is ordinarily small, except for chromium, but may increase dramatically under conditions of stress, prolonged starvation, severe trauma, major surgery, or septicemia. In plasma, all the metals are bound by protein, either by a multitude of specific proteins such as transferrin and ceruloplasmin or the nonspecific binding sites on proteins such as albumin.

It is well known that the gut is the site of several important interactions between metals. Drugs containing iron may depress the absorption of copper.[24] Zinc depresses copper absorption and vice versa.[25] Cobalt and iron have been shown to competitively inhibit the absorption of each other.[26]

While primary trace-element deficiency does occur, secondary deficiencies are more common. Deficiencies may arise because of increased metal losses from the body (i.e., zinc from small bowel drainage) or as a result of increased demand, as in infancy, surgery, or burns. The lack of availability of trace elements may be caused by chelating agents in food. Phytic acid in bread and dietary fiber have been implicated in binding zinc and minimizing its absorption. Chronic diarrhea, caused by bowel disease such as ulcerative colitis, may decrease absorption, decrease gastrointestinal transit time, or increase secretion of these metals. Malabsorption states, especially following jejunoileal bypass operations can result in trace-element deficiencies.

Protracted IV feedings without oral supplementation are an increasingly important cause of trace-element deficiency. As previously mentioned, deficiency states have been described due to lack of zinc, copper, chromium, and selenium in total parenteral nutrition (TPN) solutions. These deficiency symptoms were reversed with the inclusion of these essential nutrients in the solutions.

ZINC

Zinc is an essential nutrient in man that is a component of about 100 metalloenzymes such as carbonic anhydrase and alkaline phosphatase.[27] Zinc also functions as a catalyst in initiating the action of critical enzymes like DNA polymerase, RNA polymerase, and thymidine kinase. A zinc deficiency results in a decrease or loss of enzymatic function.[28] Zinc is also involved in the metabolism of proteins, lipids, and possibly vitamin A.[29]

The human body contains about 1 to 2.3 g of zinc, which is present in most tissues. Its highest concentrations are intracellular. Balance studies suggest that the oral dosage requirement is about 10 to 12 mg per day.[4,30] Since zinc has an intestinal absorption factor of about 33%,[31] the IV requirement for a stable adult patient is 2.5 to 4 mg.[4]

The major route of zinc secretion is through the gastrointestinal and pancreatic juices—usually 500 μg in 24 hours. However, under acute metabolic stress (starvation, sepsis, or burns), urinary excretion of zinc may exhibit a threefold increase.[8]

The zinc deficiency syndrome is characterized by diminished growth and sexual development, impairment of sensations of taste (hypogeusia) and smell (hyposmia), impaired wound healing, and anorexia.[32] Other components of the syndrome are as follow:

- Poor growth and sexual development (hypogonadism)
- Impaired wound healing
- Anorexia
- Decreased sensation of taste and smell
- Hepatosplenomegaly
- Iron deficiency anemia
- Alopecia
- Mental depression
- Acrodermatitis Enterohepatica

An acrodermatitis enterohepatica syndrome accompanied by severe chronic diarrhea, alopecia and roughed, ulcerated skin around body orifices and extremities are described due to zinc deficiency caused by long-term, trace-element-deficient TPN.[33] The response to zinc supplementation is dramatic and results in cessation of symptoms. It should be noted, however, that zinc supplementation has not been shown to be useful in treating ordinary taste and smell abnormalities.[34]

Assessment of zinc status can be made by measuring content in the serum, plasma, RBC, hair, and urine. A definitive diagnosis of a zinc-deficient state cannot be assumed based solely on low zinc blood levels. Certain other factors, such as the use of oral contraceptives, a myocardial infarction, and infection can lower serum zinc levels.

Erroneous serum zinc levels can also result from using laboratory collection tubes in which zinc is present as a contaminant in rubber stoppers.[35] At present, the critical test for zinc deficiency is a positive clinical response to zinc supplementation under controlled conditions.

COPPER

Copper is an essential nutrient in man for several metabolic functions. Copper is involved in the oxidation of catecholamines and ascorbic acid and serves an integral function in the development and maintenance of the cardiovascular system and of skeletal integrity. The human body contains approximately 100 mg of copper, with about 95% bound to ceruloplasmin—a multifunctional enzyme.[1] Ceruloplasmin facilitates the mobilization of iron from stores and catalyzes its conversion to the ferric form, which can be utilized in hemoglobin synthesis.[36]

Copper is absorbed predominantly through the upper small intestine and stomach.[1] Suggested oral requirements are about 2 mg per day for an adult. Since 30% of orally ingested copper is absorbed,[37] approximately 0.5 to 1.5 mg should be given daily via the IV route to the TPN patient.[4]

Excretion of copper occurs primarily through the bile[27]; therefore, copper should be withheld or decreased in patients with hepatic failure or biliary disease.

Copper deficiency is manifested in many ways. Generally, neutropenia, anemia, and osteoporosis are the earliest signs.[38] Other signs of copper deficiency include defective connective tissue formation, growth retardation, abnormal keratinization and pigmentation of the hair (Menke's kinky hair syndrome), and skeletal deformities.[1,13,27,36]

TABLE 18-1. Summary of Selected Trace Elements

Element	Body Content and Primary Concentration	Physiological Function	Daily Estimated Requirement (oral)	Sources	Deficiency Symptoms
ZINC (Zn)	1-2.3 g, present in almost all tissue; highest concentration in intracellular "normal" serum = 68-136 μg/dl	Metalloenzyme function, protein metabolism, lipid metabolism, vitamin A metabolism (?)	Infants and children, 3-10 mg; adult, 15 mg; pregnant, 20 mg; lactating, 25 mg	Meat, liver, eggs, seafood (esp. oysters)	Poor growth and sexual development, impairment of sensory perception (hypogeusia and hyposmia), impaired wound healing, 'acrodermatitis enterohepatica'
COPPER (Cu)	80-120 mg liver, brain, heart and kidneys; "normal" serum 70-150 μg/dl	Hemoglobin synthesis, bone mineralization, enzyme function	0.1 mg/kg children; 2 mg, adults	Nuts, shellfish, raisins, dried legumes, liver	Anemia, defective connective tissue formation, growth retardation, imperfect keratinization and pigmentation of the hair, secondary iron deficiency
CHROMIUM (Cr)	60 mg mainly in combination with transferrin	Glucose metabolism, mediates effect of insulin on membranes (?)	0.3 mg	Animal protein, grain, brewer's yeast	Impaired glucose clearance, peripheral neuropathy, ataxia
MANGANESE (Mn)	12-20 mg kidneys, pancreas, liver	Bone structure, reproduction, activator of enzyme function of CNS	10-22 mg	Green leafy vegetables, nuts, grain, tea	Impaired growth, skeletal abnormalities, ataxia, convulsions, fat metabolism abnormalities, nausea, and vomiting

TABLE 18-1. (continued)

Element	Body Content and Primary Concentration	Physiological Function	Daily Estimated Requirement (oral)	Sources	Deficiency Symptoms
IODINE (I)	8 mg thyroid gland	Synthesis of thyroid hormones, regulation of basal metabolic rate, growth, reproduction, and cellular metabolism	Children, 5 μg/kg; adults, 1 μg/kg	Seafood	Goiter
COBALT (Co)	1.1 mg	Integral part of vitamin B_{12}	Can be supplied as vitamin B_{12} approx. 0.003 mg	Varies on soil content on which food is grown	Pernicious anemia
IRON (Fe)	45 mg/kg body wt (hemoglobin, myoglobin ferritin, hemosiderin, and enzymes), "normal" serum iron 36-166 μg/ml	Constituent of hemoglobin, myoglobin and many enzymes	10-18 mg	Liver, turkey, veal oysters, clams, raisins	Anemia, disturbance of bone marrow function
SELENIUM (Se)	as low as 1.5 mg-liver, kidney, heart, spleen	Glutathione peroxidase (human red blood cell), antioxidant, maintenance of membrane function	0.05-0.2 mg	Onions, grains, varies depending on soil content	Muscle pain; growth retardation; cataract formation; aspermatogenesis

It is important to stress that trace elements are not completely innocuous substances. Toxicity, although rare, can occur. For example, chronic copper poisoning was suggested as the cause of death from cirrhosis in a 15-month-old child.[39] Copper toxicity may induce nausea and vomiting, dizziness, epigastric pain, acute hemolysis, bluish-green diarrhea stools, and damage to the renal tubules; jaundice may appear after 2 to 3 days.[40]

CHROMIUM

The importance of chromium as a nutrient was discovered as the result of observations of impaired glucose tolerance, developing within a few weeks, in rats fed diets low in trivalent chromium. Recently, hyperglycemia and glucosuria have been reported in humans receiving TPN without supplemental chromium.[17,18]

There is approximately 6 mg of chromium in the body, which is bound and transported mainly in combination with transferrin. Absorption is predominantly through the small intestine, and excretion occurs in the feces and urine.

Intravenous chromium has reversed persistent hyperglycemia in TPN patients unresponsive to insulin. It is believed to mediate the effects of insulin on cell membranes and acts as a glucose tolerance factor. Suggested IV requirements are 10 to 15 μg per day for the stable adult.[4] However, it has to be emphasized that chromium is *not* a drug for the treatment of nonspecific abnormalities of carbohydrate metabolism.

MANGANESE

Manganese is an essential mineral for man because it is an activator of several enzymes, such as liver arginase and serum alkaline phosphatase, and it is involved in the synthesis of protein and central nervous system function.[27] The precise functions of this element need to be further elucidated. An average man has about 12 to 20 mg of manganese in the body, concentrated primarily in the brain, kidneys, pancreas, and liver. Manganese is absorbed primarily through the small intestine and is excreted via the bile and, to a lesser extent, pancreatic juice. Symptoms of manganese deficiency include ataxia, convulsions, impaired growth, and skeletal and fat metabolism abnormalities.[32] These symptoms have been described extensively in animals but are extremely rare in humans. Suggested intravenous requirements for the stable adult are 0.15 to 0.8 mg per day.[4]

SELENIUM

Selenium is an essential nutrient that has received a significant amount of attention recently. It has several physiologic roles in animals, including enhancement of primary immune response, functional interrelationship with Vitamin E, maintenance of muscle structure and function, and as a possible antioxidant and anticarcinogen.[41] It is also an integral part of the enzyme glutathione peroxidase of human red blood cells, although its exact function is unknown.[23] Selenium-responsive symptoms (muscular pain) have been observed in a patient receiving TPN, indicating that this element is essential in human nutrition.[5]

Little is known about the exact metabolism of selenium, but it is excreted primarily in the urine, the skin, and the sweat.[41] Selenium levels in the blood are decreased in a number of clinical conditions such as malnutrition, burns, and some types of cancer, as well as in patients living in geographic regions with low selenium soil content (New Zealand). The exact amount of selenium and the most suitable form for its use in the parenteral nutrition patient is unknown at this time. This element deserves much more research.

GUIDELINES

Suggested guidelines for intravenous use of trace elements in TPN patients are shown in Table 18-3. Recently, single-entity solutions have been introduced (zinc, 1 mg/ml; copper, 0.4 mg/ml; manganese, 0.1 mg/ml; and chromium, 4 μg/ml) that comply with the suggested standards prepared by a panel of experts assembled by the American Medical Association Department of Foods and Nutrition.[4] This represents a significant advance in the field of clinical nutrition. However, it should be stressed that various commercially available intravenous solutions, especially amino acids, contain trace elements as contaminants. The amounts present vary from manufacturer to manufacturer and even between lots of the same brand of solution.[4]

DOSING

The dosing recommendations presented (Tables 18-2 and 18-3) are to be used only as guidelines, not as minimum or maximum doses. These recommendations must be modified to meet the individual patients' needs. The doses required vary, depending on age, losses, and clinical and metabolic status. Appropriate monitoring and clinical response are the key to safe and adequate trace-element administration. It is appropriate to routinely determine the zinc and copper status of patients receiving nutritional support (parenteral and enteral) from the onset of therapy. The status of chromium and manganese should be followed in patients receiving long-term nutrition support.

It is important to recognize that normal blood levels of trace elements do not always indicate normal tissue levels. Blood levels alone cannot be used to determine trace-element administration. The patient's losses and clinical state must also be followed. The administration of trace elements should begin from the onset of nutrition support unless blood levels and clinical state dictate otherwise. Several reports have suggested relationships between blood and hair or saliva levels of trace elements. To date there is little evidence to show any strong relationship in individuals who are ill or have acute losses.

The patient must also be monitored for losses—metabolic, functional, and disease-related. Therefore, the dose of zinc or chromium must be modified, based on renal function to prevent excess dosing. The dosing of copper and manganese must be reduced or omitted in patients with biliary tract obstruction to avoid excess retention.

The commercial trace-element solutions should be diluted before administration. It is *not* recommended to give them by bolus injection. Trace elements currently used are compatible in total parenteral solutions.

It should be noted that some calcium gluconate injections contain disodium edetate, a heavy metal chelating agent, as a stabilizer. It is possible that the disodium edetate may bind or precipitate trace elements.

CONCLUSIONS

Trace elements are essential nutrients that should be provided in parenteral nutrition solutions. Special emphasis should be placed on monitoring the requirements of zinc, copper, chromium, manganese, and se-

TABLE 18-2. Suggested Daily Intravenous Intake of Essential Trace Elements*

	Pediatric Patients	Stable Adult Patients	Acute Catabolic State Adult	Stable Adult with Intestinal Losses
Zinc	300 μg/kg + 100 μg/kg**	2.5-4.0 mg	Additional 2.0 mg	Add 12.2 mg/liter small bowel fluid loss; 17.1 mg/liter of diarrheal fluid loss
Copper	20 μg/kg	0.5-1.5 mg	?	?
Chromium	0.14-0.2 μg/kg	10-15 μg	?	20 μg
Manganese	2-10 μg/kg	0.15-0.8 mg	?	?

* AMA 1979, + = premature, ** = full term children to 5 years. From reference.[4]

TABLE 18-3. Administration of Trace Elements in Parenteral Nutrition

Element	Daily Dosing		Additional Dosing		Available as	Administration	Monitoring	
	Pediatrics	Adults	Catabolic Adults	Intestinal Losses			Serum	Urine
ZINC[4]	(300 μg/kg premature) 100 μg/kg (to 5 yrs)	2.5 to 4.0 mg	2 mg additional	12.2 mg/L additional for small bowel losses 17.1 mg/L additional for diarrhea losses	Chloride salt 1 mg/ml 10 ml vial	Dilute, do not bolus (may increase renal losses), monitor copper levels, ceruloplasmin and renal function.	80-160 mg/dl	0.5-0.8 mg/24 hrs.
COPPER[4]	20 μg/kg	0.5 to 1.5 mg			Chloride salt 0.4 mg/ml 10 ml vial	Dilute, administer with caution to patients with biliary obstruction may depress zinc levels when given without zinc.	88-150 μg/dl	5-25 μg/24 hrs.
CHROMIUM[4,17]	0.14-0.2 μg/kg	10 to 15 μg	150 μg/day to treat deficiency symptoms for 2 weeks (ref. 17)		Chloride salt 4 μg/ml 10 ml vial	Dilute, do not bolus (may increase renal losses), monitor serum levels, glucose tolerance (and insulin response), and renal function.	0.5-9 μg/dl	5-10 μg/24 hrs.
MANGANESE[4]	2-10 μg/kg	0.15 to 0.8 mg			Chloride salt 0.1 mg/ml 10 ml vial	Dilute, administer with caution to patients with biliary obstruction	0.4 μg/dl	5-11 μg/24 hrs.
SELENIUM[5,41]	Undetermined	100 μg for 21 days[41] (case report)	See references 5 and 41 for information		Selenomethonine not commercially available	See reference 41	21 μg/dl (seleniferous areas	8 μg/24 hrs. on TPN[41]

+ These are values from the literature, use the values for the laboratory making the determination.

lenium in patients receiving prolonged intravenous feedings (home TPN patients).

Requirements for parenteral trace elements vary among patients, depending on age, and clinical and metabolic status. Additional zinc should be given to those patients with large gastrointestinal losses and those in acute catabolic states. Suggested guidelines for parenteral trace elements are given in Tables 18-2 and 18-3. It should be pointed out that only guidelines are presented—not minimum or maximum dosages—which should be modified as individual needs dictate.

With the recent introduction of commercially available trace-element formulations, there is no reason to omit these critical nutritional components for the prevention and treatment of trace-element deficiencies.

BIBLIOGRAPHY

1. Reinhold, J.G.: Trace elements—a selective survey. Clin. Chem., *21:*476, 1975.
2. Ulmer, D.D.: Trace elements. N. Engl. J. Med., *297:*318, 1977.
3. Cotzias, G.C.: Importance of Trace Substances in Environmental Health as Exemplified by Manganese. *In* Proc. 1st Ann. Conf. Trace Substances, Environmental Health. D.D. Hemphill, ed. Columbia, MO, University of Missouri, 1967, p. 5.
4. A.M.A. Dept. of Foods and Nutrition: Guidelines for essential trace element preparations for parenteral use. JAMA, *241:*2051, 1979.
5. Van Rij, A.M., et al.: Selenium deficiency in total parenteral nutrition. Am. J. Clin. Nutr., *32:*2076, 1979.
6. Arakawa, T., et al.: Zinc deficiency in two infants during total parenteral alimentation for diarrhea. Am. J. Clin. Nutr. *29:*197, 1976.
7. Hankins, D.A., et al.: Whole blood trace element concentrations during total parenteral nutrition. Surgery, *79:*674, 1976.
8. Kay, R.G., et al.: A syndrome of acute zinc deficiency during total parenteral nutrition in man. Ann. Surg., *183:*331, 1976.
9. Wolman, S.L., et al.: Zinc in total parenteral nutrition: Requirements and metabolic effects. Gastroenterology, *76:*458, 1979.
10. Srouji, M.N., Balisfreri, W.F., and Caleb, M.H.: Zinc deficiency during parenteral nutrition—Skin manifestations and immune incompetence in a premature infant. J. Ped. Surg., *13:*570, 1978.
11. Okada, A., et al.: Skin lesions during intravenous hyperalimentation: Zinc deficiency. Surgery, *80:*629, 1976.
12. Prasad, A.S.: Zinc deficiency in man. Am. J. Dis.Child., *130:*359, 1976.
13. Karpel, J.T., and Peden, V.H.: Copper deficiency in long term parenteral nutrition. J. Pediatr., *80:*32, 1972.
14. Vitler, R.W., et al.: Manisfestation of copper deficiency in a patient with systemic sclerosis on intravenous hyperalimentation. N. Engl. J. Med., *291:*188, 1974.
15. Hull, R.L., and Cassidy, D.: Trace element deficiencies during total parenteral nutrition. Drug Intell. Clin. Pharm., *11:*536, 1977.
16. Dunlop, W.: Anemia and neutropenia caused by copper deficiency. Ann. Intern. Med., *80:*470, 1974.
17. Jeejeebhoy, K.N., et al.: Chromium deficiency, glucose imbalance and neuropathy reversed by chromium supplementation in a patient receiving long-term TPN. Am. J. Clin. Nutr., *30:*531, 1977.
18. Freund, H., Atamian, S., and Fischer, J.E.: Chromium deficiency during TPN. JAMA, *241:*496, 1979.
19. Solomons, N.W., et al.: Plasma trace metals during total parenteral alimentation. Gastroenterology, *70:*1022, 1976.
20. Lowry, S.F., et al.: Abnormalities of zinc and copper during total parenteral nutrition. Ann. Surg., *189:*120, 1979.
21. Goodhart, R.S., and Shils, M.E., (eds.): Modern Nutrition in Health and Disease, 6th Ed. Philadelphia, Lea & Febiger, 1980.
22. Good, R.A., Fernandes, G., and West, A.: Nutrition, immunity and cancer—a review. Clin. Bull., *9:*3, 1979.
23. Prasad, A.S.: Trace Elements and Iron in Human Metabolism. New York, Plenum Publishing Corp., 1978.
24. Seely, J.R., Humphrey, G.G., and Matter, B.J.: Copper deficiency in a premature infant fed an iron fortified formula. N. Engl. J. Med., *286:*109, 1972.
25. Evans, G.W.: Copper homeostasis in the mammalian system. Physiol. Rev., *53:*535, 1973.
26. Thompson, A.B., Valber, L.S., and Sinclair, D.G.: Competitive nature of intestinal transport mechanisms for cobalt and iron in the rat. J. Clin. Invest., *50:*2384, 1971.
27. Burch, R.E., Hahn, H.K.J., and Sullivan, J.F.: Newer aspects of the roles of zinc, manganese and copper in human nutrition. Clin. Chem., *21:*501, 1975.
28. Kirchgessner, M., Roth, H.P., and Weigand, E.: Biochemical Changes in Zinc Deficiency. *In* Trace Elements in Human Health and Disease. Vol. 1. A.S. Prasad, ed. New York, Academic Press, 1976.
29. Smith, J.C., et al.: Zinc: A trace element essential in vitamin A metabolism. Science, *181:*954, 1973.
30. Shils, M.E.: Minerals in total parenteral nutrition. Drug Intell. Clin. Pharm., *6:*385, 1972.
31. WHO Expert Committee Report: Trace elements in human nutrition. WHO Tech. Rep. Ser., *532:*1, 1970.
32. Odne, M.A., Lee, S.C., and Jeffrey, L.P.: Rationale for adding trace elements to total parenteral nutrient solutions—A brief review. Am. J. Hosp. Pharm., *35:*1057, 1978.
33. Tucker, S.B., et al.: Acquired zinc deficiency: Cutaneous manifestations typical of acrodermatitis enterohepatica. JAMA, *235:*2399, 1976.

34. Henkin, R.I., et al.: A doubleblind study of the effects of zinc sulfate on taste and smell dysfunction. Am. J. Med. Sci., *272:*285, 1976.
35. Ralstin, J.O, Schneider, P.J., and Blackstone, L.: Serum zinc concentrations: Contamination from laboratory equipment. JPEN, *3:*179, 1979.
36. Dowdy, R.P.L.: Copper metabolism. Am. J. Clin. Nutr., *22:*887, 1969.
37. Cartwright, G.E., and Wintrobe, M.M.: Copper metabolism in normal subjects. Am. J. Clin. Nutr., *14:*224, 1964.
38. Hambridge, K.M.: Trace elements in pediatric nutrition. Adv. Pediatr., *24:*191, 1977.
39. Walker-Smith, J.A., and Blomfield, J.: Wilson's disease or chronic copper poisoning? Arch. Dis. Child., *42:*108, 1973.
40. Fliss, D.M., and Lamy, P.P.: Trace elements and total parenteral nutrition. Hosp. Formul., *14:*698, 1979.
41. Van Rij, A.M., McKenzie, J.M., and Robinson, M.F.: Selenium and total parenteral nutrition. JPEN, *3:*235, 1979.

Chapter 19

Subclavian Catheterization

Richard M. Vazquez, M.D.
Nutritional Support Service
Northwestern Memorial Hospital
Chicago, Illinois

Central venous catheterization by percutaneous puncture of the subclavian vein is a popular and useful technique for gaining access to the greater veins. The early application of the procedure was directed toward use of the catheter for determining the right atrial filling pressure. Such information sometimes aids the health care team in making decisions concerning the adequacy of the relative blood volume of patients who are suspected of having acute blood volume abnormalities. The relative "ease" with which these catheters can be placed has led to their widespread use, but unfortunately, has also led to some overuse of the technique, especially for resuscitation.

The suitability of this method of venous access for intravenous hyperalimentation was not recognized until 1967. At that time, Stanley Dudrick suggested that hyperosmolar solutions of protein hydrolysate and hypertonic glucose could safely be administered through the subclavian vein.[1] The hyperosmolarity of the solution precluded its infusion into peripheral veins. However, hypertonic glucose was the only available source of sufficient nonprotein calories to support growth and anabolism. An isotonic intravenous fat emulsion was available in the United States for a brief time in the 1960s but was removed from the market because of frequent untoward reactions. From 1968 until 1973, when 10% Intralipid was introduced into the U.S., no available isotonic intravenous nonprotein calorie source could satisfy the majority of the daily caloric requirements of patients. For this reason, IVH, which relied on hypertonic glucose as the primary source of nonprotein calories, became the mainstay of nutritional support in the United States. This necessitated the popularization of the subclavian catheterization technique.

Early experience with subclavian puncture left much to be desired. The incidence of both technical and septic complications was excessively high. Technical and septic complication rates of 10% and 27 to 56% respectively were reported in literature from 1971 to 1974.[2–5] One author published an opinion that the technique was unsafe and should be abandoned entirely.[6] Application of knowledge concerning the proper technique for insertion and care of these catheters, coupled with extensive experience, has been responsible for a decrease in complication rates in the hands of many operators. Complication rates for both types of complication of less than 3% are currently being published with increasing frequency.[7] It is to be hoped that, through application of the surgical techniques found here and in the many other manuscripts about subclavian catheterization, surgeons and their trainees will continue to experience a low complication rate with this useful procedure.

Several other routes of access to the central venous system have been proposed as safer alternatives to subclavian puncture. Each of the techniques was suggested in the hope of avoiding some of the infrequent but serious complications of subclavian puncture. The suggested alternative methods are venous cutdown or puncture of the ex-

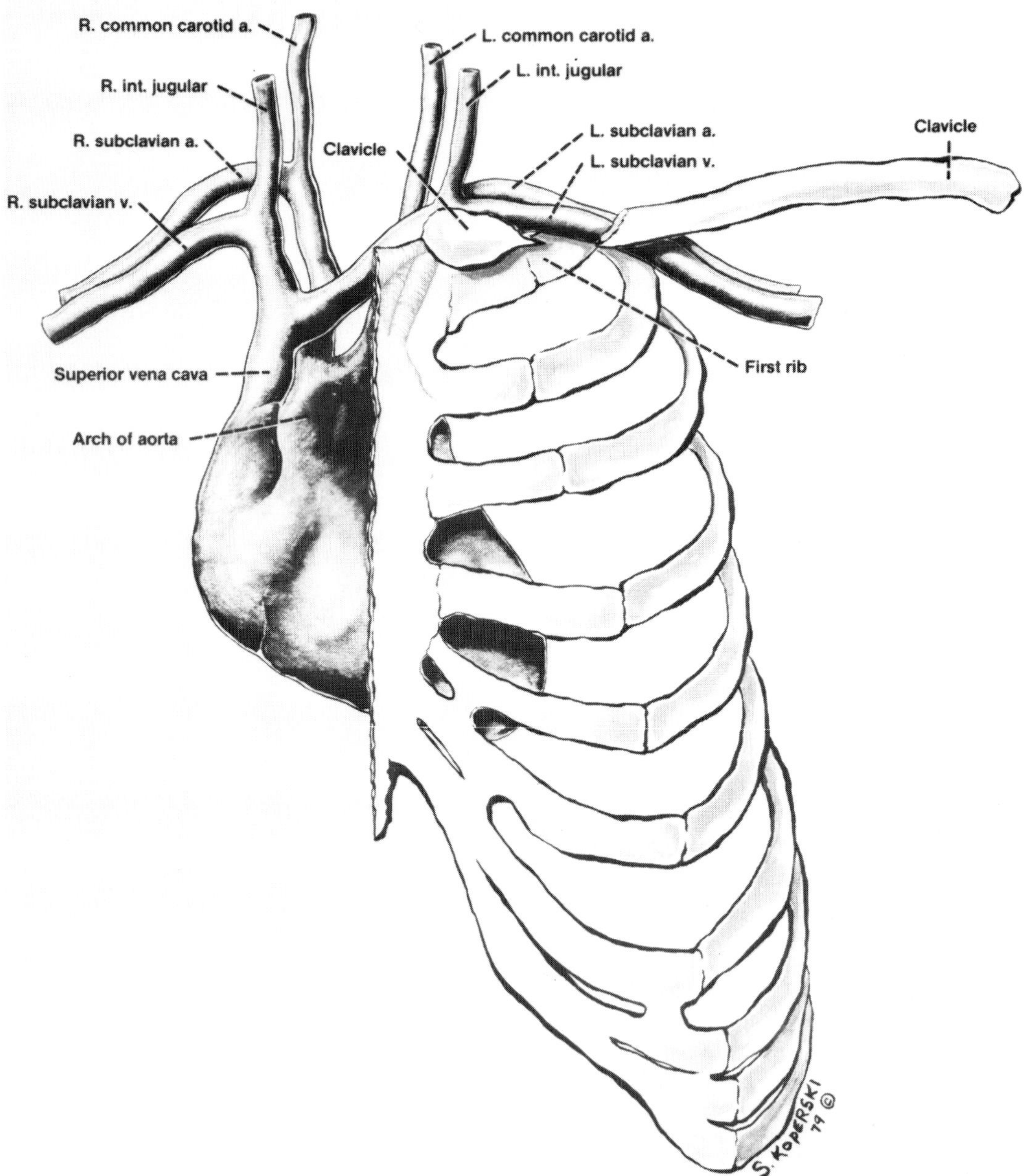

Figure 19-1. Note the position of the subclavian vein which is posterior to the clavicle, superior to the first rib, and anterior to the subclavian artery.

ternal jugular vein or a peripheral vein, the internal jugular puncture, or the supraclavicular approach to the subclavian vein. In each instance, a catheter of sufficient length is threaded from the point of venous entry to the superior vena cava (Figure 19-1). Experience gained with each of these techniques revealed that each method had its own associated problems and was certainly not devoid of complications. Each of the other techniques are best suited to special applications. For example, puncture of the internal jugular vein can safely be accomplished by an anesthesiologist during many surgical procedures.

Since central venous catheters placed by the subclavian approach are relatively easy to care for after insertion, this approach continues to be suggested as the workhorse of central venous access. The technique carries some definite risk of morbidity and even mortality and should be reserved for those patients who manifest clear indication that they may benefit from the procedure. Those patients with relative or absolute contraindication to the procedure need to be determined before subclavian catheterization is attempted.

This discussion of central venous catheterization is meant to apply predominantly to patients who are catheterized for the purpose of intravenous hyperalimentation (IVH). Many of the comments made are directly applicable to situations for which the catheter is being placed for monitoring purposes; however, catheters placed for monitoring purposes are intentionally short-lived and usually are removed as soon as the problem for which they were inserted has been resolved. Such catheters are prone to infection due to the multiplicity of uses assigned to them, such as monitoring functions, administration of drugs, and blood replacement therapy. Catheters inserted for IVH are generally intended to be long-lived and are reserved for use only for nutritional support. Aseptic technique during catheter insertion and during postinsertion catheter care is mandatory regardless of the reason for which the catheter is placed.

INDICATIONS FOR SUBCLAVIAN CATHETERIZATION

The indications for subclavian catheterization include hyperalimentation, the absence of other acceptable venous access sites, administration of solutions poorly tolerated by peripheral veins, and some emergency situations. During cardiac arrest, subclavian puncture cannot be safely performed and may interfere with other aspects of the resuscitation. During hemorrhagic shock, low venous pressure with central venous collapse makes subclavian catheterization potentially hazardous; however, circumstances may require catheter placement regardless.

ANATOMY

Knowledge of the anatomy of the upper thoracic and lower neck regions is necessary for the safe and proper placement of subclavian catheters. Figure 19-1 depicts the relationship between bony and vascular structures of concern.

Anatomic Landmarks

The subclavian artery is posterior to the subclavian vein. The arterial pulse may be palpated in most patients and provides a good landmark for the procedure of subclavian catheterization (SC). When one palpates the subclavian artery pulse as it passes beneath the clavicle, the subclavian vein is located just medial and anterior to that point. The vein is approached through a skin wheal of anesthetic raised in the area medial to and anterior to the subclavian artery. The location of the vein estimated by palpation of the artery fairly well coincides with the popular guide of using the junction of the medial and middle thirds of the clavicle as the point of entry. The relationship of the vein to the artery is rather constant, so that when one uses the vascular relationship to estimate the location of the subclavian vein rather than the bony landmarks method, the frequency of unintentional puncture of the subclavian artery is diminished. The more medial approach one can make to the vein, the more likely a successful and complication-free catheter placement will occur. The more lateral the approach, the more likely that the artery will be punctured and the vein missed. The limiting factor medially is the distance between the clavicle and the first rib; for if one attempts catheterization too far medially, the bony structures will prevent access to the vein.

Anatomic Details of the Left Neck

Figure 19-2 demonstrates the relationships of the neurovascular system and the thoracic duct to the clavicle, first rib, and scalenus anticus muscle. The thoracic duct returns lymph to the venous system. This duct is sometimes injured during subclavian puncture. Because of the presence of this duct on the left, supraclavicular puncture on

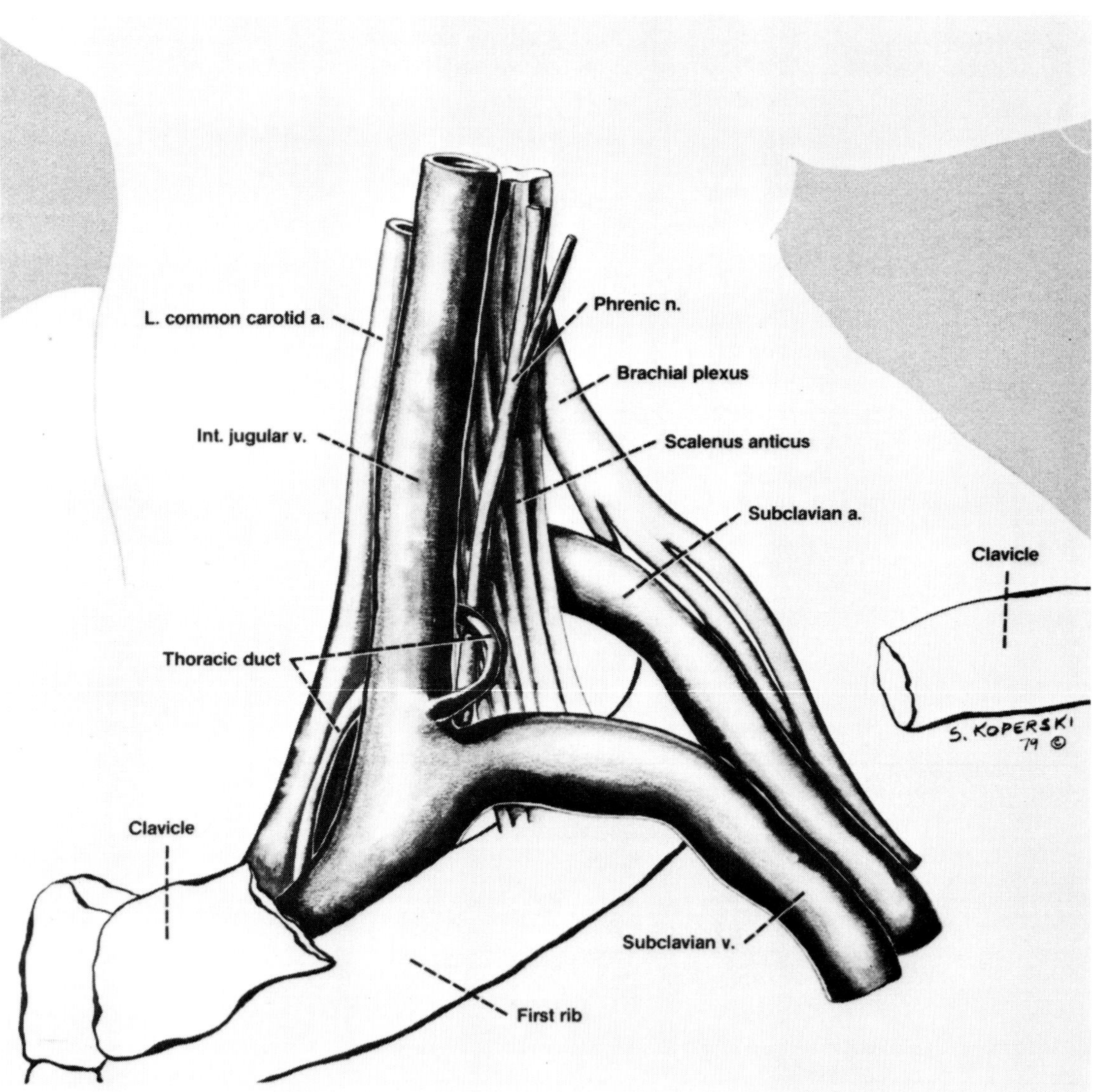

Figure 19-2. The brachial plexus, a far posterior structure, is infrequently injured during subclavian vein catheterization. The supraclavicular approach to the subclavian vein is generally not used on the left side in order to avoid injury to the thoracic duct.

the left side by the junctional approach is generally not recommended.

TYPES OF CATHETERS

Catheters made of several different materials are available in kit form for this procedure. Teflon, polyvinyl chloride, and silicone rubber catheters have all been successfully used. These devices are currently available with essentially two different types of introduction methods for central venous puncture.

In one type, the catheter is placed through a large bore needle; whereas in the other, the catheter is placed through an introducer catheter. Using the first technique, it is possible to puncture or completely tear the catheter during placement if the operator attempts to retract the catheter through the needle during the catheterization. Although the physician is usually aware that such a maneuver may sever the catheter, the error is sometimes made. Embolus of the severed catheter to the heart has been reported and is a serious complication.

With the other type of introduction device, the vein is entered with an over-the-needle introducer catheter (Figure 19-3). The needle is removed, leaving the intro-

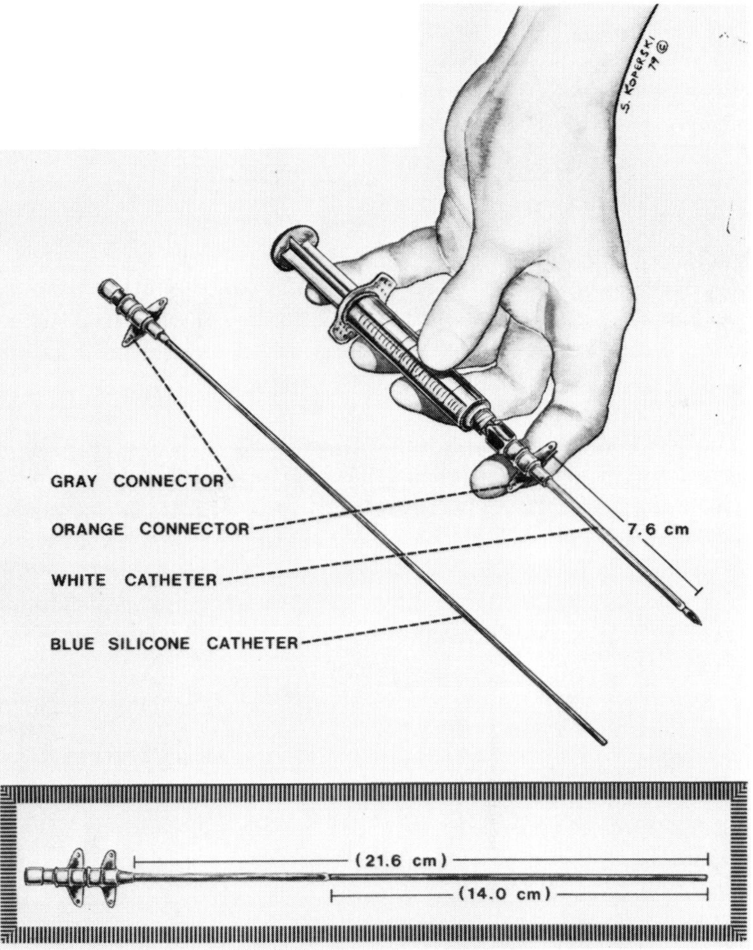

Figure 19-3. This system of central venous puncture allows the operator to place a silicone catheter through a teflon introducer rather than a large bore needle.

ducer catheter in place in the vein. The IVH silicone rubber catheter is then placed through the introducer catheter. Ultimately, the white introducer catheter is removed to a position external to the patient. The guide wire which stiffens the silicone rubber catheter is removed just prior to connecting the newly installed catheter to the IV solution.

Other methods of catheter introduction are basically variations of these two. There is some evidence that the incidence of venous thrombosis is decreased with the use of silicone rubber catheters.[8] The physician will generally use the device with which he is most comfortable unless he desires to change techniques or master a new one. Several of the technical details of the use of an introducer type of delivery system are referred to in the set of figures.

PERIPHERAL INSERTION OF CENTRAL VENOUS IVH CATHETERS

On occasion, it may be necessary to administer central venous IVH to a patient in whom a subclavian central venous puncture cannot be performed. If a subclavian puncture cannot or should not be performed, then one should utilize a peripherally placed central venous catheter if possible. Indications for the placement of a peripherally inserted long silicone rubber central venous* catheter include the following:

1. The unavailability of a skilled surgeon for the placement of a percutaneous subclavian catheter.
2. The presence of any absolute or relative contraindication to the performance of central venous puncture such as a coagulopathy, bilateral radical neck dissection, or other cause for anatomic distortion.
3. An uncooperative patient who might cause a complication during central venous puncture.
4. The elderly patient with severe curvature of the spine (kyphosis), who is unable to thrust his or her shoulders back for safe SC puncture.

This catheter, as do all silicone rubber catheters, has an affinity for particulate matter. The operator must be sure to rinse his or her gloved hands with sterile water so as to remove all of the starch from the surface of the gloves. Even with such precaution, the patient sometimes develops aseptic phlebitis in the vein housing this device. A low grade temperature elevation with tenderness over the vein but no signs of systemic toxicity may develop. These findings may resolve with several days of application of warm packs to the affected area; however, the reaction may not subside until the catheter is removed.

INITIAL APPROACH TO THE PATIENT

During the history and physical examination of the patient, information should be obtained concerning any findings that might contraindicate central venous puncture. A past history of eventful IVH, such as sepsis, swelling of the arm during therapy on the same side as the IVH catheter, or the development of a collateral venous pattern around the shoulder, suggest a past history compatible with subclavian vein thrombosis. In the event that such a complication is expected, bilateral upper extremity venography is indicated. The radiographically normal-appearing side is chosen for catheterization. Another absolute contraindication to use of a subclavian vein is recent severe local trauma with clavicular fracture and/or upper anterior rib fracture on the side under consideration for catheterization. Such injuries may distort the anatomy, or the vein may actually have been injured.

Surgical procedures may also distort the anatomy. Radical neck or breast surgery alter the anatomy on the side of the surgical procedure. Such distortion makes subclavian vein catheterization unsafe. Other contraindications include abnormal coagulation, previous radiation therapy to the immediate area, or an uncooperative patient.

---

* Intrasil catheter—Vicra Division, Baxter Travenol Laboratories.

Patients with altered coagulation should have their coagulopathy corrected if at all possible. Those with thrombocytopenia should have platelet infusions started just prior to central venous puncture. These precautions will minimize the risk of hemorrhage from the SC puncture or an unintentional puncture of the subclavian artery.

The patient with severe kyphosis is unable to thrust his shoulders backward. The situation is similar to the normal patient who has not had a rolled towel placed under the spine, as may be seen in Figure 19-4b. The operator is unable to achieve a proper trajectory parallel to the horizontal plane with the catheter introduction device because the patient's shoulder is in the way. Elderly patients with this severe curvature of the spine should be catheterized by the supraclavicular approach or with a peripherally placed long silicone rubber catheter (Intrasil).[9]

The nurse and the physician should review the most recent chest x-ray before a catheter insertion is performed. The review of the chest radiograph is performed with

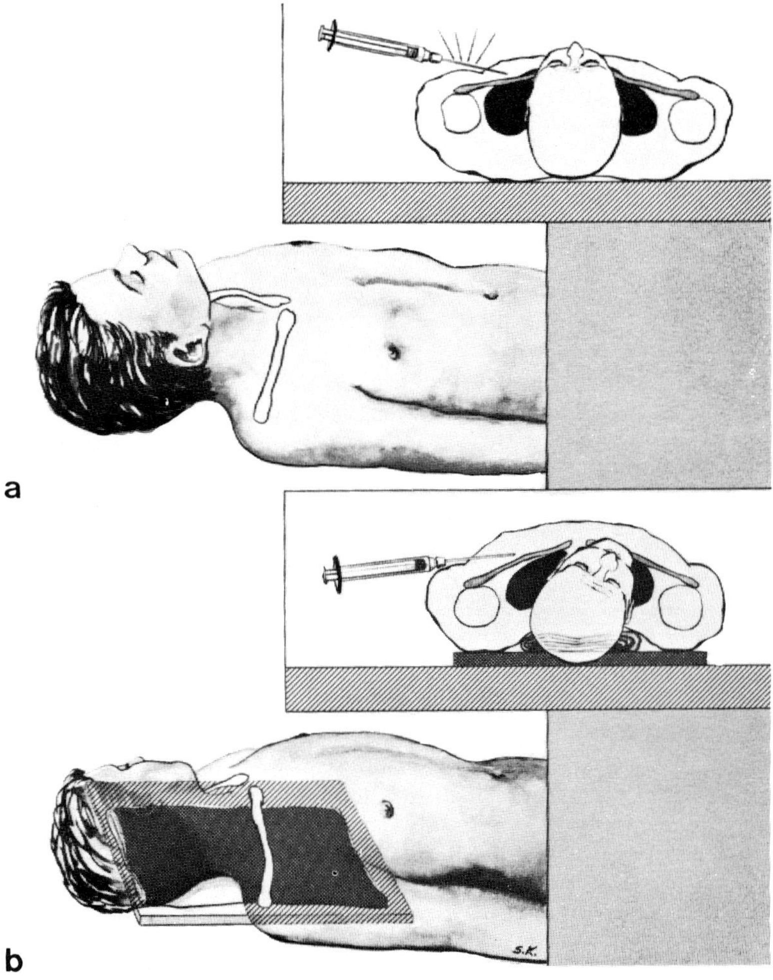

Figure 19-4a. If the patient cannot assume the "military position" with shoulders thrust posteriorly the subclavian approach should be abandoned in favor of a supraclavicular approach to catheterization. 4b. A rolled towel or sheet placed beneath the vertebral column allows the shoulders to fall posteriorly and the operator to assume a needle trajectory away from the cupula of the lung.

special attention to anatomy or a disease process that might alter the approach to the patient.

Patient Education

An often neglected aspect of subclavian catheterization is education of the patient. It is important for the patient to understand why the central venous catheter needs to be used. The patient also needs to know the risks associated with catheter placement. In many institutions, an informed consent for the procedure is obtained to the benefit of all concerned parties. The nurse clinician or physician should tell the patient about all of the expected occurrences during catheterization, such as the head-down position of the bed, the preparation of the skin, the surgical draping, any pain they may anticipate, and above all, the reason for taking a chest x-ray at the end of the procedure. Many uninformed patients will assume that the chest x-ray is being taken with stat portable technique because something went wrong. The nurse should tell the patient what is expected of him or her during the catheterization and demonstrate breath holding at end inspiration and a valsalva maneuver.

With respect to patient education, the roles of the physician and nurse are redundant. The physician should explain the rationale for the procedure and discuss the potential benefits and risks. Inevitably the patient forgets most of what the physician has said, and repetition by the nurse is desirable and necessary. Also, by the time the nurse actually begins to prepare the patient for the SC procedure, the patient has had additional time to think of more questions concerning the procedure.

The pharmacist's role in the educational process places emphasis on the use of the catheter rather than on the technical details of catheter placement.

Patient Preparation

Subclavian catheterization may be performed in the patient's room or in the operating room. Some hospitals have special procedures rooms in which these catheters may be inserted. At whichever site is chosen, strict asepsis must be provided. If the patient is being catheterized in his hospital bed, then the headboard should be removed to allow the physician to place a catheter by the supraclavicular approach. Also, draping the patient is easier if the headboard is out of the way.

The patient should be located toward the same side of the bed that has been chosen for catheterization. That is, the patient should be at the right edge of the bed for right subclavian vein catheterization and at the left side for left subclavian catheterization. The patient should also be moved near the head of the bed. The bed must be the type that can be placed in the Trendelenburg position. Attention to all these details by the nurse allows a safer and easier operative approach to the patient.

Some assessment of the patient's volume status should be made, since central venous catheterization is less difficult when the patient is adequately hydrated. The patient should be placed in the supine and/or the Trendelenburg position and observed for venous distention of the external jugular vein. If the vein remains collapsed in both of these positions, the patient may be hypovolemic. Catheterization may be easier and safer to accomplish after an additional day's hydration.

THE PROCEDURE

We have found it useful to have all the supplies for the placement of a subclavian catheter on one cart. This facilitates not only the actual procedure, but also makes record keeping and charging for supplies used by the staff easier. If a consent is to be obtained, this is done before any formal preparation of the patient begins. For the majority of the prepping and draping process, the bed may remain in flat position to allow the patient as much comfort as possible. The patient is then positioned along the edge of the bed on the same side as is being catheterized. The patient should turn his face away from the nurse who is preparing the field or the patient should wear a mask as does everyone else in the room. Occasionally, the patient may require a cap to keep hair away from the field. Hair on the chest is clipped closely or shaved so as not to interfere with the dressing process.

A wide operative field is then prepared with acetone/alcohol swabs or freon. This cleanses and defats the skin thoroughly. The field should extend from the trapezius muscle and lower edge mandible superiorly to the seventh anterior intercostal space, and from the ipsilateral anterior axillary line to the other contralateral margin of the sternum. This allows for some margin of safety, and allows the physician to use an alternate site of access on the prepared side should an alternate site be required. The same area is then washed with an iodophor soap solution, rinsed with sterile-water-moistened gauze pads, and then painted with an iodophor solution. At this point, the prepared field is covered with a sterile drape. A padded but rigid flat surface and rolled towel are then placed under the pa-

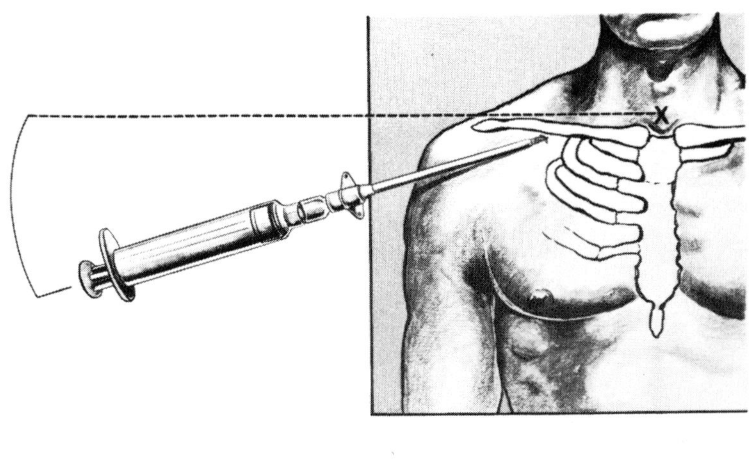

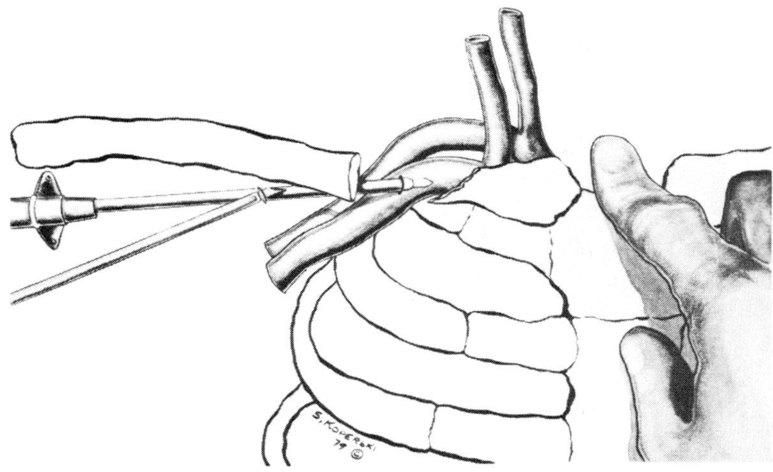

Figure 19-5. The needle-introducer set assumes the same trajectory as the needle and syringe used to infiltrate the area with local anesthetic. The needle is marched posteriorly along the clavicle then advanced toward a point one finger breadth above the suprasternal notch while maintaining gentle negative pressure on the syringe plunger. After free flow of venous blood is obtained, the introducer is advanced into the vein over the needle.

tient if the subclavicular approach is to be used (Figure 19-4). The sterile drape is removed from the operative field just as soon as the physician is gowned, gloved, and ready to drape the area. After the area is draped and the local anesthetic for the catheterization has been infiltrated, the patient is placed in the Trendelenburg position until external jugular venous distention can be observed. The positive venous pressure created by the Trendelenburg position distends the subclavian vein and helps to decrease the possibility of an air embolism.

Figures 19-5, 6, and 7 demonstrate the technique of puncture of the subclavian vein with the over-the-needle introducer. After catheterization is completed and the "keep open" solution flows readily, indicating that the catheter is patent, the patient is taken out of the Trendelenburg position. This aids the patient's comfort and lessens the likelihood of backbleeding around the catheter. Figure 19-8 demonstrates the position of the operator and patient for the supraclavicular approach should that approach be necessary.

Our service has used OP-SITE dressing material for all IVH catheters inserted and cared for by us. The dressing material is a clear polyurethane film with a hypoallergenic adhesive backing. It is permeable to water but impermeable to bacteria. The initial dressing is placed by the physician. Several modifications in the anchoring method of the catheter have proven useful with this dressing technique.

Previously, we sutured IVH catheters in place to prevent their dislodgement. The presence of an additional foreign body, the nonabsorbable suture material, penetrating the skin in proximity to the catheter puncture site seemed worth avoiding.

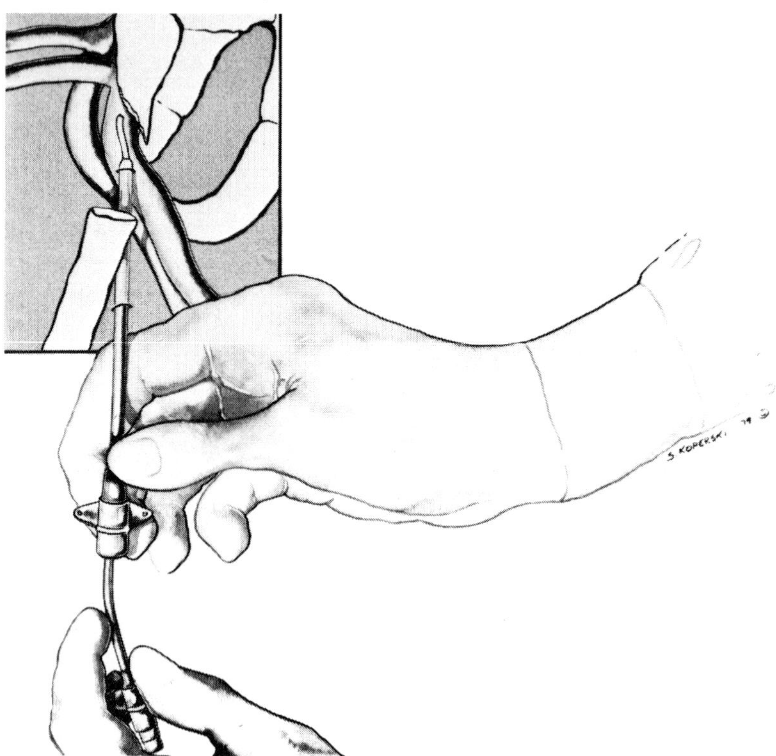

Figure 19-6. The 8½" blue silicone elastomer catheter containing its stiffening guide wire is advanced through the white introducing catheter as far as possible assuring a central venous placement.

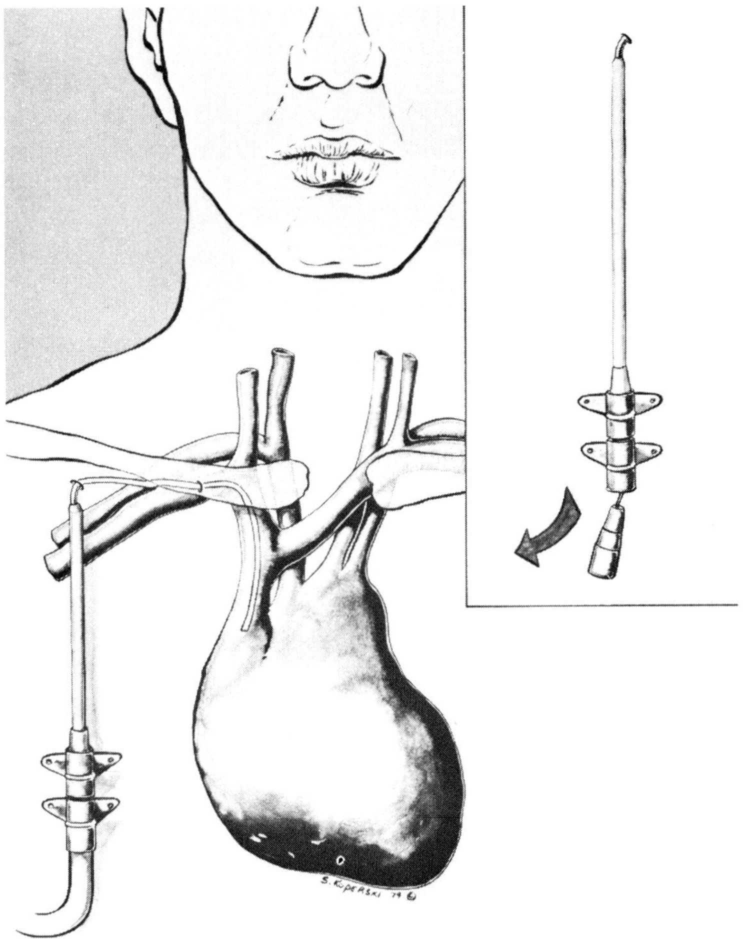

Figure 19-7. The guide wire is removed and a sterile primed extension tubing is connected to the gray connector. After the intravenous solution begins to flow, the white introducer is withdrawn until the blue catheter can be seen in an external unkinked position.

For the past 18 months, we have secured all catheters inserted by our service with ½″ × 1½″ sterile tape closures. The self-adhering dressing further buttresses the catheter-anchoring effect of the tapes. Unintentional catheter removal has been a rare occurrence with this method of dressing. Only 4 of 75 catheters have been unintentionally removed by patients during periods of confusion or disorientation. However, no catheters have been accidentally removed by the nursing personnel during routine catheter care utilizing this dressing technique.

Dressing Technique

The skin immediately adjacent to the IVH catheter is coated with sterile tincture of benzoin. After the benzoin compound becomes tacky, the sterile tapes are applied to hold the catheter in place (Figure 19-9). A sparing amount of iodophor ointment is applied to the catheter insertion site. The clear dressing material is then applied from about 2 inches above the catheter insertion site to about 1 inch below the junction of the extension set with the IVH catheter. Care is taken to protect the patient's skin from pressure necrosis secondary to contact with

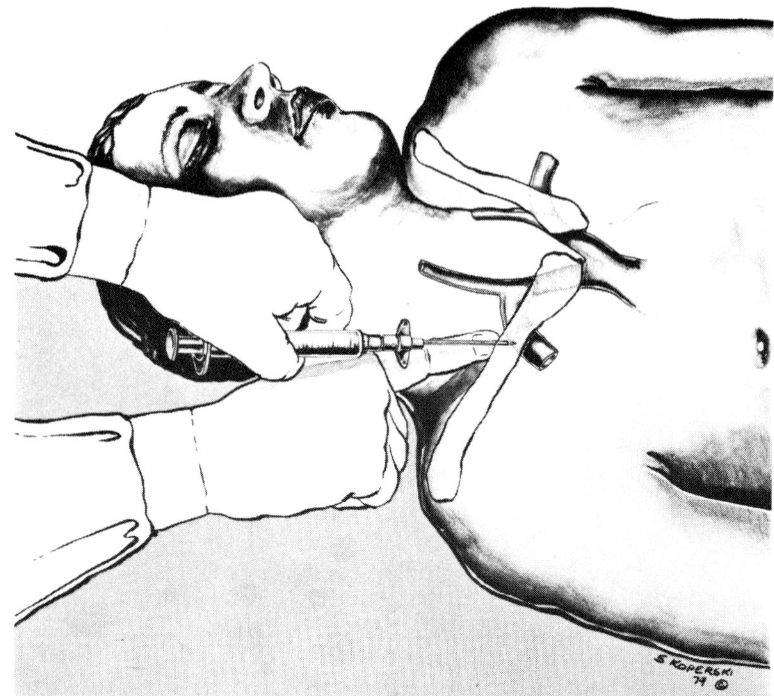

Figure 19-8. In the supraclavicular approach, the patient is placed in a supine position with the neck slightly flexed and rotated to the opposite side. Flexion relaxes the anterior scalenus muscle, and rotation tenses the sternocleidomastoid muscle, thus, facilitating differentiation of the two muscles.

the rigid plastic parts. Small pads of gauze dressing material (Telfa) serve this purpose (Figure 19-9). We do, however, use suture material to fasten the two plastic hubs of the Centrasil catheter to one another (not shown in figure).

A stat portable upright chest x-ray is then obtained to ascertain the position of the catheter and to detect any possible technical error related to catheter insertion.

TECHNICAL COMPLICATIONS

Pneumothorax is the most common technical complication of subclavian catheterization and represents about one third of all the technical mishaps.[10]

A pneumothorax is a collection of air in the pleural space, the space between the lung and the chest wall. Treatment of the pneumothorax is not always necessary, and observation of the patient may be all that is required. If no respiratory distress occurs and the pneumothorax is not under "tension," then it may slowly resolve without evacuation of the air. If the size of the pneumothorax increases on later chest x-rays or if the findings of respiratory distress or progressively increasing subcutaneous emphysema occur, the possibility of a persistent air leak from the injured lung is suggested. Subcutaneous emphysema is diagnosed by the observation of swelling in the subcutaneous tissue which feels spongy and crackles with fine crepitation on palpation. The floor nurse or IVH nurse may be the first observer to note these changes because they are frequently delayed events. If any of these findings are present, a new stat chest x-ray should be ordered and the operating physician should be notified. The patient should be accompanied by a nurse or physician for the x-ray and instability of vital signs suggests the need for a portable technique x-ray. If the patient is hypotensive, a supine film should be obtained,

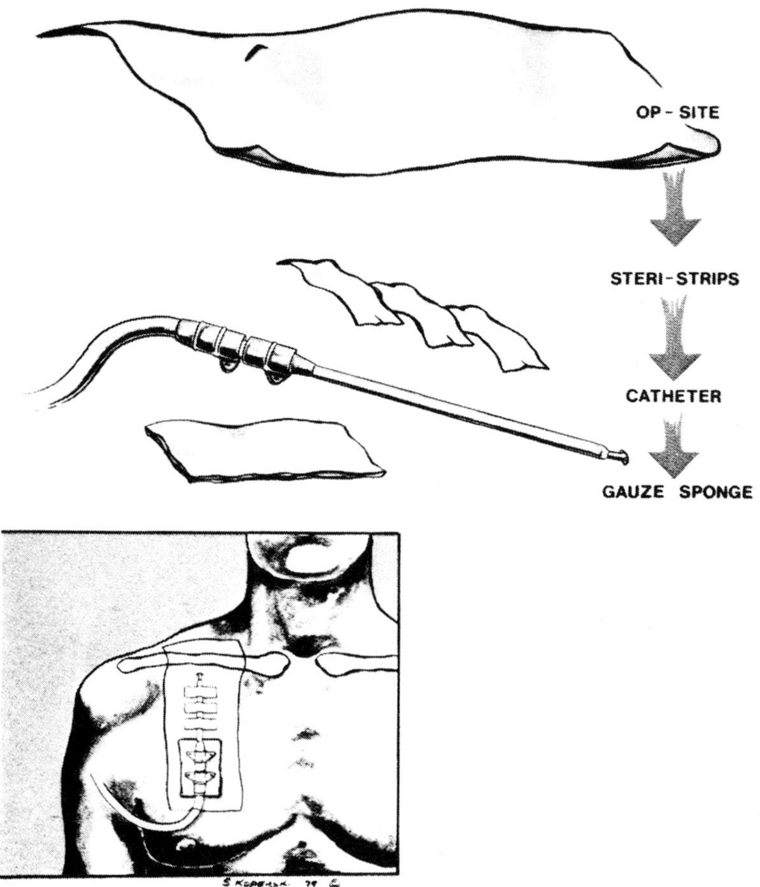

Figure 19-9. The catheter and introducer may be affixed with tincture of benzoin and sterile skin closure tapes. The patient's skin is protected from the hard plastic surfaces with a pad of sterile dressing. An occlusive dressing is applied over the entire assembly. A self-adhering polyurethane dressing technique is demonstrated.

since an upright position may cause further hypotension and result in cardiac arrest. The placement of a chest tube to control the pneumothorax may be required. When a chest tube is required, the IVH catheter, if it has been successfully positioned, may not have to be removed if it does not externally physically interfere with chest tube insertion.

Subclavian artery puncture is the next most frequent complication. Usually, the immediate problem is resolved by withdrawing the needle and applying digital pressure to the puncture site. Care should be taken never to catheterize the subclavian artery since any air or debris which enters the artery may embolize to the brain and result in a central neurologic deficit. Laceration of either the subclavian artery or vein can occur with a resultant hemothorax or large local hematoma. A hemothorax is a collection of blood in the pleural space. Both pneumothorax and hemothorax may be either immediate or delayed complications. Both conditions can be diagnosed on a chest x-ray.

If the immediate postcatheterization radiograph shows good catheter position in the superior vena cava and the patient goes on to develop symptoms of these complications, a new chest x-ray should be obtained and compared to the earlier one.

Catheter Malposition (Extravascular)

During the process of passing a catheter into the subclavian vein, it is possible to have the needle or introducer through which one is working slip out of the vein. Passage of the catheter becomes difficult and the catheter may actually be positioned outside the vein and come to lie in the pleural space or the mediastinum. To avoid this complication, one should never force the catheter into or through the introducing device. After the catheter is judged to be in place, the operator should be able to freely aspirate blood through the catheter. The old trick of lowering the IV bottle to observe for a "flashback" is not likely to be useful, since many IV sets are now equipped with valves to prevent any fluid from going back toward the bottle. "In line" filters in an IV set may also prevent the possibility of a flashback. Should the catheter tip come to rest in the pleural space and the infusion of IVH solution or other fluid is started, a hydrothorax (fluid in the pleural space) will result. Hydromediastinum occurs when the catheter tip comes to lie in the mediastinum and an infusion is allowed to run into this space where the heart and great vessels are located. Such malpositioned catheters must be withdrawn and replaced.

Catheter Malposition (Intravascular)

Intravascular malposition of the catheter is a commonly reported catheter complication and requires repositioning of the catheter.[11] A coiled catheter must likewise be repositioned, since it may penetrate the vessel and also will be likely to cause venous thrombosis. It is said that having the patient turn his head toward the side being catheterized increases the acuteness of the angle between the subclavian vein and the internal jugular vein. This decreases the likelihood of the catheter assuming a position in the internal jugular vein rather than the superior vena cava. Also, rigid catheters that come to lie in the right atrium should be retracted to the superior vena cava to avoid cardiac dysrhythmia.

Chylothorax and Chylous Fistula

Injury of the thoracic duct on the left side may result in chylothorax (the collection of lymph in the pleural space). Because of the anatomic position of the thoracic duct, the left supraclavicular approach to the subclavian vein should be avoided if possible (Figure 19-2). Control of lymphatic leak from the thoracic duct to the skin is usually difficult to stop; likewise, a chylothorax may be difficult to control.

Cloudy material leaking from around an IVH catheter suggests the possibility of chylous fistula. Any fluid leaking from the IVH catheter should be aseptically collected and checked for glucose content. A low glucose suggests the fluid is a body fluid, whereas a high glucose content suggests the fluid is leaking IVH fluid. If the IVH catheter is leaking, the catheter may have to be repaired or replaced.

Others

Any structure in the upper chest or root of the neck can be and has been injured. The other complications of catheterization, especially neurologic ones such as brachial plexus injury or phrenic nerve injury, cannot be directly diagnosed on chest x-ray. The frequency of their occurrence can be minimized by careful insertion technique.

The most difficult to detect, but most life-threatening complication, is pericardial tamponade caused by penetration of the atrium by the catheter. Cardiovascular collapse with neck vein distention, a narrow pulse pressure, and hypotension, with or without symptoms of congestive heart failure, suggest the possibility of this catastrophe. The complication is usually delayed since, in order to cause it, blood or IVH solution must leak into the pericardial space. Symptoms suggestive of pericardial tamponade require emergency intervention by the physician. Suspicion that this uncommon complication exists is necessary to avoid patient fatality. Beveling of the rigid catheters, whether long and placed through the arm or short and placed by subclavian puncture, enhances the likelihood of vascular penetration and the development of pericardial tamponade, hydrothorax, or hydromediastinum. The beveling creates a sharp leading edge on a stiff catheter, therefore predisposing the patient to vascular penetration. The treatment for pericardial tamponade is aspiration of the pericardial sac, which is usually done with a 22 gauge spinal needle from just below the xyphoid process of the sternum. The catheter should be withdrawn and replaced after resuscitation is complete.

Air Embolism

Air embolus is the passage of air into the heart, resulting in an intracardiac air lock at the pulmonic valve. This prevents the ejection of blood from the right heart. Fortunately, this complication occurs rarely. The clinical steps recommended for suspected air embolus are to remove the causative factor and to position the patient so as to minimize the hemodynamic consequences of the embolus.

The patient should be placed in the left lateral decubitus Trendelenberg position. This keeps the amount of air in the pulmonary outflow tract to a minimum by trapping it in the right heart chambers and great veins proximal to the pulmonic valve. Cardiothoracic surgical consultation should be obtained immediately since emergency cardiopulmonary bypass may be required.

On rare occasions, a patient with an intracardiac right-to-left shunt may require subclavian catheterization. A right-to-left shunt refers to an abnormal communication between the chambers of the right side of the heart with those on the left. That is, blood may pass from the right atrium or ventricle to the left atrium or ventricle without passing through the lungs. If air enters the great veins in any amount, it may pass through the cardiac shunt and embolize to the brain, resulting in immediate neurologic deficit which may be permanent. In a patient with such a shunt, extreme caution with all intravenous lines is warranted, and central venous IVH should be avoided in favor of a peripheral TPN regimen if at all possible. The use of 0.22 micron filters as air lock devices for all IVs in this group of patients is indicated.

USE OF IVH CATHETER

The dedicated use of the IVH catheter for nutritional support purposes has in part been responsible for the reduction in catheter associated sepsis now being reported by the medical community. A more lenient approach to the use of the catheter has been suggested by one group, but this seems to be an approach that can be successful only under rigidly controlled circumstances. In general, such an approach should be avoided.

Infusion of Lipid Emulsions Through Central IVH Catheters

Most IVH patients require infusion of lipid calories each week to prevent an essential-fatty-acid deficiency from developing, whereas others may have 40 to 60% of their daily caloric requirement given as fat. In either event, we have found it useful to install a sterile "Y" connector at the junction nearest the IVH catheter for the simultaneous infusion of lipid and IVH solutions. If the patient receives the lipid infusion once daily, then the "Y" connector is installed for the lipid infusion and the daily tubing set change is performed at the conclusion of the lipid infusion. The IVH solution would then be infused with a standard set until the next bottle of lipid is hung and a new "Y" connector is installed. The process is repeated daily or more often as required. Electronic infusion control devices should be used for both the lipid emulsion and aqueous solutions.

Technical Problems with IVH Catheters

CATHETER OCCLUSION

This problem seems largely avoidable, but has a propensity for occurring under mysterious circumstances on someone else's shift. When the infusion control device begins to alarm "occlusion," several potential causes for the alarm must be considered. The least likely cause for the alarm is a faulty electronic device; the most likely cause is user error or catheter malfunction. All of the IV tubing should be inspected for kinks and obstructions. If an 0.22 micron filter is being used, it should be inspected for integrity, the presence of trapped air, or other obstruction. Should these steps not reveal the cause of the alarm, it would seem wise to change the infusion control device before proceeding to inspect and aspirate the catheter. If these manuevers fail to reveal the cause for the alarm, the catheter under the dressing must be inspected. If an occlusive dressing has been used, then it must be aseptically dismantled and changed. If a clear dressing is in place, the catheter may be easily inspected by looking through the dressing. At this point, the best approach is to aspirate the catheter to retrieve any thrombus material. If the thrombus cannot be aspirated, the catheter should be removed and a new catheter inserted at a new site. Irrigation of the catheter or the passage of a guide wire to clear the line are not acceptable methods of dealing with this infrequent problem. Forceful irrigation of a silicone catheter should *never* be performed, since the catheter may be disrupted should the obstruction not be overcome.

LEAKING IVH CATHETER

By far, the most common cause of a leaking catheter or a saturated IVH dressing is either a break in one of the components of the IV tubing or a separation of the IV extension tubing from the IVH catheter hub. If neither of these defects can be discovered, then one should closely inspect the IVH catheter for leaks.

Catheters inserted through a needle may be damaged during insertion by the needle tip. A small leak may develop which slowly saturates the dressing material. Such a condition sets the stage for catheter sepsis and should be handled by removal of the suspected faulty catheter or by repair under aseptic conditions. Change of the catheter over a guide wire is also acceptable and is described in the section on potential catheter sepsis.

Catheter Embolus

Catheter embolus may be discovered at the time of catheter insertion, during therapy, or at the conclusion of therapy. If the technical mishap is suspected during catheter insertion, the potentially damaged catheter should be inspected for integrity. Should the catheter appear shortened, the

Technical Complications of Subclavian Catheterization

	Immediate	Delayed	Detectable on Chest Radiograph
Pneumothorax	Yes	Yes	Yes
Hemothorax	Yes	Yes	Yes
Arterial Puncture	Yes	No	Yes*
Chylothorax	No	Yes	Yes
Hydrothorax	No	Yes	Yes
Hydromediastinum	No	Yes	Yes
Pericardial Tamponade	No	Yes	No
Brachial Plexus Injury	Yes	No	No
Phrenic Nerve Injury	Yes	No	Yes**
Air Embolus	Yes	Yes	No
Catheter Malposition			
Intravascular	Yes	Yes	Yes
Extravascular	Yes	No	Yes

* If hematoma forms. ** Indirect evidence elevated hemidiaphragm.

catheterization procedure should be interrupted and a stat portable chest x-ray should be obtained. The sheared off catheter may be lodged in the great veins, the right heart, or the pulmonary outflow tract. Hopefully, such an event will not take place in a patient with an anatomic intracardiac right-to-left shunt. In most instances, the catheter may be retrieved with a specially designed snare. The procedure involves the intravenous passage of the snare under fluoroscopic control to remove the catheter from its aberrant position. If the radiologist does not meet with success, thoracotomy may be required to remove the embolized catheter. A sheared off catheter may be observed on a chest x-ray performed days after the catheterization. Precatheterization chest x-rays should be inspected so that it can be determined if the embolic catheter was present prior to the current catheterization. Though uncommon, such an event is not unheard of. Removal of the catheter in the latter instance is likely to require thoracotomy due to the deposition of fibrous tissue around the catheter.

Occasionally, the IVH nurse or house officer may be in the process of removing a central venous catheter and notice that the tip of the catheter appears to be missing. If any such device is modified by the operator placing the catheter, then a note should be made in the patient's record, describing the modification. Better yet, any portion of the catheter removed prior to insertion should be fastened to the patient's chart for future reference. If uncertainty exists about the integrity of the removed catheter, a chest x-ray should be obtained after catheter removal to establish whether or not a portion of the catheter has remained in the patient.

USE OF EMERGENCY PLACED CATHETERS FOR IVH

Occasionally, the question arises as to whether or not a catheter placed for resuscitation in the emergency room should be used for IVH. In general, a good rule of thumb to follow is that all catheters placed under emergency conditions should be changed within 24 to 48 hours after placement because of the high probability that they are contaminated. Such a catheter could be used temporarily for IVH if no sign of catheter sepsis existed with the understanding that the catheter would be changed as soon as possible. However, the catheter should be changed over a guide wire, as described later in the text, or preferably, should be removed and replaced at a new site.

POTENTIALLY CONTAMINATED CATHETER

The development of a new significant elevation in the thermogram of the patient receiving central venous IVH requires a thorough investigation. A significant elevation in the thermogram of a patient with a previously normal temperature has been arbitrarily set at 101.6°F. IVH catheters are frequently inserted in patients with spiking fevers. If there is no significant change in the previous thermogram, a work-up for catheter sepsis is usually not warranted. For example, if a patient has been spiking fevers daily to 102°F and repeats this same fever spike after the IVH catheter is inserted, a new fever work-up is not indicated just because the patient has been recently catheterized. However, if the patient begins to spike an even higher fever, to perhaps 103°F or 104°F, a work-up for potential catheter sepsis is indicated.

In general, when one begins the work-up of a patient with potential catheter sepsis, the bottle of IVH solution currently being administered should be discontinued and replaced with a fresh bottle. The old solution is sent for culture. However, "bottle fever" is rarely the cause of sepsis. A search, including all the other frequent sources of temperature elevation, is then performed. Cultures of the peripheral blood, as well as cultures of blood aspirated through the IVH catheter, are obtained. The IVH catheter puncture site should be inspected. Tenderness or erythema, especially with cloudy material around the catheter site, increase the suspicion that the patient may have catheter sepsis. Any material draining from or located near the puncture site should be sent for culture and sensitivity. Tenderness at the insertion site in the immediate post-insertion period is not uncommon and is probably related to the amount of tissue trauma caused by the insertion process. After all these possibilities are evaluated, changing the catheter over a guide wire is an acceptable alternative to removal of the suspect catheter and its replacement at a new site. The procedure for changing a catheter over a guide wire is as follows.

The patient is prepared as for a dressing change on the side of the catheter in question. A wide sterile field is set up around the catheter insertion site, which excludes the IV extension tubing, and the dressing is carefully removed. Any fluid at the puncture site should be cultured. A guide wire of the appropriate size is chosen. The size varies with the type of catheter being changed. An 0.018 inch, 50 cm length, flexible tip stainless steel wire is used for the Centrasil catheter. The wire is passed through the catheter immediately after an assistant disconnects the IV tubing from the IVH catheter. The old catheter is withdrawn and submitted to the laboratory for culture and sensitivity. If a new silicone rubber catheter is going to be placed through the old insertion site, a tissue dilator and short 5 Fr. introducer are required. Before the tissue dilator is passed over the wire, local anesthetic should be infiltrated into the skin and subcutaneous tissues surrounding the guide wire. The tissue dilator and introducer set are placed over the guide wire. The physician takes care to always have control of the guide wire so as not to lose it in the vein. The introducer set is advanced into the vein, and the tissue dilator and guide wire are removed. The new IVH catheter is then placed through the introducer. The introducer is withdrawn to a position external to the patient, the catheter is attached to a "keep open" infusion, anchored to the skin, and a dressing is applied in the usual fashion. The use of this technique saves the patient from exposure to the potential complications of a percutaneous insertion of a new catheter, while it allows adequate sampling of the old IVH catheter for possible contamination.

After changing a catheter over a guide wire, the decision as to whether or not to remove the catheter is made as follows. If the catheter culture comes back positive or, while the laboratory results are pending, the patient deteriorates, the newly placed exchange catheter is removed. However, if the blood cultures, either peripheral or central, are positive but the catheter culture is negative, then catheter-induced sepsis is unlikely and the exchange catheter is allowed to remain in place. If one takes the time to exchange or replace IVH catheters for potential catheter sepsis, then all intravascular catheters should be changed simultaneously. Arterial monitoring catheters, peripheral IV catheters, and Swan-Ganz catheters have all been the sources of sepsis in patients with or without IVH catheters in place. Another acceptable alternative is removal of the central line and maintenance of the patient with a peripheral TPN regimen until the issue of catheter sepsis can be satisfactorily resolved.

SUBCLAVIAN VEIN THROMBOSIS

If thrombosis of the subclavian vein is expected, studies should be done to confirm the diagnosis. The physician will probably choose noninvasive flow studies. If doubt exists concerning the status of the vein's patency, a period of observation followed by repeat flow studies or bilateral simultaneous upper extremity venography may be indicated. Confirmation of the diagnosis necessitates removal of the causative catheter and anticoagulative treatment of the patient, preferably with heparin. If IVH therapy needs to be continued, the new catheter should be placed, just prior to anticoagulative treatment of the patient, at an uninvolved site. Preferably, the patient can be maintained with peripheral TPN and central venous catheterization avoided.

Check List for Subclavian Catheter Insertion

Chart review for pertinent information
History of previous hyperalimentation
Coagulation problems
Altered anatomy from
  Past surgery
  Congenital e.g., Atrial septal defect, persistent left superior vena cava
  Trauma, non-operative
  Chronic pulmonary disease
  Old age (Kyphosis)
  Subclavian thrombosis
  Hypovolemia
Precatheterization chest x-ray review
Patient education completed
Consent obtained

OTHER CONSIDERATIONS

The addition of heparin to IVH solutions has been proposed by various authors as a preventive measure to decrease the incidence of catheter sepsis and subclavian vein thrombosis. If a polyethylene or teflon catheter is used, 2000 to 3000 units of heparin should be added to each liter of IVH solution. Heparin is probably not useful for those patients who have a silicone rubber catheter in place.[11]

SUMMARY

The management of patients with central venous catheters who are receiving IVH has been gradually improving throughout most of the medical community over the past decade. Attention to all of the details of catheter insertion and aseptic care of the catheter after insertion continue to assure both the patient and the members of the nutritional support team of the best results possible with respect to safety for the patient during this useful form of therapy.

BIBLIOGRAPHY

1. Dudrick, S.J., Rhoads, J.E., and Vars, H.M.: Growth of puppies receiving all nutritional requirements by vein. Fortschritte der Parenteral Ernahrung, *2:*16, 1967.
2. Bernard, R.W., and Stahl, W.M.: Subclavian vein catheterizations: A prospective study, I. Non-infectious complications. Ann. Surg., *173:*184, 1971.
3. Bernard, R.W., Stahl, W.M., and Chase, R.M.: Subclavian vein catheterizations: A prospective study, II. Infectious complications. Ann. Surg., *173:*191, 1971.
4. Curry, C.R., and Quie, P.G.: Fungal septicemia in patients receiving parenteral hyperalimentation. N. Engl. J. Med., *285:*1221, 1971.
5. Ryan, J.A., Jr., et al.: Catheter complications in total parenteral nutrition. N. Engl. J. Med. *290:* 757, 1974.
6. Shapiro, M., and Stern, W.Z.: Hazards of subclavian vein cannulation for central venous pressure monitoring. JAMA, *201:*327, 1967.
7. Lumb, P.O., et al.: Aggressive approach to intravenous feeding of the critically ill patient. Heart and Lung, *8:*71, 1979.
8. McDonald, A.S., Master, S.K.P., and Emerson, A.M.: A comparative study of peripherally inserted silicone catheters for parenteral nutrition. Canad. Anaesth. Soc. J., *24:*263, 1977.
9. Hoshal, V.L.: Total intravenous nutrition with peripherally inserted silicone elastomer central venous catheters. Arch. Surg., *110:*644, 1975.
10. Mitchell, S.E., and Clark, R.A.: Complications of central venous catheterization. AJR, *133:*467, 1979.
11. Deitel, M., and McIntyre, J.A.: Radiographic confirmation of the site of central venous pressure catheters. Can. J. Surg., *14:*42, 1971.
12. Blackburn, G.L.: Hyperalimentation in the critically ill patient. Heart and Lung, *8:*67, 1979.

Chapter 20

Developing Nutrition Screening/Assessment Forms

Abby S. Bloch, M.S., R.D.
Head Clinical Diet/Nutrition Specialist
Clinical Nutrition Support Kitchen
Memorial Sloan-Kettering Cancer Center
New York, New York

To nutritionally assess a hospital population effectively several decisions must be made prior to developing a form. An initial evaluation should provide a means by which patients at risk or potentially at risk are identified early in their hospitalization and managed appropriately.

If the goal of a program is screening of every patient, then a prescreening questionnaire could be filled out by the patient or a family member during admission or just prior to admission.[1] One must be careful and diligent in creating this type of questionnaire. The questions should be direct, succinct, and unambiguous. The advantage of this type of form is that it minimizes staffing requirements and can be done in a setting less threatening to the patient. Family members can help communication between the patient and hospital personnel if language is a problem. Problems with this method are that questions may not be interpreted correctly by the patient or that the information may not be totally accurate or completely answered.

An alternative to a prescreening questionnaire could be a combination of patient response and dietitian interview.[2] This has the advantage of assuring more reliable answers, but requires somewhat more staffing demands. The dietitian also establishes rapport with the patient at the time of admission. This initial interview sets up a basis for future interaction when discharge planning or counseling with the patient are required.

A third alternative is a rapid, concise, initial screening form which would be completed by the dietitian or other member of the staff skilled and knowledgeable in using the form.[3] The goal of this screening procedure would be to identify those patients who are deemed at risk nutritionally or who have the potential for becoming nutritionally depleted.

Each institution and health care facility must decide on the profile of their particular patient population.* If your setting is an inner city population, then drug–alcohol abuse and/or their effects on nutritional status might need to be considered. For a suburban hospital with a predominantly affluent patient population, an assessment that incorporates cholesterol and triglyceride values or overweight risk factors may be of help. In our hospital, a specialty cancer center, the focus of initial screening is a nutritional profile appropriate for a cancer patient. Each setting requires its own indi-

---

* A working group of the Section on Public Health, N.Y. Academy of Medicine is addressing these issues. The goal of this group is to develop standards and guidelines which could serve as models for appropriate screening and assessing of patients.

vidual form based on patient type and relevant risk factors.

When we were designing a rapid assessment form, we looked at many parameters before selecting those which would give us effective determinations.† In a 3½-month pilot study conducted at Memorial Hospital in January 1978, an Initial Nutrition Assessment Form and a Follow-up Form were tested (Figures 20-1 through 20-3).[3,4] In designing these forms, many considerations went into the decision of the questions we chose. We felt that primary diagnosis in our center would be the specialty diagnosis of cancer, and other diagnoses would be secondary. In our particular setting, treatment plan is critical and was included. Depending on the nature of the general population in a clinical setting, treatment plan may be either obvious or secondary in a nutrition screening assessment.

The third area we gave consideration was the patient's weight change over given periods of time. Preillness weight needed to be established. This is not always as easy a question as it seems nor were the answers always accurate. Many patients know the weight they should be, the weight they would like to be, or the weight they thought they were. If patients are in their 50s, 60s, or 70s, their weight may have changed each decade. Another problem is that many patients fluctuate 20 or 30 pounds in a given time frame. Therefore, you cannot just ask one simple question, "What was your preillness adult weight?" You may need to ask other questions, such as, "How much did you weigh when you were married? What is your dress size/belt size and how many wardrobes do you own? What sizes? How much did you weigh 10 years ago? How much did you weigh 5 years ago?" or whatever other markers based on the patient's age, status, and condition seem appropriate. It may be helpful to get a frame of reference of weight at some period relatively close to the time of admission, be it 1 month, 6 weeks or 2 months. This gives an idea as to whether or not the weight change has been a slow progression or a rapid change over months or weeks.

Admission weight is important; however, one should be aware of inaccuracies of admission weights and must scrutinize them carefully. For example, many patients are weighed with shoes, jackets, with heavy items in the pockets, and other items that skew the actual weight. Patients with a prosthesis may have to define whether or not the weight is with or without the prosthesis.

In selecting the standards the patient would be compared against, one must again make decisions. Several height/weight tables are currently available. Based on your patient population and what your goal is, you may want to pick ideal or desirable vs. average or minimum standards. It will make a difference in the percent admission weight to standard weight of your patient population. Height, sex, and age must also be taken into account in assessing a patient's nutritional status.

In our pilot study, laboratory data were also part of the initial form. We were not sure whether many of the criteria previously cited by other clinicians were valid criteria as flagging or screening tools. Therefore, a screening profile of meaningful laboratory data that may relate to nutritional status was included in the form. Interestingly, the results of our study showed that most of the laboratory data were not significant as tools for screening patients and identifying patients who might be at nutritional risk. It is important for a dietitian or nutritionist, not just the clinician, to be familiar with the patient's electrolyte and hematologic values as a tool for further clinical management of the patient. Knowledge of baseline laboratory values is helpful in working with dietary management. However, we felt that, based on the available lab data, these were not valid criteria for use in flagging a patient at nutritional risk. If a clinician is evaluating renal, cardiac, dia-

† Nutrition Assessment of the Cancer Patient, Report of a Pilot Study: Shils, M.E., Coiro, D., et al., Unpublished data.

MEMORIAL SLOAN-KETTERING CANCER CENTER
Initial Nutrition Assessment Form

1. a) What is your usual weight? ______ pounds.
   b) What is your height? _____feet _____inches.
   c) In the last two months, have you gained weight?
   No _____ Yes _____. If yes,how many pounds? _____.
   Lost weight? No ____ Yes ____. If yes,
   how many pounds? ______.

2. Is your present appetite usual? _____ better? _____ or worse? _____ than normal.

3. a) Do you have a problem related to eating? No _____ Yes _____. If yes, check the appropriate reason(s): Sore Mouth _____. Swallowing _____ Chewing _____ Choking _____ Salivation _____ Change in taste _____ Food aversion _____ Nausea _____ Vomiting _____ Diarrhea _____ Constipation _____ Other ______________________________
   b) Do you need help in eating? No ____ Yes ____.

4. Do you wear dentures? Upper _____ Lower _____ None _____.

5. a) Were you previously on a special diet? No ____ Yes ____. If yes, specify: ____________
   b) Do you take vitamins or minerals? No ____ Yes ____.
   c) Do you have any personal or religious dietary restrictions? Kosher ____ Vegetarian _____ Other (specify): ______________________________

6. Do you have any allergies or intolerances for food? No ____ Yes ____. If yes, please list:

7. Do you take any other special food regularly? No ____ Yes ____. If yes, please list:

8. Do you have any major food dislikes? No ____ Yes ____. If yes, please list: ____________

9. What is the reason for this admission? ______________________________

DO NOT WRITE BELOW THIS LINE - FOR DIETITIAN'S USE ONLY

Date of Initial Visit: ____________________
1. Diagnosis: ____________________

2. Expected Treatment Plan: Surgery _________
   RT _________ Chemo ________Other _________

3. Abnormal Lab Data (list): ____________

4. Metabolic and other problems:
   Diabetes_______ Hyperlipidemia _____
   Other Endocrine _____ Malabsorption
   Hypertension_____ Type ____________
   Heart Disease_____ GI Obstruction
   Persistent Fever_____ Partial _________
   Severe Trauma/Burns____ Complete _________
   Alcohol/Drug Abuse ____ GI Fistula _________
   Renal Disease _____
   Liver Disease _____

5. Present Medications: ____________

6. Ht: _____cm. Adm. Wt: _____kg Avg Std._____kg
   Pre-illness Wt: ____lbs. _____kg
   Percentage Wt Change (%): _______
   (pre-illness - Adm/Pre-illness X100)

7. Anticipated problems due to illness or treatment plan? No _____ Yes _____

8. Edema/Ascites: (Site) Degrees-0-4+)
   Ascites: _________ Sacral _________

9. Nutritional Care Plan:
   a) No apparent problem ____________
   b) Diet Rx ____________
   c) Supplements Rx ____________
   d) Date to Reevaluate ____________
   e) Nutrition Team Consult ____________

10. Discharge Plan/Comments: ____________

DIETITIAN: ____________________

Figure 20-1.

MSKCC
NUTRITION ASSESSMENT FORM: INITIAL

Date: ____________ ____________
(of Admission (of Assessment)

A. PRIMARY AND OTHER DIAGNOSES; (treatment & dates)

B. TREATMENT PLAN: ____________

C. WEIGHT-HEIGHT (to nearest Kg-Cm)
1) Pre-Illness Wt: ______ Kg
2) Wt 1 month ago: ______ Kg
3) Admission Wt: ______ Kg
4) Height: ______ Cm
5) Loss or gain* ______ %
6) Adm wt/Avg Std: ______ %
*(Pre-ill - adm/Pre-ill)

D. LABORATORY DATA: Date: ______

Hgb ______	BUN ______	Glucose ______
MCV ______	Creatinine ______	Fe ______
WBC ______	Na ______	TIBC ______
Platelets ______	K ______	Bilirubin ______
	CO_2 ______	Albumin ______
	Cl ______	SGOT ______

E. WEIGHT AND METABOLIC STATUS:

		0	1	2
WT. +	+			
CHANGE _	0-5			
%	>5-9			
	>9-12			
	>12-20			
	> 20			

0=Normal temperature range.
1=Persistent fever ≤ 39.0.
2=Persistent fever > 39.0 w/or without trauma.

F. PRESENT MEDICATIONS: ____________

G. KNOWN OR PROBABLE METABOLIC PROBLEMS:

Diabetes ______	Liver Disease ______
Heart Disease ______	Hyperlipidemia ______
Hypertension ______	Malabsorption ______
Other Endocrine ______	Type ______
Renal Disease ______	______

H. PREVIOUS DIET PRESCRIPTION: ____________

I. EDEMA/ASCITES: (Site/Degree - 0-4+)

Ascites: ______

Sacral: ______

J. IMPAIRED FOOD INTAKE: Yes ____ No ____
If yes: Mild ____ Mod. ____ Severe ____

K. NUTRITIONALLY RELEVANT ASSOCIATIONS:

1) Anorexia ______
2) Altered Taste ______
3) Nausea ______
4) Vomiting ______
5) Sore Mouth ______
6) Dysphagia ______
7) Pain ______
8) Obstruction ______
a) partial ______
b) complete ______
9) Fistula ______
site: ______
10) Post-Op ______
11) RT-past ____ Site: H&N ______
Present ____ Chest ______
Abdomen ______
12) Current Chemotherapy ______
13) Altered bowel habit ______
a) Diarrhea ______
frequency/day ______
watery, brown ______
yellow ______
b) Constipation ______

L. PATIENT AT NUTRITIONAL RISK: Yes ____ No ____
If yes; on basis of E ____ and/or K ____

M. RECOMMENDATION: Oral- Regular Diet ____ Special Diet ____ Supplement ______
Tube formula:MSKCC ____ Special ____ Consultation ______

*Nutritional risk: As defined by E, obstruction, serious malabsorption or persistent inability to be fed enterally; albumin ≤ 2.5g%

Signature: ____________

32
NUTRITION

Figure 20-2.

MSKCC
NUTRITION ASSESSMENT - FOLLOW UP FORM

Follow-up date ________

Adm. Wt. ______kg Date ________

Initial % Wt. Change ________%

Current Wt. _____kg Date ______ Edema/Ascites:

% weight change from admission _______%

Impaired Food Intake Yes ___ No ___
If yes: Mild ____ Moderate ____ Severe _____

Ambulatory ( )
Bedridden ( )

Factors associated with interval change:

	Yes	No		Yes	No		Yes	No
surgery . . . . If yes - date and type	___	___	chemotherapy	___	___	vomiting . . .	___	___
fistula . . . . If yes - site	___	___	radiation . .	___	___	dysphagia . .	___	___
obstruction	___	___	mucositis . .	___	___	diarrhea . .	___	___
progress of disease	___	___						

Previous diet therapy:

Oral - Regular Diet _____ Special Diet _____ Supplement _____

Tube Formula - MSKCC ____ Special _____ TPN ______ PPN ___

Present Medications (indicate changes only): ______________

WEIGHT AND METABOLIC STATUS:

%Wt.Loss Change*	0	1	2
+			
0-5			
>5-9			
>9-12			
>12-20			
>20			

*From Preillness Weight

0=Normal temperature range.
1=Persistent fever < 39.0.
2=Persistent fever > 39.0
w/or without trauma

PATIENT AT NUTRITIONAL RISK: Yes ____ No ____

*Nutritional risk defined by Wt-metabolic status, serious malabsorption, persistent inability to be fed enterally, albumin ≤ 2.5 g%.

RECOMMENDATION: Oral - Regular Diet _____ Special Diet _____ Supplement ________

Tube formula: MSKCC ____ Special ________ Consultation ______

Signature: ______________________

32a
NUTRITION

Figure 20-3.

Date of consultation____________________
Diagnosis: Same as on admission____________________
additional or modified____________________
(indicate)

Anthropometric data:
a) Present Wt.________ Kg.
(nearest Kg.)
b) Triceps skin fold________ cm. % standard______
c) Mid-arm circumference ________cm. % standard ______
d) Muscle________ cm. % standard ______
e) Edema & degree (1–4) ________Ascites______ ______
Site(s) ________________ (yes) (no)

Additional Lab Data:
Fe/TIBC________ Mg______
Ca______ P______ Art. Ph______
PCO_2______ CO_2______ O_2______
Other________________

Previous radiation therapy to abdomen____________________
(rads and dates)
Previous alimentary tract surgery and dates____________________

Absorption data:
Xylose________________
Fat________________
B_{12}________________
Other________________

Gastrointestinal status________________
Metabolic status________________
(0–3)

Nutritional diagnoses:____________________

Etiology of nutritional problem:____________________

Plan of nutritional therapy:____________________

Clinical Diet/Nutrition Specialist________________
Physician________________

Figure 20-4.

betic, or other nutritionally related medical problems, those indices which are appropriate should be incorporated into the form.

Another area that was included in our form was the use of medications. There are many drugs that will either produce a drug-nutrient interaction or specific side effects such as nausea, vomiting, diarrhea, or depressed appetite. It is important for the clinician assessing the patient who is having problems with poor nutrition intake to be aware of such medication and whether or not the medication plays a role in the patient's deteriorating nutritional condition.

If the clinician is not otherwise screening for metabolic problems, it would be of help to note whether or not there are other possible problems such as diabetes, hypertension, liver disease, hyperlipidemia, malabsorption or other known medical problems which would adversely affect the nutritional status of the patient. Again, this information is supplementary rather than critical as the flagging technique for identifying patients at risk.

The next area for consideration was whether or not the patient had edema or ascites. This is critical in that the patient who has marked edema and/or ascites will need to have the weight findings reevaluated. Stable body weight may in fact reflect lean body weight loss with superimposed fluid gain.

Identification of impaired food intake is also of importance. In this regard, our team found that an in-depth nutrition history or diet recall interview was not as expedient as determining nutritionally relevant associations such as anorexia, nausea, vomiting, altered taste, problems in chewing and swallowing, and altered bowel habits. A patient indicating problems in this area was more readily flagged as being at or potentially at nutritional risk. These questions, rather than a diet history, become meaningful when assessing the patient's present status. False information occurring in the use of recall or diet histories results from oversight by patients in accounting for every mouthful of food consumed, forgetting additions, such as butter, sugar, dressings, mayonnaise, or other items.

Perception of portion sizes varies. What is considered a large portion for the patient may be inadequate for the healthy individual. Also, one must elicit what was actually eaten vs. what was served. Combination dishes present problems since ingredients are not always known and proportions are impossible to estimate. Calculating a diet also creates errors and guesses. The time and effort involved in retrieving the data must be carefully weighed against the validity of the information received.

Calorie counts and documentation of habits may be appropriate and useful for establishing trends or rough averages while the patient is in the hospital or for discharge planning. Such discussions may best be done at a later date. The initial time commitment could then focus on determining whether or not the patient has a nutritional problem.

In order to have a visual method of flagging patients at risk, we developed a grid which plotted percent of weight change on the vertical axis against temperature and metabolic status on the horizontal axis (Figure 20-2, E). An area of predetermined risk was marked out, and any patient who fell below this area was deemed at risk and in need of more aggressive nutritional therapy.

At this point, a more in-depth nutrition screening is appropirate for those patients identified as being at risk.[5] Diagnostic studies could be requested, further blood tests might prove helpful in ascertaining nutritional deficiencies, and calorie counts or a specific dietary history could be useful in identifying the extent and cause of the nutritional problem. It has been our experience that the majority of patients are not malabsorbing or having metabolic difficulties, but rather are demonstrating compromised food intake. Various reasons could account for this inability to achieve the needed intake.

Physical limitations frequently are responsible for poor eating habits: the patient who is unable to obtain food, manipulate utensils or equipment, or who is too weak or lacks motivation to prepare meals if left alone for long periods during the day. If pain is present, many patients find eating secondary to their primary problem, dealing with pain. Patients who want to eat or enjoy foods but have negative reactions as a result of eating, such as cramping, diarrhea, nausea, vomiting, frequently make a decision not to eat rather than experience the effects of the food.

The emotional response to the medical problem may also cause a patient to lose his appetite. Preoccupation with the illness, treatment alternatives, financial concerns, and family responsibilities all play a role in the patient's ability to cope. Knowing what is at the bottom of the patient's poor intake may remove some if not most of the nutritional obstacles the patient is creating.

In approaching a realistic method of assessing or screening patients as soon after admission as is feasible, our team elected not to use some of the popularly known techniques such as anthropometrics, cellular immunity skin testing, or nitrogen balance studies. We believe that to implement a realistic, rapid screening technique, only the most relevant, easily identifiable parameters should be included. With the questionable accuracy, validity, and consistency involved in the technique of measuring tricep skin fold, arm muscle circumference, and mid-arm muscle circumference, compounded by the time and staffing required to perform the measurements, we felt that the information did not warrant the time and effort involved. Several recent articles[1–6] have documented some of the problems in these procedures.

Biochemical parameters are helpful, but not usually included in normal admission screening requests. Patients would be billed for additional blood tests arbitrarily even if they are at no nutritional risk or if they are being admitted for a simple elective procedure. Some of the biochemical parameters are questionable in patients with specific medical problems; for example, a low albumin may be due to many other medically related causes, not necessarily nutritionally related. Creatinine can be affected by renal disease. All biochemical indices will be affected by the fluid status of the patient, be it dehydration or fluid overload.

Although biochemical indices are useful and necessary for management of the patient during hospitalization, their use as a screening tool in flagging patients at risk may be unnecessary.

Skin testing for anergy also seems inappropriate for every patient on admission. This is a costly, time consuming and personnel demanding procedure. The benefits gleaned from the results are far from assured. Many patients who have been chronically debilitated, such as those with cancer, COPD, rheumatoid arthritis, or IBD, will be relatively anergic due to their medical status, not their nutritional status. This method would be inappropriate for assessing all incoming patients in a general hospital setting.

Each center must identify those nutritional factors relevant to their patient population. With these factors in mind, a meaningful nutrition screening form should be designed. If the form is correctly constructed, patients will be identified as to whether or not they are nutritionally at risk. The information taken from the form has to be meaningful and interpretable by those using the data. The key point may be a weight change or another nutritionally relevant factor, but it should be significant in that setting to allow a decision to be made about the patient and his management and nutritional manipulation from admission to discharge.

An effective follow-up form, using similar criteria could be adapted to evaluate patients at realistic intervals during hospitalization. In this way, patients who are stable at admission but deteriorate while hospitalized can be identified and supported before too much weight loss and malnutrition develop.

As has been said so often, it is much easier to maintain a patient nutritionally than to renourish a severely debilitated patient. Our goal should be to prevent malnutrition before it occurs.

REFERENCES

1. Behnke, A.R., Katch, F.I., and Katch, V.L.: Routine anthropometry and arm radiography in assessment of nutritional status: Its potential. JPEN, *2:*4, 1978.
2. Bray, et al.: Use of anthropometric measures to assess weight loss. Am. J. Clin. Nutr., *31:*769, 1978.
3. Burgert, S.L., and Anderson, G.F.: An evaluation of upper arm measurements used in nutritional assessment. Am. J. Clin. Med., *32:*2136, 1979.
4. Gray, G.E., and Gray, L.K.: Validity of anthropometric norms used in the assessment of hospitalized patients. JPEN, *3:*5, 1979.
5. Heymsfield, S., et al.: A radiographic method of quantifying protein calorie malnutrition. Am. J. Clin. Nutr., *32:*693, 1979.
6. Nixon, D.W., et al.: Protein-calorie undernutrition in hospitalized cancer patients. Am. J. Med., *68:*683, 1980.

Chapter 21

Nutrition Support: Team Approach

Murray H. Seltzer, M.D., Director
Bernadette A. Slocum, R.N., B.S.N.
Emma L. Cataldi-Betcher, R.D., M.S.
David W. Bedell, R.Ph.
Florine R. Wright, L.P.N.

Nutrition Support Service
Saint Barnabas Medical Center
Livingston, New Jersey

HISTORICAL PERSPECTIVES OF NUTRITION SUPPORT

The mid 1960s represented an exciting era at the hospital of the University of Pennsylvania in Philadelphia. During those years, the development of what was ultimately to be known worldwide as hyperalimentation was taking form in the Harrison Department of Surgical Research at the University of Pennsylvania. Dr. Murray H. Seltzer, one of the authors, attended medical school and completed a surgical internship and residency at Penn during the years 1961 to 1971. Watching history unfold and being a part of it was a memorable experience. Dr. Jonathan E. Rhoads, then chairman of the department of surgery, had devoted a significant portion of his academic career over many decades to the concept that proper nutritional support was vital for the well-being of the surgical patient. Through his encouragement and that of Dr. Harry Vars of the Harrison Department of Surgical Research, Dr. Stanley Dudrick and others first demonstrated that sufficient nutrients could be given intravenously to Beagle puppies to support normal growth and development. Eventually, this technique was carried on to both infants and adults and now represents a milestone in medical history.

Initially, the pharmacy at the hospital at the University of Pennsylvania had to prepare the intravenous solutions, beginning with basic materials. As word of success spread, the most severely debilitated, moribund patients were transferred to the University Hospital to see if this new miracle treatment could save their lives. These frequently were patients with serious gastrointestinal disorders, multiple gastrocutaneous fistulae, and severe sepsis. The pronounced gratification of watching patients who were starving to death gradually turn around, gain weight, heal their wounds, and eventually be discharged is indescribable. Naturally, all was not quite so smooth. Many of the potential complications were previously undescribed and much of the success came by trial and error. Several house staff, following on the heels of Dr. Dudrick, were able to participate in the growth of this new therapeutic modality. To include but a few, Dr. Douglas Wilmore, Dr. William Currieri, Dr. Ted Copeland, Dr. James Long, Dr. Ezra Steiger, Dr. Bruce MacFadyen, Dr. Howard Silverman, Dr. Bob Ruberg, and many others were present during these developmental years. They subsequently carried forth techniques, and in many instances, made significant advances themselves in the field of nutritional support.

In 1969, as part of the University's residency program, Dr. Seltzer had a 6-month rotation at Lancaster General Hospital in Lancaster, Pennsylvania. As would be expected in a hospital of approximately 500 beds, situations arose in which patients needed intravenous nutritional support. Commercially available products were limited at that time. The technique was just beginning to achieve notoriety. It was with Dudrick's original article in hand,[1] that one of the hospital pharmacists and Dr. Seltzer, without benefit of air-flow hoods or sophisticated techniques, were able to combine protein hydrolysates with hypertonic glucose to prepare hyperalimentation fluid. Appropriate electrolytes and vitamins had to be added. The concept of inserting a subclavian catheter in a patient was relatively new and was considered to be a radical invasion of the body. Carefully selected patients were treated, and although it was known that careful attention to asepsis was required, it was not infrequent that patients would spike a 104° fever because of an inadvertent contaminant during the preparation of the solutions. During the remainder of Dr. Seltzer's training years at the Hospital of the University of Pennsylvania, hyperalimentation became a standard form of treatment, the merits of which were not disputed. Of the many physicians who had the privilege of observing the immediate and dramatic successes of therapy, the impressions were so overwhelming that there did not appear to be a need for randomized prospective studies to prove the merits of intravenous nutritional support. It could be viewed similarly to the curative power of appendectomy for appendicitis. The overwhelmingly obvious nature of the success precluded the need for statistical evaluation. Moreover, morally, it was unacceptable to allow any patient to participate in a controlled study in which he was deliberately allowed to starve. Having become a firm believer in this therapeutic modality, it was then disappointing for Dr. Seltzer to enter the military in 1971 and no longer have intravenous nutritional support at his disposal. Having been stationed at the Walson Army Hospital at Fort Dix, New Jersey, it became apparent that the patient spectrum included individuals seriously ill enough to merit intravenous nutritional support. With the encouragement of an interested Chief of Surgery, Lt. Col. Edward P. Quarantillo Jr., M.D., and with an eager and enthusiastic pharmacy department, it was not difficult to establish hyperalimentation as a treatment at Walson Army Hospital. Solutions were similarly prepared; and this standardization of solutions was advantageous for practicing physicians. Conditions were always arranged so that if a formula needed changing, it could be done rather easily.

Upon leaving the military in 1973, and entering the private practice of surgery at the Saint Barnabas Medical Center, Livingston, New Jersey, Dr. Seltzer was once again encouraged by the then-chairman of the department of surgery, Dr. Louis R. M. Del Guercio, and the then-director of pharmacy, Mrs. Anna Catena, to establish appropriate methodology within the institution to make intravenous hyperalimentation readily available to all patients in need. In viewing the problems of transition from a University Hospital to a Military Hospital and then to a private practice voluntary Medical Center, it was felt that simplification of techniques would be necessary to allow a significant number of physicians to provide appropriate hyperalimentation to the greatest number of patients. It did not appear practical to hand tailor each solution de novo for the specific patient, nor did it seem reasonable that the busy physician, house staff, or private practitioner would be able to devote sufficient time on a daily basis to redesign the patients' solutions. The transition to amino acid solutions, both essential and nonessential, in combination with hypertonic dextrose, as contrasted with the previous use of fibrin hydrolysate, was beginning to occur in the early 1970s. The standardization of techniques for initiating, ordering, and monitoring intravenous nutritional support enabled a diversity of physicians to provide such treatment for a wide spectrum of patients.

It was felt that the performance of all hyperalimentation by only one or two physicians with a monopoly on care might provide a slightly higher quality of care, but in the long run, because of the nature of private practice institutions, would minimize the number of patients able to benefit from such treatment.[2] The standardization of techniques has enabled as many as 50 different physicians on the staff to give and monitor hyperalimentation to their own patients.

The nutrition support committee of the surgery department functioned as an administrative coordinator and initiator in the departments of surgery and pharmacy to facilitate the purchasing, preparation, and standardization of the materials necessary for hyperalimentation. It also served as an educational vehicle for the hospital family, enabling them to improve their expertise. A team concept gradually evolved, initially without specific design. In the early days, Al Coco, R.Ph., Ed Lucchino, R.Ph., and David Bedell R.Ph., in conjunction with the director of the pharmacy, Anna Catena, R.Ph., paid meticulous attention to the pharmacy preparation of solutions and participated as "team" members in the "unofficial team."

It became readily obvious that if standardization of dressing changes could be accomplished and if this chore could be removed from the house staff duties, the incidence of complications could probably be greatly reduced. Florine Wright, L.P.N., better known to many as Flo Wright (an ironic name for someone involved with intravenous solutions), assumed the task of changing subclavian dressings. Almost immediately, there was a marked decrease in complication and infection rates as one person became responsible for the meticulous care of the dressings.

In 1978, Bernadette Slocum, R.N., recognizing the development of a new nursing specialty, i.e., nutrition support nursing, joined ranks with us, initially in a research capacity, but very shortly thereafter in a clinical hyperalimentation nursing role. The team was gradually assembling itself, without quite realizing it was actually a team, and starting to function rather harmoniously. Through the years, it became equally obvious that nutrition support was not to be restricted to intravenous feedings alone, but in an equally important fashion, could be administered enterally, using proper materials and proper supervision. Not truly having a formal team but recognizing the need for dietetic expertise, Cecilia Fileti, R.D., assistant director of dietetics, was available so that we could draw upon her abilities as a resource person in the area of enteral support. We, thus, had assembled a Nutrition Support Team without having such a designation within the hospital.

Acceptance of this group, consisting of a physician, pharmacist, registered nurse, licensed practical nurse, and registered dietitian, was generally good throughout the hospital. The group tended to work quietly behind the scenes while encouraging the entire hospital family to assume responsibility for seeing that patients received proper nutritional support. They proved the merits of having a team, whether official or otherwise, by improving the quality of patient care, while at the same time, instituting cost-saving maneuvers. The hospital administration, under the direction of Joseph Lindner, M.D., president of the medical center, formalized the Nutrition Support Service in August, 1979. No longer was the majority of the group to be essentially volunteering much of their spare time or donating bits and pieces of their professional time from their other duties to make nutrition support effective. The team was formed and was allowed to institute appropriate measures in the areas of clinical care,

Orders for Insertion of Subclavian Catheter

Please have the following materials available
by________ (time).

1. Acetone
2. Betadine Ointment
3. Betadine Solution
4. Deseret Intracath #16 gauge
5. Cut down tray
6. 2″ X 2″ and 4″ X 4″ pads
7. 2″ adhesive tape
8. Tincture of Benzoin
9. Sterile gloves
10. Two 3 cc. syringes with one #22 1-1/2″ needle
11. Xylocaine 1%
12. 1000 cc. 5% D/W
13. Macrodrip IV administration set and 1 extension set (sterile)
14. Chucks
15. Disposable razor
16. Face Masks

Thank you,

____

(signature)

Figure 21-1.

teaching, clinical research, and intrahospital administrative functions. Shortly after the formalization of the team, Mrs. Fileti moved to Michigan and Emma Cataldi, R.D., M.S., joined the Nutrition Support Service at the Saint Barnabas Medical Center.

During the course of this team's official and unofficial activities, a grass roots approach was taken and promulgated in publications concerning a simplified standardization hyperalimentation formula,[3] an instant nutritional assessment,[4] and a standardized approach to the insertion of subclavian catheters.[5] Preprinted order sheets for subclavian catheterization, initiation of hyperalimentation, and monitoring of parenteral and enteral nutrition were instituted. (Figures 21-1, 21-2, 21-3.) This gradual transition from informality to formality appeared natural and appropriate over the period of 6 years. Drawing on the benefits of the historical development of our Nutrition Support Service, it is the purpose of this article to assist others in developing a logical sequence for the formation of Nutrition Support Services within their hospitals. One must recognize the need for an evolutionary development of a team as opposed to the radical institution of a full support service where no rudimentary beginnings of a team previously existed.

NUTRITIONAL ASSESSMENT

Malnutrition is a term related to nutrition support, which is frequently used in the literature without being defined. In the most literal of senses, one would say that malnutrition means bad nutrition. The problem then begins in attempting to define bad nutrition. One can possibly think of bad nutrition being defined as a state in which certain

Hyperalimentation Order Sheet

A standard preset formula for hyperalimentation is used.

500 cc. Amino Acid 8.5% + 500 cc. 50% Dextrose
Na 40 mEq.
K 40.5 mEq.
Mg. 8 mEq.
Acetate 40.6 mEq.
Chloride 33.5 mEq.
Phosphate 15 mM.
Calcium 5 mEq.
Gluconate 5 mEq.
MVI 5 cc. will be added to the first liter daily

1. After insertion of catheter, please order portable chest x-ray STAT in sitting position.
2. Run 5% Dextrose at KVO rate until position of catheter is ascertained.
3. Starting at 3:00 p.m., run_______ liter(s) of hyperalimentation solution per day (to run at a steady rate).
4. Additional orders________________________________.
5. Vitamin B_{12} 1000 micrograms IM today.
6. Folic Acid 5 mg. IM once a week.
7. Aquamephyton 20 mg. IM Tuesdays and Fridays.
8. Subclavian line not to be used for any purpose other than hyperalimentation *except* in an extreme emergency.

Thank you,

____

(signature)

Figure 21-2.

aspects of the body's composition are below normal, or perhaps, one may consider malnutrition to be those instances in which abnormal body composition affects the functioning of the body. One may feel that malnutrition more importantly relates to specific components of the body such as protein in which there is either a deficiency of visceral or skeletal, or both visceral and skeletal proteins. Others may feel that components other than protein are equally important. Some, in the most literal sense, believe the composition of the body to be the ultimate aspect of malnutrition; whereas others feel that to be clinically relevant, even though composition is probably the most accurate in the purest sense, functional malnutrition may be more important and more in need of definition. Thus, it does not help clinicians to merely know whether all the body's components are intact. It is of much greater assistance in the care of patients to be able to predict ultimate outcome in terms of recovery, complications, and deaths as related to specific nutritional factors. Thus, one can see the myriad of problems inherent in merely trying to define malnutrition without embarking upon the topic of how it should be assessed.

Methods for nutritional assessments range from the most simple types described previously by our support team[4] to the most sophisticated of assessment parameters as described by Blackburn.[6] It is not the pur-

Specialized Nutritional
Support Monitoring Orders

The orders listed below are to be followed while the patient receives specialized nutritional support. Please D/C orders when patient no longer receives specialized nutritional support.

1. Strict I & O
2. Weight daily and record on graphic sheet.
3. Laboratory tests:
   a. CBC, Electrolytes and Blood Sugar ×3 days and then Monday, Wednesday and Friday.
   b. SMA_{12}, PT, PTT, Platlet Count, Retic. Count, Magnesium, Total Iron Binding Capacity, Osmolarity, Triglyceride, Ammonia, Cholesterol in AM, repeat in 7 days, and then weekly.
4. 24 hr. urine for: urea nitrogen and creatinine. } to run simultaneously
   24 hr. calorie count
   To be done twice a week:
   1. start Monday 7:00 a.m.–end Tuesday 7:00 a.m.
   2. start Thursday 7:00 a.m.–end Friday 7:00 a.m.
5. Fractional urines for S&A q6h:
   4+ Sugar________ units of Regular Insulin subcutaneously + notify physician
   3+ Sugar________ units of Regular Insulin subcutaneously
   2+ Sugar________ units of Regular Insulin subcutaneously
   1+ Sugar________ units of Regular Insulin subcutaneously

Thank you,

____
(signature)

Figure 21-3.

pose of this chapter to review the various forms of nutritional assessment, but rather to comment on nutritional assessment in general. When an institution is attempting to establish those parameters by which it will assess the nutritional state of its patients, it must design a system that is totally practical. The majority of hospitals in the United States do not have sophisticated assessment and financial resources at their disposal to perform complicated evaluations. Routine evaluations can be performed by using proper weight and nutrition histories; evaluating visceral proteins via albumin or transferrin measurements; anthropometrics; and immunocompetency determinations, when indicated, by skin testing or, in certain instances, by use of total lymphocyte counts.

PATIENTS VULNERABLE TO MALNUTRITION

The problems of malnutrition are not restricted to any one medical specialty, nor is any one medical specialty excluded from the potential of being required to care for malnourished patients. It is, therefore, important that when an institution designs its methodology for the identification and subsequent care of the malnourished that it keep these activities in perspective so that all specialties may avail themselves of the services. It was initially felt that the problem primarily existed in seriously ill patients. There has been ample documentation that surgical patients merely represent a part of the total malnourished population in hospitals.[7,8] Rounds on medical floors frequently reveal severely malnourished patients, some of the worst being renal failure patients.[9] Cardiac cachexia is being more widely recognized,[10] and attention is being given to the nutritional state of the cancer patient.[11] Gastroenterologists have long been aware of the various deficiency states associated with gastrointestinal disease and today, more seriously than ever, are involved in assessments and nutritional repletion of their patients. The areas of neonatology and pediatrics have for some time recognized the nutritional deficiency and needs of the pediatric group. Thus, just as antibiotics may be indicated in any specialty in medicine, so it appears that attention to the nutritional status of the patient will be a serious consideration in all specialties and for all hospital patients in the future. This does not mean that all will require assessment or specialized attention. It merely means that ignoring the potential for such need will be considered deficient care.

MATERIALS

Over the course of the past decade, the armamentarium of products available for the specialized treatment of nutritional deficiency in hospitalized patients has grown significantly. While it is acknowledged that we are still in a rather primitive state, somewhat similar to that of antibiotic development in the 1940s, it is important to note that the modalities of therapy available for intravenous and enteral use today are proving so complex that many practitioners are unable to adjust. Whether formal Nutrition Support Teams exist or whether groups of interested individuals participate with each other, it has become apparent that to effectively use parenteral and enteral products, a physician, nurse, pharmacist, and dietitian will have to interact at some level with each other. At the present time, the most used intravenous solution is that commonly known as hyperalimentation, consisting of hypertonic dextrose (25%), a 4 to 5% amino acid solution, and appropriate vitamins, electrolytes, and minerals. Some have advocated, for certain situations, the use of peripheral intravenous amino acids alone, known as protein-sparing. Lipids have been used not only for fatty-acid deficiency, but also in conjunction with carbohydrate and amino acids peripherally as a short-term source of calories. Second generation intravenous nutrition support solutions are being developed. Renal failure solution is now currently available, and solutions of branched-chain amino acids for hepatic failure will most likely be available in the near future. It is not unreasonable to assume that over the course of the next decade, many specific intravenous nutritional solutions will be developed to address specific illnesses.

In the area of enteral products for specialized nutrition support, we have seen many products evolve in three broad categories. The first, the defined formula diet also known as the elemental diet, was one of the earliest developed during the space exploration program. The materials used are more costly than other forms of enteral replacement and, not infrequently, are less well tolerated by the patient. Approximately 10 such commercially available products are on the market. Meal replacement formulas represent a more balanced enteral replacement than the defined formula diets and are therefore in greater use. They are of lower cost and greater patient acceptability, with perhaps 20 or 25 such products on the market. We also have a variety of enteral supplements, again numbering perhaps 25 or 30 products, which although not complete nutritional replacements, serve the purpose of replacing a specific component. Thus, the available armamentarium comprises, at the present time, approximately 40 or 50 different products.

NUTRITION SUPPORT TEAMS

One begins to see a paradox evolving in our discussion. Few persons in the United States would not acknowledge the importance of nutrition. They further would agree that in the disease state it may be even more important to pay attention to nutritional deficiencies. One must wonder why, over the course of the 1970s, the majority of hospitals in the United States did not develop strong nutrition support methodology within their walls. It is estimated that in 1980, only a small percentage of hospitals had a Nutrition Support Team. In fact, in a survey of the State of New Jersey performed by our Nutrition Support Team, only 10% of hospitals had an organized team. It was further noted that perhaps an additional 40% of hospitals were making an effort to use various nutrition support materials.

One of the prime reasons that there has not been more rapid growth in the development of Nutrition Support Services is a cultural complacency. Americans, believing that we are the best nourished nation on Earth, tend to deny the extent of malnutrition present in our patients. Gradually, this denial is being eroded by fact, and perhaps by 1985, we will note approximately 75% to 80% of American hospitals paying serious attention to the nutrition support of their patients.

Another reason that hospitals have not forged ahead as might have been expected in the field of nutrition support is the lack of appropriate professional expertise. The only individual within the walls of the hospital who has had respectable education in nutrition is the dietitian. Unfortunately, in many institutions the dietitian does not interact clinically with the remainder of the hospital family. Physicians, nurses, and pharmacists receive virtually no formal nutrition education and, in the course of preparing for their respective careers, acquire so little expertise that they are unable to function in a satisfactory manner to provide good patient nutrition. It is not unreasonable to assume that as the field of nutrition support expands, in a manner analogous to that of antibiotics, there will be, perhaps by 1990, Board Certified physicians who devote themselves exclusively to nutritional support of both hospitalized and outpatients. Since we have not progressed to that point, it is the responsibility of all practicing physicians today to become familiar with the need for supporting their patients, and it becomes the responsibility of all hospitals to provide some organizational structure to assist them in such care. Another area accounting for the lack of progress is the feeling of being overwhelmed by the problem and being frustrated. Although not terribly sophisticated, there are numerous products, materials, and devices currently existing, with a variety of conflicting therapeutic theories, so that the average busy practitioner feels unable to grasp the concepts and implement them on a day-to-day basis. This frustration frequently spills over to the concept of organizing nutrition support teams. Much of the effort that would be better spent in trying to provide minimal nutrition support care to patients is not infrequently diverted to the massive administrative task of developing an entire Nutrition Support Service where none previously existed.

In most areas of endeavor, we do not expect to go from complete incompetency to complete competency without a long, arduous training and experience phase. Thus, it does not seem logical to assume that individuals or institutions providing virtually no nutrition support care should, as their first endeavor, embark upon a full multidiscipline Nutrition Support Service. Unfortunately, in their zeal to rectify the situation of providing no care, there has been much overreaction towards requesting or demanding the immediate development of such teams in many institutions. It is not unreasonable to ask physicians, pharmacists, nurses, or dietitians to consider walking before they actually run. It is not necessary and perhaps, at times, unadvisable to assemble with great effort and with great expense a team that has not previously been tried in the field of clinical nutrition support.

In initially thinking about providing nutrition support within an institution, it is desirable that one physician at least be identified as interested in addressing the medical and administrative problems. Once identified, this physician can make absolutely no progress whatsoever unless a pharmacist is similarly identified. This does not mean that either individual should be addressing their full careers to nutrition support, but a mutual agreement must exist between the two to explore the use of intravenous nutrition support products. They should realize that minimal, rather than maximal, equipment and hardware should be used in the early stages and should recognize that an interested dietitian, if available, could provide invaluable services.

It is at this point that an institution, unless it develops realistic goals that are not discouragingly complex, will have difficulty in the gradual development of a responsible program.

Recognizing the fact that so few institutions have progressed to a satisfactory level of providing nutrition support in the United States, this chapter presents different phases or levels of expertise, ranging from number I to VII, requiring as little as zero time to as much as perhaps 30 months for development. It is hoped that for those institutions and individuals who have an overwhelming feeling concerning where to start, the sequence here described will carry them either from nonexistent or minimal nutrition support activities to the highest level desired within their institution, even approaching that of the complete Nutrition Support Service.

PHASES OF DEVELOPING NUTRITION SUPPORT SERVICES IN THE HOSPITAL SETTING

As it is difficult for many institutions to embark upon an organized, intelligent nutrition support program involving parenteral and enteral nutrition within the confines of the hospital, it would appear reasonable to approach this problem by gradually phasing in complex skills simultaneously. We, therefore, propose seven different levels of expertise by which hospitals can progress from the most rudimentary of nutrition support capabilities at Level I, to the most sophisticated capabilities at Level VII (Figure 21-4).

Level I

Most hospitals in the United States have a dietitian on their staff, thus, zero time would be required for the development of a dietitian alone as the only person interested in nutrition support. At Level I, it is assumed that there is no physician, nurse, or pharmacist in a given hospital interested in providing nutrition support. Under these circumstances, the dietitian has professional training and can easily acquire the necessary skills to assess patients within the institution who are at high risk for malnutrition. The dietitian then could bring the status of the patient to the attention of the physician either by direct contact or by written communication. In general, most hospitals have fairly intricate rules concerning who may make written entries into which part of the patient's hospital records. Thus from an expediency point of view, it would seem most reasonable for the dietitian to make personal verbal contact with the physician when malnutrition is encountered. This serves the purpose of not only rapidly making the physician aware of existing malnutrition in the patient, but also serves on a personal level to identify the

Phases of Developing Nutrition Support in the Hospital Setting:

Level I (0 months)*
Dietitian alone—no other resources
a. assess High Risk patients for malnutrition
b. provide Enteral Support when possible
c. make hospital family aware of more sophisticated centers for advanced Nutritional Support.

Level II (0–6 months)
Minimum of one (1) Physician and one (1) Pharmacist interested in nutrition support.
a. Stock one (1) Hyperalimentation solution only (Standardize formula)
b. Stock 2 or 3 Enteral products only utilizing Dietitian's recommendation
c. Pharmacist responsible for preparation and inventory of above with Dietitian, when available
d. Physician responsible for overseeing all aspects of clinical Nutrition with individual Physician caring for own patients.

Level III (6–12 months)
Plus part-time member of nursing service
a. Responsible for proper dressing changes and IV surveillance
b. In combination with *interested* dietitian when available

Level IV (12–18 months) Unofficial Team now formed.
Conscious Assessment of High Risk Patients with Primitive Assessment.
a. i.e., weight loss, albumin, total lymphocyte count, anthropometric measurements.
b. increase materials to include:
1. Hyperalimentation plus Lipids.
2. Increase Enteral products to 6–8 products.
c. Start formal record keeping of complications and patients treated.

Level V (18–24 months)
Continue sophistication of Resources by adding:
a. Nephramine, Protein Sparing
b. Additional Enterals, Pumps
c. Various tubes and supplies, etc.

Level VI (24 months)
Designate formal Team.
The Need Documented by:
a. Records of usage and complications in hospital
b. Advantages of using full time personnel
c. formal request to administration

Level VII (30+ months)
Formal Team.
Role of Team.
a. Clinical
b. Teaching
c. Administration
d. ± Research

Coordinate with other Specialty Committees in hospital.

* indicates estimated time for development and implementation.

Figure 21-4.

dietitian as someone interested in providing ongoing assistance.

The dietitian without any other resource individuals has the capability of utilizing enteral support materials for the patient's benefit and has the capability of advising physicians as to which materials might be useful for their patients.

Lastly, the dietitian working alone without other support team members can easily, via professional organizations such as American Dietetic Association or American Society for Parenteral and Enteral Nutrition, make the hospital family aware of sophisticated nutrition support techniques being performed at other institutions and can even make the hospital family aware of the location of these centers performing advanced nutritional support. Thus, although Level I is the most rudimentary of levels, requiring no development time, it is important to note than an interested dietitian already employed by an institution can make significant impact within the institution, if so motivated.

Level II

To progress from Level I to Level II may require a time framework of zero to 6 months. Please note that the various levels are cumulative, and although more specific methodology and expertise will be described at each level of development, they naturally include that which was described in the preceding level.

Level II requires at least one physician and one pharmacist interested in providing nutrition support. These two individuals can agree on the use of a specific central hyperalimentation solution. The simplicity of stocking one solution and becoming familiar with it as opposed to similar products produced by many companies is self-evident. The physician, with the assistance of the pharmacist, can easily learn what formulations are being used at other institutions. It is then highly desirable to formulate a standardized central hyperalimentation solution which can be used on a daily basis without having to write all of the specific ingredients on an order sheet (Figure 21-2). While this approach is certainly academically impure and could not be argued as being the most appropriate for all patients, it will allow practical application of central venous hyperalimentation to many more patients than if specific itemized orders had to be written on a daily basis. It is to be hoped that it will also allow more physicians than just the one initially interested to care for patients with hyperalimentation. Naturally, despite a standardized formula and despite the use of only one hyperalimentation product, the formula could be tailored by the physician's orders whenever necessary. By including a hyperalimentation solution and by identifying an interested physician and pharmacist, any institution, by combining Level I and Level II, can now start to provide both parenteral and enteral nutritional support. It is recommended today that an air-flow hood be acquired by a hospital pharmacy prior to the preparation of central hyperalimentation fluids. The approximate cost of such a 6-foot hood is $2500. At this level, specific attention should be directed to pharmacy procedures.

PURCHASING

Product selection criteria are used in purchasing nutrition support products. Four criteria for selection should be considered. First, what products are going to be used in your institution. A pharmacy department beginning an intravenous nutrition support program will probably start with the basic central venous hyperalimentation (C.V.H.) solution. The cost of this solution is the next criteria. At present, there is no evidence to indicate that the C.V.H. solution made by any one manufacturer is clinically more effective than any other. Therefore, contracts or group purchasing may play a larger role in product selection than clinical performance. The time required for preparation of C.V.H. solutions is a third criteria in purchasing nutrition support products. The companies have numerous solutions, each with an intended purpose. Solutions can be bought separately, in kits with and without electrolytes. The clinical applications of the solutions must be considered before deciding which products will be ordered. The pharmacy must take into consideration the use of standardized or individualized formulations of solutions. The use of electrolyte additives, transfer sets, syringes, filters, and the like will effect preparation time and ultimate cost. Hospital pharmacies that develop an intravenous nutrition support program may benefit by starting with standardized C.V.H. formula.

Presently, there exists a great divergence among the manufacturers in delivery methods of nutrition support products to hospital pharmacies. Some companies have their own warehouses and delivery systems, while others utilize private or public delivery systems. The manufacturers may have separate nutrition divisions which are contacted for purchasing. Day-to-day dealings with the companies and representatives may influence choice of products independent of time and cost.

STORAGE

Storage of large volume parenteral solutions is always a concern of hospital pharmacists. Independent of storage in the receiving department, store room, or pharmacy, the intravenous nutrition support products must be inspected for damage or excessive abuse. The pharmacy department has the ultimate responsibility to assure the quality and integrity of these products by exercising appropriate handling and storage techniques.

Defects in nutrition support products fall into four general categories. Mishandling of products may cause damage leading to crystallization on the outside of containers, cracks in glass, which may not leak, and denting of hardware. Products may also be incomplete due to missing labels, hangers, or tamper-proof seals. Labeling should be appropriate, and reasonable expiration dates should be on all products. Lastly, gross deterioration, exemplified by discoloration or mold growth, may occur.

All products should be protected from extremes of heat and cold, and storage conditions should include rotation of stock. Satisfactory light and space should be available for general handling and inspection of products.

PREPARATION

Facilities and equipment for preparation of intravenous nutrition support solutions should include, but not necessarily be limited to, a separate "clean room" and laminar flow hood. The clean work area or "clean room" should be isolated from heavy traffic or stored supplies. The hood should be the size appropriate to accommodate expected needs. The laminar flow hood requires inspection and certification by qualified inspectors every 6 months. Daily care of the hood should include cleaning with an appropriate germicide before preparation of solutions. It is also cleaned at the end of each day. The hood should be run for at least 30 minutes prior to beginning work. Solutions should be prepared 6 inches within the hood to avoid contaminated air from entering into the work area. The laminar flow hood should supplement good technique in preparation, not replace it.

Preparation technique for the intravenous nutrition support solutions should follow the manufacturers' recommendations. The manufacturers' built-in quality control should be adhered to as far into the preparation routine as possible. In addition, a surgical detergent should be used for handwashing before beginning the preparation of solutions. Specific techniques and procedures for preparation have been outlined for sterile products. These references give detailed descriptions for most operations that may be encountered when preparing solutions. It is advisable for a hospital pharmacy to develop its own specific guidelines for preparation of solutions. Figure 21-5 is an example of a procedure for the preparation of central venous hyperalimentation solutions.

Labeling and record keeping are important in the daily preparation of all solutions. Labels for bottles should include the contents of the solutions, the preparation and expiration dates, the preparers' name, and patient information provided by a computer print-out or other information system used within a given hospital. A log book should contain all information for intravenous nutrition support solutions prepared each day. It should include the patient's name and hospital identification number, solutions prepared and additives used (Figure 21-6). Daily totals of all solutions prepared and patients treated are important statistics. The totals can be compiled into monthly reports to the director of the Nutrition Support Team, the director of pharmacy and the hospital administration.

SAINT BARNABAS MEDICAL CENTER
Livingston, New Jersey

PREPARATION OF AMINO ACID HYPERALIMENTATION SOLUTION

Materials and Equipment

1. Laminar Flow Hood
2. Amino Acid, Dextrose solution
3. One vial of electrolyte concentrate 25 ml.
4. One vial of Sodium Phosphate 45 mM. (3 mM. P/ml.)
5. One 30 ml. syringe, two 5 ml. syringes and three 18 gauge needles.
6. Alcohol Prep Swabs.

Procedure

.... Clean hands thoroughly
.... Wipe all injection sites with alcohol swabs.

1. Place all equipment under Laminar Flow Hood and remove metal top of Amino Acid solution 8.5% and Dextrose 50%, and plastic top of Hyperlyte and Sodium Phosphate.
2. Using 30 ml. syringe and 18 gauge needle, inject 25 ml. of electrolyte (entire vial) through the large hole of the Amino Acid solution.
3. Using the 5 ml. syringe and 18 gauge needle, add 2 ml. of Sodium Phosphate (Approx. 10 mEq. Na and 5 mM. $Po_4\equiv$) to the Amino Acid solution.
4. To the first liter for each patient each day, add 5 ml. MVI using the other 5 ml. syringe and 18 gauge needle.
5. Remove the rubber seal from the Amino Acid solution and place the end of the transfer set with the drip chamber into the large hole. Shut off stop-cock and place the needle on the end of the tubing.
6. Invert and inject Amino Acid 8.5% solution through large hole of Dextrose 50% bottles shutting off the stop-cock before air is allowed to enter the line. SHAKE
7. Cap the bottle, complete the label and place inverted over the Dextrose 50% label.
8. Place the small label from the computer printout of the order on the bottle.

Preparation of Amino Acid Hyperalimentation Solution

9. Record in Intravenous Nutrition Support Daily Log.
10. Dispose of needles, syringes, bottles and other waste properly. Clean Laminar Flow Hood area.

NOTE:
The final solution contains that which appears on the Quantitative-Qualitative Breakdown record of the Amino Acid Hyperalimentation Solution

Figure 21-5.

CONTROL

Various mechanisms of control are used in an intravenous nutrition support program. The pharmacist reviews the physician's order, which is written every 24 hours. This is of particular importance in programs where individualized electrolyte formulations are prescribed. It may be beneficial for a hospital pharmacy to begin an intravenous nutrition support program with a standardized electrolyte formula. In any case, the pharmacist preparing solutions must clearly understand exactly what the physician desires. Once prepared, the solutions are delivered to the nursing units to start infusing at 3:00 P.M. each afternoon. Nurses check to be sure that all solutions have been delivered for each patient for a 24-hour period. Solutions not being immediately administered are refrigerated. All solutions not used within 24 hours are returned to the pharmacy. Destructive and nondestructive microbiologic testing can be performed on those solutions returned. The testing can be done periodically and should be relatively simple, rapid, reliable, and inexpensive. Quality control should be used in cases of a suspected problem.

SAINT BARNABAS MEDICAL CENTER
Livingston, New Jersey

QUANTITATIVE—QUALITATIVE BREAKDOWN OF AMINO ACID HYPERALIMENTATION SOLUTION

On liter Amino Acid Hyperalimentation solution contains:

COMPONENT	%	Gm	mEq	mMoles
Amino Acids	4.25	42.5(39)		
Dextrose	25	250.0		
Sodium (Na^+)			40	
Potassium (K^+)			40	
Magnesium (Mg^{++})			8	
Calcium (Ca^{++})			5	
Chloride (Cl^-)			33	
Acetate (Ac^-)			40	
Phosphate ($Po_4^{\equiv}$)				15

The first liter of hyperalimentation solution for each patient each day contains 5 cc multivitamin infusion:

5cc MVI contains:

	mg.	I.U.
Ascorbic Acid (vitamin C)	250	
Vitamin A		5,000
Vitamin D (Ergocalciferol)		500
Thiamine HCl (B_1)	25	
Riboflavin (B_2)	5	
Pyridoxine Hcl (B_6)	7.5	
Niacinamide	50	
Dexpanthenol	12.5	
Vitamin E (di-Alpha Tocopheryl Acetate)		2.5

Total Nitrogen provided by
Amino Acids = 6.25 Gms

Total calories provided by
Amino Acids = 156.0 cal.

Total calories provided by Dextrose = 850 calories (3.4 cal./Gm dextrose)

Osmolarity = 1687 mOsm

Total calories = 1006 cal./liter ph = 5.8

Figure 21-6.

At Level II, the dietitian can make recommendations concerning the specific enteral support products to be stocked within the hospital. Depending on the cost centers within the institution, such products may originate from either the pharmacy or the dietary services. The dietitian should recommend a few products in each of the three categories, i.e., defined formula diets, meal replacements, and supplements. If a limited number of products is stored and utilized by the medical staff, familiarity will become rapid and utilization will increase. If an overabundance of products is stocked, confusion will exist and misuse will result.

It is to made clear to the hospital family that the pharmacist will retain complete responsibility for the preparation of all intravenous nutrition support fluids and that additives will not be given on the floors or at the bedside by nurses. The pharmacist will also assume responsibility for the inventory of products, while the dietitian assumes responsibility for the enteral products. The physician involved should assume responsibility for overseeing all aspects of clinical nutritional support for the patients whom he is treating or should correlate care if the individual treating physician is different from himself. The interested physician who will coordinate nutrition support techniques can easily formulate the standardized order sheets for ordering hyperalimentation solutions, for introducing subclavian catheters, and most importantly, for monitoring the various parameters in parenteral and enteral nutrition. Examples of such order sheets used at the Saint Barnabas Medical Center in Livingston, New Jersey, have previously been noted in Figures 21-1, 21-2, and 21-3.

In routine practice, it is the physician's responsibility to see that the various biochemical parameters are maintained within normal limits, and it is the floor nurse's responsibility to notify the physician of abnormal laboratory studies.

It is desirable at Level II (within the first 6 months of development) for the responsible physician and pharmacist to visit a nearby center performing more sophisticated nutritional support and to establish a liaison with that institution, so that a free flow of educational material and dialogue can exist during the development of Level II through Level VII. Frequently, such communication can be via telephone once the initial in-person contact is made. It is hoped that eventually all advanced centers in the United States offering sophisticated nutritional support to their patients will outreach to a variety of institutions at lower levels of development within their geographic locale to assist them in upgrading their services.

Level III

It is anticipated that after Levels I and II have been reached (requiring perhaps 6 months), during the next 6 months a member of nursing service could be introduced to work in conjunction with the existing interested physician, pharmacist, and dietitian. It becomes readily apparent that nursing involvement can become essential to the proper administration of nutrition support. In the initial phases of nursing involvement, the first area of proven benefit is the standardization of subclavian dressings. The responsibility for changing these dressings should be delegated to one member of the nursing service. This will decrease the complication rates associated with subclavian catheters. It will also serve as an impetus to physicians to provide intravenous nutritional support, if they themselves are not responsible for the time-consuming dressing changes. A variety of approaches has been taken towards dressing changes in various institutions. Some feel that this activity can only be performed by a registered nurse; others, such as ourselves, have found the services of a licensed practical nurse perfectly satisfactory for the changing of the dressings. The nurse who initially joins the team, probably as a part-time member, can also be an important resource person in regard to intravenous pumps and can, in conjunction with the dietitian, assist the hospital in the acquisition of appropriate hardware such as pumps, filters (if desired), feeding tubes, and various enteral appliances.

Gradually, over a period of one year, without a significant expenditure of money, it is possible to assemble an interested physician, pharmacist, dietitian, and member of the nursing service. Thus, it is possible at the end of one year to have defined an intravenous hyperalimentation solution, a few enteral products, and certain materials necessary for the provision of parenteral and enteral nutrition. It is recognized that not all modalities of intravenous nutrition support nor enteral support are available at this time. If the group looks back to the point its institution was one year before, it will find that significant strides have been made.

Level IV

Despite the fact that individuals may not be working fulltime, it could be assumed that over a 6-month period (taking this now unofficial team from its first year to its first 1½ years), nutritional assessment techniques of high-risk patients could be performed at a fairly simple level.

While it is acknowledged that the most appropriate nutritional support parameters are hotly contested, there are at least sim-

ST. BARNABAS MEDICAL CENTER
NUTRITION STATUS EVALUATION

Patient Name______________________________Attending__________

Diagnosis________________________________Date__________

Criteria Evaluated:	**Value**	**Findings**	
		Normal	**Abnormal**
1. Involuntary weight loss 10 lbs. or over during last 6 months. If yes, record amount.			
2. Albumin (Norm = 3.5 gm. or greater)			
3. Total Lymphocyte Count (Norm = 1500 m^3 or greater)			
4. Anthropometric Arm Measurements, (Norm = 70% of standard or greater) Triceps Skinfold Arm Circumference			

Nutrition Status:______________________________

Nutritional Status Key:
None Abnormal—Adequate Nutrition
Any 1 Abnormal—Possible Malnutrition
Any 2 Abnormal—Mild Malnutrition
Any 3 Abnormal—Moderate Malnutrition
Any 4 Abnormal—Severe Malnutrition

Provided by: Nutrition Support Service

Figure 21-7.

ple measures that the unofficial team could look for and bring to the attention of the hospital family. These include weight loss of either greater than 10 pounds within a 6-month period or 10% of body weight. It could include evaluation of the patient's serum albumin, total lymphocyte count, and anthropometric measurements such as mid-arm circumference, lean body mass, and tricep skin-fold, measuring body fat (Figure 21-7).

During this time period from 1 year to 18 months, the parenteral and enteral materials stocked can be expanded. Assuming the group has sufficient expertise and comfort with intravenous hyperalimentation, it does not take much additional effort to stock and utilize a lipid solution. The lipid solution can either be used as a replacement for fatty acids or as part of a peripherally administered lipid based calorie system, including carbohydrate and amino acids.[12] At this point, the option is open to the members of the hospital family to provide calories not necessarily via a central line, but under certain circumstances, peripherally.

At the same time, the stocked supply of enteral products can be increased to a total of six or eight, with the individuals involved becoming familiar with the new additions. It is appropriate, at this point, for the unofficial team to start formal record keeping of patients treated, materials used, and complications encountered (Figures 21-8 and 21-9). Records of this type will form the early phases of quality control for a future support service. It is also of value for this group to start defining specific disease entities where major impact can be made with proper nutritional support. Thus, patients

Saint Barnabas Medical Center

ENTERAL DATA SHEET

DX. #1.

#2.

Height__________IBW__________Wt.Hx.__________

MEDS:

Spec. Treat.

DATES:

Enteral									
p.o. diet									
Route									
tube									
weight									
energy int.									
pro. int.									
temp.									
Ca/Phos.									
BS/BUN									
U.A./Chol.									
T.P./ALB									
Hep Enz.									
Creat									
Na/K									
Wbc/lymph									
Hg/Hct									
Mcv/Mch									
S&A									
TIBC									
N-bal									
other									

Problems:

Recommendations:

initial alb.__________

Diet Orders:

TLC__________

COMPLICATIONS:

Figure 21-8.

SAINT BARNABAS MEDICAL CENTER

Nutrition Support Service
Parenteral Monitoring Form

Patient__________ Admission Height__________

Hosp. No.__________ Admission Weight__________

Physician__________ Therapy Started__________

Date							
Temp./Weight							
Parenteral Product Ordered							
Amount infused							
Nitrogen Study: Nitrogen In Nitrogen Out Balance 24 hr. Creat.							
S&A							
Ca/Inor. Phos.							
B.S.							
BUN/U.A.							
Chol.							
T.P.							
Alb.							
T.B./Alk. Phos.							
Na/K							
Cl/Co_2							
Iron/TIBC							
Mq/Ammonia							
Mg							
Osmo.							
Platelet/Retic.							
WBC/L							
Hq/Hct.							
Hg							

Comments:

Figure 21-9.

can be specifically identified in the high-risk areas of the surgical intensive care unit, burn unit, coronary care unit, oncology floor and renal failure floors. Probably 50% of patients, at a minimum, in each of the categories noted will be malnourished. By carefully educating the nursing staff and associated physicians, increased nutritional support and better therapeutic results can be obtained.

To recapitulate, in reaching Level IV, approximately 18 months will have elapsed from the point where no organized nutrition support was provided to the point where a group of interested individuals (a physician, pharmacist, dietitian, and member of the nursing service) have assembled for the purpose of acquiring appropriate materials. They will be able to act in their institution in the areas of identifying malnutrition and providing the elements of parenteral and enteral nutrition support. By this time, materials including carbohydrates, amino acids, lipids, vitamins, minerals, and a variety of enteral products should be available. In addition, some form of standardization of the subclavian dressing change procedure should be formulated, as well as the standardization of orders. Minimal record keeping should be developed. In this way, an unofficial team functions without any members of the team necessarily performing their tasks on a full-time basis. After 18 months of study and practice, the group is ready to increase the resources available to it over the next 6 months.

Level V

After 1½ to 2 years of functioning, the group should now be in a comfortable position to add an appropriate renal failure solution, consisting of essential amino acid solution, to its armamentarium. It is important to remember that most of the other items necessary for use with essential amino acid solutions are already stocked in the pharmacy. Peripheral amino acid solutions for use in protein-sparing can be acquired and stocked. The hospital family can be instructed in the use of these two additional intravenous solutions.

At the same time, it is appropriate that the supply of enteral materials be increased, and the utilization and acquisition of pumps and administration kits be refined. It is also appropriate that, at this level, decision trees for use by the hospital family be disseminated. If this is not done, the materials will be incorrectly used. It is appropriate to consider first whether the patient's gut is working and can be used. If indeed, the gut is working, an enteral diet should be selected. In selecting the enteral diet, it must be determined whether it is acceptable for the patient to form any fecal residue or not. If, because of the nature of the medical situation, the patient is unable to have fecal residue, then a defined-formula diet is indicated. If the formation of feces is acceptable and the patient has no other caloric source, a meal replacement formula should be used. In fact, if the patient is eating and the diet being consumed is not complete, then one of the appropriate supplements should be selected.

If, by the same token, the patient is unable to utilize his gastrointestinal tract for enteral support, then the decision must be made to provide intravenous nutritional support. If the patient is severely ill, catabolic, and/or septic and is going to require intravenous support for more than 5 or 10 days, it is advisable to use central venous hyperalimentation fluids. If a previous fatty-acid deficiency exists or if the patient requires intravenous hyperalimentation for more that 14 days, it is advisable to administer intravenous lipids. The utilization of peripheral amino acids without carbohydrates as "protein-sparing solutions" is suggested by some for short term use (5 to 7 days) in patients who are not initially nutritionally depleted. Once again, the merits of this form of therapy are somewhat controversial. By the same token, many have advocated the use of the peripheral route for the administration of lipids, carbohydrates, amino acids, and vitamins in that individual who is not yet malnourished and who may in 7 to 10 days be able to take adequate oral nutrition. The administration of essential amino acids in renal failure is primarily discussed in terms of patients not receiving dialysis treatment. For the patient receiving dialysis, many feel that conventional central venous hyperalimentation may be either equally as appropriate or more appropriate for the patient than the provision of essential amino acids only. While the preceding is primarily meant to serve as a guideline, each institution should accordingly advise its members of the indications for use of the various modalities available. It is an important concept that while any group is forming over the period of the first 2 years, it should maintain liaison with a more sophisticated group for educational purposes. The group, when it acquires its own levels of sophistication, can start to serve as a resource for other outlying institutions of lesser expertise.

Level VI

Once the group has functioned for approximately 2 years, a significant level of expertise will have been acquired. The rough spots within a given institution will have been defined, and hopefully, the hospital administration will have come to respect the efforts of the unofficial Nutrition Support Team in providing patient care and in carefully controlling the acquisition of new products and materials. At this time, utilization of resources within the institution should have progressed to a point of need for a formal Nutrition Support Team. Having previously demonstrated expertise in this area, the unofficial group should make a formal proposal to the hospital administrators and Board of Trustees that certain individuals be employed full-time to formalize a team. This team should consist of a pharmacist, dietitian, registered nurse, and possibly, a practical nurse, depending on the institution's philosophy. It is important to note that, in general, the physicians are not salaried or full-time on Nutrition Support Teams and that it is the nurse clinician (registered nurse) who really functions, particularly in a private practice setting, as the administrative coordinator of the Nutrition Support Service. In institutions where the physicians are involved in private practice, the physician does not have the appropriate time to devote to the varied administrative duties of the Nutrition Support Service. Of the other members of the team, it is the nurse and dietitian who possess the professional expertise to review clinically the course of patients and to oversee the Nutrition Support Service.

In designating the need for a formal team, the group should be prepared to provide records of material usage and of complications in the hospital, the advantages of using full-time personnel, and a coherent expression of why a team is needed. The following few paragraphs represent an abstract of our own proposal, initially presented to our hospital administration.

> There is a need to formalize a Nutrition Support Service at Saint Barnabas Medical Center such that a R.N., L.P.N., R.Ph. and R.D. may devote their full efforts to assisting physicians in assessing the nutritional status of patients and providing specialized nutritional support to malnourished patients. Sophisticated means for providing specialized nutritional support to hospitalized patients have become available. These materials and techniques are currently employed at Saint Barnabas Medical Center. It has been well documented in the Medical literature that 40-50% of hospitalized patients suffer from malnutrition. Utilizing a superficial form of Instant Nutrition Assessment, a minimum of 7.6% of admissions sampled at Saint Barnabas Medical Center were found to be nutritionally deficient. A survey of the Cancer Unit revealed a 50% malnutrition rate.
>
> Complication and death rates are markedly increased in malnourished patients.
>
> Such complications and deaths contribute to the suffering of the patient and to the overall increase in the cost of health care. It has been shown that many of the complications and deaths are preventable when patients are given specialized nutritional support.
>
> In 1973, Murray H. Seltzer, M.D., was appointed Chairman of the Surgical Nutrition Committee. This multidiscipline committee was able to provide quality treatment to patients by standardizing solutions and monitoring techniques, and unifying trends within the Hospital to control usage and costs. In 1977, a $30,000 reduction in unit price of Hyperalimentation fluid was effected by the cooperation of the Committee and Pharmacy. The

Committee has attempted to instruct hospital Physicians and other personnel on standards of care and avoidance of waste. At the current time various individuals within the hospital by volunteering their time have been able to keep Saint Barnabas Medical Center ahead of the nation, and able to provide specialized nutrition support. It is felt that in the next year or two, we will be surpassed by many institutions of lesser capability if we do not organize properly.

At the present time, Ms. Wright, who changes the subclavian dressings, is the only individual salaried by the Hospital for the specific purpose of tending to patients.

To continue top quality efficiency in the future, there is a need for the following personnel and materials at hospital expense:

1. A full-time Registered Nurse.
2. A full-time Practical Nurse for dressing changes.
3. A full-time Pharmacist.
4. A full-time Dietitian.
5. Part-time assistance from Dr. Engler in Surgical Research.
6. Small office space for records.
7. Secretary.

Physician input and supervision would continue to be on a voluntary non-hospital reimbursed status. The benefit to patients is unquestionable and the long term academic and financial benefit to the hospital would make such a Department worthwhile.

The financial benefits to the Hospital are numerous. Some benefits include marked economy in the utilization of material, economy in negotiating purchases of materials used, restriction in the variety of material available, etc.

Formation of a Nutritional Support Service at the Saint Barnabas Medical Center is proposed to enhance the quality of patient care, to institute maximal cost containment in this area, to attract research funding and to comply with present and future government demands for increased attention to nutritional support of the hospitalized patient.

The early assessment of patients' nutritional status and careful attention to their specialized nutritional needs will provide a higher quality patient care while at the same time allowing better cost containment within this area.

It should be noted that the team unofficially had been functioning from Levels 0 to Level VI for a period of approximately 6 years prior to the initiation of a formal team. However, since the state of the art has developed so rapidly in recent years, it seems not unreasonable to condense Levels I to VI to a period of 24 months prior to initiation of a formal team.

Level VII

Assuming a team has been successfully formed, it may take an additional 6 months to acquire office space, secretarial assistance, and materials, and develop more sophisticated record-keeping systems. By approximately 2½ years from inception, the institution should have progressed to Level VII, where a formal team exists. Upon reaching this level, a variety of philosophic questions should be addressed to determine the role of the team. Some feel that, having acquired such expertise, this team should now provide all of the parenteral and enteral nutrition to the patients who are in need of this therapy. While it would certainly be logical to have those individuals with the greatest knowledge and expertise rendering the care, such is not the way of the real world. Of the approximately 6000 hospitals in the United States involved in acute care medicine, the majority are engaged in the private practice of medicine. Recognizing that the ever increasing number of patients will require specialized nutritional support, it becomes questionable whether any team, without endless expansion of personnel, will be able to assume the ever increasing burden of caring for the patients. Thus, it seems logical to suggest, in a manner analogous to the development of antibiotic usage, that each physician be responsible for the basic nutritional support of his own patient, and that he draw upon the team as a resource for expertise when needed but that the team not have the primary responsibility for patient care. Thus, we would suggest that there not be a monopoly within a given institution. By so doing, the team can coordinate policy and oversee the quality of care without inhibiting the free usage of parenteral and enteral nutrition. If inhibition is avoided, more physicians will utilize nutritional support and more patients will ultimately benefit, despite the fact that the expertise of the individual physician may not truly approach that of the given team. The team should address itself to four primary areas, including clinical care, teaching, administration, and research. The nature of clinical care has been described throughout the previous levels. The team can make clinical rounds within the hospital. It can be involved in the teaching of all members of the hospital family. It can interact clearly with the administration and can form a close working harmony with the administrators in the complex areas of cost negotiations and product acquisition. The team can perform research without sophisticated facilities. The team in individual institutions can decide, i.e., from a clinical level to a sophisticated research level, what questions about this new evolving field it would most enjoy studying. As the team becomes steadily more sure of itself, it must then coordinate with other specialty areas within the hospital and, if desirable, meet periodically with physicians from the major specialties to evaluate the needs of their patients related to nutrition support. Obviously, having reached Level VII, it is important to remember when the Institution was at Level I. Recognizing that surrounding institutions may be at Level I, it is desirable to communicate with individuals in those institutions and make them aware of the fact that in approximately 2½ years, your institution has progressed to a Level of expertise such that you are prepared to assist them.

At the present time, approximately 1000 patients are dependent on home intravenous hyperalimentation or home enteral nutritional support. The logistics required to provide such outpatient care are complex and involved. Despite the attainment of Level VII as a formal team, it will most likely be the responsibility of the most sophisticated regional centers to accept responsibility for home care. Thus, it is not recommended that every formal team attempt to manage home T.P.N. patients.

While the described seven Levels may seem somewhat tedious, an institution is more likely to build a solid team on the first six levels than if it attempted to proceed directly to Level VII. By providing gradations of expertise, it is hoped that this chapter will serve as a logical framework for hospitals to expand their facilities for providing appropriate parenteral and enteral nutrition to their patients.

SUGGESTED READINGS

1. Recommendations of the National Coordinating Committee on Large Volume Parenterals. American Society of Hospital Pharmacists.
2. Turco, S., and King, R.E.: Sterile Dosage Forms, Their Preparation and Clinical Application. 2nd Ed. Philadelphia, Lea & Febiger, 1979.
3. King, J.C.: Guide to Parenteral Admixtures. St. Louis, Missouri, Cutter Laboratories, Inc., 1971.

REFERENCES

1. Dudrick, S.J., et al.: Long-term parenteral nutrition with growth, development and positive nitrogen balance. Surgery, *64:*134, 1968.
2. Seltzer, M.H., et al.: Letter to the Editor: Establishing a hyperalimentation team. JPEN, *3:*182, 1979.
3. Seltzer, M.H., et al.: The use of a simplified standardized hyperalimentation formula. JPEN, *2:*28, 1979.
4. Seltzer, M.H., et al.: Instant nutritional assessment. JPEN, *3:*157, 1979.
5. Asaadi, M., and Seltzer, M.H.: Subclavian intravenous catheterization. Resident and Staff Physician, *26:*53, 1980.
6. Blackburn, G.L., et al.: Nutritional and metabolic assessment of the hospitalized patient. JPEN, *1:*11, 1977.
7. Bistrian, B.R., et al.: Protein status of general surgical patients. JAMA, *230:*858, 1974.
8. Bistrian, B.R., et al.: Prevalence of malnutrition in general medical patients. JAMA, *235:*1567, 1976.
9. Abel, R.M., et al.: Improved survival from acute renal failure after treatment with intravenous essential L-amino acids and glucose. N. Engl. J. Med., *288:*695, 1973.
10. Kyger, E.R., III, et al.: Adverse effects of protein malnutrition on myocardial function. Surgery, *84:*147, 1978.
11. Deitel, M., Vasic, V., and Alexander, M.A.: Specialized nutritional support in the cancer patient: is it worthwhile? Cancer, *41:*2359, 1978.
12. Silberman, H., et al.: Parenteral nutrition with lipids. JAMA *238:*1380, 1977.

Nutrition Support Nomenclature

1. **Air Embolism:** Obstruction of a blood vessel by an air bubble; symptoms include dyspnea, chest pain and disorientation leading to collapse and coma. Air embolism usually occurs when there is negative intrathoracic pressure relative to the pressure of the open catheter.
2. **Albumin:** A serum protein considered useful in the assessment of visceral protein status.
3. **Amino Acid:** The smallest unit of protein which contains an amino (NH_2) and carboxyl (COOH) group. Essential amino acids cannot be synthesized by the body while nonessential amino acids can be manufactured provided the necessary precursors are available.

4. **Anergy:** Absent or impaired ability to react to specific antigens and may be indicative of protein deficiency.
5. **Anthropometrics:** Measuring the human body and its parts by height, weight, skin-fold thickness and arm, head or wrist circumference. It is important for the nutrition status assessment.
6. **Bolus feeding:** Volume feeding of enteral formula at one time (100cc-400cc).
7. **Calorie/Nitrogen Ratio (C:N):** A ratio of kilocalories consumed to the amount of nitrogen contained within the total. Under normal conditions the ratio should be approximately 300:1. For a catabolic patient the C:N range is 140-180:1.
8. **Cannulation:** Insertion of one tube into another, i.e.: catheter insertion into a vein.
9. **Catheter embolism:** Obstruction of a blood vessel when the catheter is broken off in the venous tree due to faulty technique. Symptoms include thrombosis, cardiac arrhythmias or may lead to sepsis.
10. **Catheterization:** Use of an intravenous tube to deliver special I.V. nutrition fluids.
11. **Central Hyperalimentation:** See Hyperalimentation.
12. **Central Venous Hyperalimentation:** See Hyperalimentation.
13. **Cyclic Hyperalimentation:** The administration of Hyperalimentation fluid over a designated time period, i.e. 12 hours, alternated with the administration of Hyperalimentation fluid devoid of dextrose over a similar time period. The intent being to offer the liver a respite from glucose and hopefully diminish fatty infiltration and hepatic enzyme alteration.
14. **Defined Formula Diet (DFD) or Elemental Diet:** Classification of enteral diets designed to aid impaired absorption conditions. Nutrients are prehydrolyzed for minimal digestion and rapid absorption; can be taken orally or by tube.
15. **Enteral:** Pertaining to or using the intestines and gut, i.e. for feeding purposes.
16. **Esophagostomy (Cervical):** A surgically created opening for feeding into the esophagus at the cervical level.
17. **Essential Fatty Acid:** Fatty acids which cannot be synthesized by the body and are required for growth and development—linoleic, linolenic and arachidonic acids.
18. **Feeding Tube:** A small silastic tube with a mercury weighted tip, designed to decrease complications of large rubber tubes for enteral feedings. Tubes range in diameter (5-14 French) and length (36-43 inches) depending on the size of the patient and the desired point of destination (stomach or intestines).
19. **Filtration:** A device used on the infusion line to remove microorganisms and debris from intravenous fluids.
20. **Gluconeogenesis:** The formation of glucose in the liver from non-carbohydrate sources, i.e. proteins, when body stores are depleted.
21. **Glucosuria:** Glucose in the urine.
22. **Hepatic Failure Solution:** An intravenous nutrition support fluid consisting of amino acids (fortified with branched chain amino acids), glucose, vitamins, electrolytes and minerals (when added) for use via a central catheter in patients with hepatic failure.
23. **Home Parenteral Nutrition:** A term applied to chronic intravenous nutritional support, usually using Hyperalimentation fluid through a permanently implanted superior vena cava catheter.
24. **Home Total Parenteral Nutrition:** Same as home parenteral nutrition except that nutrient intake by mouth does not occur.
25. **Hyperalimentation:** A solution containing 25% glucose, 4-5% amino acids, electrolytes, vitamins and minerals (when added) used for intravenous nutritional support and administered through a catheter placed in the superior vena cava. This term is synonymous with Central Hyperalimentation, Intravenous Hyperalimentation and Central Venous Hyperalimentation.
26. **Infusion rate:** The rate of delivery of I.V. nutrition support solutions. A constant rate is desired to prevent metabolic complications from hypertonic dextrose administration. "Catch-up" volumes are contraindicated.
27. **Internal jugular vein:** A neck vein through which catheterization of the superior vena cava can be performed for Hyperalimentation.
28. **Intravenous Hyperalimentation:** See Hyperalimentation.
29. **Intravenous Lipids:** Fatty acids in glycerol suitable for intravenous use to replace essential fatty acids or to provide fat as a calorie source.
30. **Intravenous Lipid Nutrition Support System:** A combination of lipids, dextrose, amino acids, vitamins, electrolytes and minerals (when added) suitable for administration through a peripheral vein.
31. **Jejunostomy:** A surgically created opening into the proximal jejunum designated for enteral feedings. Formula must be administered at room temperature and 24 hour continuous drip to prevent undesirable side effects.
32. **Kilocalorie (kcal):** The amount of heat necessary to raise 1 Kg of water 1° centigrade. Food energy values are calculated in kcals.
33. **Kwashiorkor:** An African term meaning "red boy" from the depigmentation of suffering children's hair, kwashiorkor or protein malnutrition (PM) is characterized by depressed visceral proteins and edema.
34. **Lactose:** Sugar derived from milk requiring the intestinal enzyme lactase for digestion into glucose and galactose.
35. **Laminar flow hood:** A semienclosed work area producing a circulation of sterile air to decrease air born contamination, used during the preparation of I.V. nutrition support solutions.
36. **Lipid (fat):** A group of organic compounds insoluble in water. Fats provide a source of energy (9 kcals per gram), provide essential fatty acids, carry fat-soluble vitamins and are stored in the body as adipose tissue.
37. **Marasmus:** A Greek term meaning "to waste away," marasmus or protein calorie malnutrition (PCM) is characterized by severe muscle wasting from deprived nutrient intake.
38. **Meal replacement:** One of many enteral products taken orally or by tube containing all of the re-

quired nutrients. To meet nutritional needs specific volumes must be administered with intact digestion and absorption required.

39. **Medium-chain triglyceride (MCT):** An easily digested and absorbed lipid indicated when fat malabsorption is present. MCT provides 8 kcals per gram and chain lengths vary from 6-10 carbons.
40. **3-Methylhistidine:** A by-product of metabolism measured in the urine. Increased urinary levels are seen following major trauma or starvation indicative of rapid wasting and breakdown of skeletal muscle mass.
41. **Mid-arm circumference (MAC):** A measurement useful to determine both energy and protein stores and to calculate arm muscle circumference by nomogram. MAC levels are markedly depressed in the more severe forms of PCM.
42. **Modular diets:** The combination of specific nutrients (carbohydrates, fat, potassium, etc.) in an enteral feeding tailored to meet the patient's individual nutritional needs.
43. **Nitrogen balance:** A calculation determined by 24 hour urine collection for urea nitrogen to measure the difference of nitrogen ingested via protein to that excreted each day. A factor of 4 is added for non-urine nitrogen losses via skin, feces, etc.

    $$\text{N. in} - (\text{N. out} + 4) = \text{N. balance}$$

    The goal for repletion is +4 to +6 gms; for maintenance 0 to + 1 gm is acceptable.
44. **Nutrition:** The sum total of all processes involved with the ingestion, digestion, absorption, metabolism and body utilization of nutrient substances. Growth, repair and maintenance of body activities are accomplished in part or wholly by nutrition.
45. **Nutrition assessment:** Evaluation of an individual's nutrition status by determining anthropometric, biochemical and historical factors.
46. **Nutrition Support Team:** A group of health care professionals trained in the assessment, development, implementation and evaluation of nutrition support therapies. Members consist of physician, dietitian, pharmacist and nurse and are usually hospital based.
47. **Parenteral Nutrition:** Administration of nutritional support by a route other than the gastrointestinal tract, i.e. via the intravenous route.
48. **Peripheral Intravenous Nutrition Support:** Provision of intravenous nutrition support through a peripheral vein; usually refers to protein sparing therapy and lipid nutritional support system.
49. **Pneumothorax:** A complication of catheter insertion by which air or gas enters the pleural space.
50. **Protein Sparing:** An intravenous solution for nutritional support consisting of amino acids, vitamins, electrolytes and minerals. The omission of glucose is thought to enhance lipolysis with resultant use of endogenous fat as a calorie source, thus sparing endogenous protein.
51. **Recommended Daily Allowances (RDA):** A *guide* of nutrient requirements designed to plan meal patterns for groups of people.
52. **Renal Failure Solution:** A solution of essential amino acids and hypertonic dextrose (70%) containing vitamins, electrolytes and minerals (when added) for use via a central catheter in treating patients with renal failure.
53. **Respiratory Quotient:** A ratio of carbon dioxide produced to oxygen consumed during the metabolic process. The quotient differs depending upon the energy substrate.
54. **Skin-fold thickness:** An estimate of the amount of subcutaneous fat measured with calipers at the triceps. The determined value is compared to prepared tables for the percent of standard.
55. **Skin testing antigens:** The use of recall antigens to measure the host immune response.
56. **Somatic protein:** Body proteins contained in the muscles or "building proteins."
57. **Subclavian vein:** That vein leading to the superior vena cava most commonly used for administration of Hyperalimentation fluids.
58. **Supplement:** One of many enteral products supplying one or more specific nutrients to complement a deficient oral diet.
59. **Thrombophlebitis:** Inflammation of a vein.
60. **Total Iron Binding Capacity (TIBC):** The capacity of iron that can be carried in the plasma by transferrin. Elevated levels of TIBC are seen in iron deficiency while decreased levels indicate iron overload or protein deficiency.
61. **Total Lymphocyte Count (TLC):** Total number of lymphocytes per cubic millimeter of blood (total white blood cell count times percent lymphocyte). TLC is considered the "poor-man's" measure of immune competence.
62. **Total Parenteral Nutrition (TPN):** Administration of *all* nutrients by a route other than the gastrointestinal tract. While in the purist sense, TPN can refer to either a central or peripheral route; by convention, TPN is usually synonymous with Hyperalimentation and was originated by those who objected to the linguistic inaccuracy of the term Hyperalimentation.
63. **Transferrin:** Carrier protein for iron and a very sensitive indicator of visceral protein status due to its rapid turnover time of 8 days.
64. **Trendelenburg position:** A position where the legs and hips are elevated higher than the head. It is used when inserting a subclavian catheter.
65. **Valsalva maneuver:** An attempt to forcibly exhale without releasing any air. This causes increased intrathoracic pressure and a decreased return of blood to the heart. It is useful to decrease the risk of an air embolus.
66. **Visceral protein:** Body proteins which function to regulate body processes estimated by measuring proteins produced by the liver.

Part III

Establishment of a Home Nutritional Support Program

The Western Pennsylvania Hospital is a 600-bed metropolitan Medical Center serving Pittsburgh and the Western Pennsylvania area. The institution is fully accredited and has an active Department of Medical Education which supports a large residency and post-graduate training program. The hospital has a long-standing commitment to progressive community health services and to that end has aggressively developed both in-hospital and home nutritional support programs during the past 5 years.

These programs are based on an integrated and well coordinated effort involving numerous disciplines within the hospital environment. Both programs are under the direction of the Nutritional and Metabolic Support Committee and the hospital administration. These programs have gained wide acceptance among the members of the various medical specialities, and their patient referral patterns now encompass many disciplines. At the present time, approximately 20 patients per day are undergoing some form of in-house venous nutritional support. A larger number of patients are receiving enteral support. As our degree of expertise with in-house nutritional support increased, we felt comfortable expanding our commitment to include home nutritional support. Subsequently, approximately one year ago, we embarked upon a program for the development of a home nutritional support service. It is the expressed intent of the editors that this chapter should relate the experience of a community hospital in establishing a home nutritional support program. To that end, we have attempted not only to outline steps to be followed in establishing this outpa-

tient modality, but also to "bare our souls" with respect to the various logistic errors and problems we encountered.

No attempt has been made to provide the reader with the definitive treatise on this topic. Rather, our goal has been to assemble a multidisciplinary collection of practical concepts as they apply to the establishment of a Home Nutritional Support Program. We have attempted to illustrate some of the pitfalls a community hospital may expect to encounter in initiating a similar program. We hope that this information will prove useful in the sense that it will allow other hospitals to avoid our mistakes and to improve where we had weaknesses. In a similar fashion, we hope that our experience and our strong points will serve as building blocks for the creation of similar programs.

STEVEN A. CAYWOOD, M.B.A.

I. WILLIAM GOLDFARB, M.D.

Prepared by The Nutritional and Metabolic Support Committee

The Western Pennsylvania Hospital
Pittsburgh, Pennsylvania

EDITOR

I. William Goldfarb, M.D.

Chairman, Nutritional and Metabolic Support Committee
The Western Pennsylvania Hospital
Pittsburgh, Pa.

CONTRIBUTORS

The Members of The Nutritional
and Metabolic Support Committee
of The Western Pennsylvania Hospital

Frank Breggar, M.D.
Angela Cavalier, R.N.
Maureen DeCourcy, R.N.
Lester Dunmire, M.D.
Lesley Eyman, R.D.
Ethel Gandy, R.N.
Joyce Grater, G.S.W.
Joseph Johnson, M.D.
Paul Kim, M.D.
Mr. Pat Mutch, M.P.H.
Monica Obsheatz, R. Pharm.
Mr. Michael Rose, M.B.A.
James Sandala, R. Pharm.
Harvey Slater, M.D.
Gwen Webb, R.D.

Chapter 22

The Administrative Perspective on the Establishment of A Home Nutritional Support Program

Pat Mutch, M.P.H.

Michael Rose, M.B.A.

Members of The Nutritional and Metabolic Support Committee of The Western Pennsylvania Hospital

The establishment of a Home Nutritional Support Program (HNSP) requires a multidisciplinary effort involving physicians, nurses, allied health professionals, support service personnel, and administrators. The administrative decision to initiate and develop such a program must be carefully made after a thorough consideration of patient need, the availability of staff, overall institutional cost, anticipated reimbursement, and other factors. While the process a hospital goes through to establish a home nutritional support program is similar to the process used to develop other new programs, the diversity of the staff involved in the program and the fact that the service is ultimately provided at home and not in a hospital necessitates a more carefully planned and extensively investigated effort.

At the Western Pennsylvania Hospital, approximately 4 months of research, discussion, and analysis were needed before an institutional commitment was made to HNSP. As of March, 1981, 10 patients have participated in the program, and continued increases are expected in the number of patients served by the program. Utilization of the program is available to all medical and surgical specialties, and the present patient population is diversified in terms of underlying disease and referring departments.

WHY ESTABLISH A PROGRAM?

Why should a hospital consider developing a home nutritional support service as a hospital resource? The answer to this question will obviously vary from hospital to hospital. For most hospitals whose primary emphasis is patient care and community service, the single most important reason is patient need.

From a clinical perspective, the significance of an individual's nutritional status has been clearly established. Estimates indicate that as many as 5% of patients who expire in hospitals in the United States do so from starvation. It is also estimated that malnutrition is either the cause of, or contributing factor to, over 200,000 deaths annually and a complication for an additional 350,000 patients.

The nutritional status of patients when entering the hospital and during their stay in the hospital has been shown to be an important consideration affecting a large number of patients. Malnutrition can significantly increase average length of stay, morbidity, and the costs of hospitalization.

To more effectively deal with this problem, hospitals have been expanding their nutritional support services on a more formally organized basis.

The development of an HNSP is a logical extension of an already existing in-hospital program. The medical and surgical indications for home nutritional support are detailed in Chapter 23. When deemed clinically appropriate by a physician, the provision of nutritional support in a home environment rather than in a hospital setting has significant advantages for the patient, the patient's family, and the general community. A patient on home therapy is better able to participate in family affairs and is likely to be less dependent on family members than while in the hospital. While on home therapy, a patient might very well be gainfully employed and/or actively participate in community affairs.

In addition to patient need, several reasons for the establishment of a home therapy program relate to financial consider-

WPH THE WESTERN PENNSYLVANIA HOSPITAL
4800 Friendship Avenue, Pittsburgh, PA 15224 Phone (412) 682-4200

CONSENT TO PARTICIPATION
IN HOME VENOUS FEEDING PROGRAM

1. I have met with Dr.____________________ who has explained to me that because I already have an artificial tube (catheter) in a vein in my chest, I am eligible to participate in a special home care nutrition program. I will be responsible for putting high powered liquid foods (hyperalimentation) into my tube (catheter) at home. The doctor told me this gets important and helpful foods into my body since my medical condition,____________________, keeps me from getting all the nourishment I need.

2. My physician has explained the following risks and possible problems with home vein feeding:____________________

3. The doctor explained that if I can't go into this program, I might have to keep coming back to the Hospital or doctor's office every time I need these foods, or I might have to wait until a nurse can visit me at home, or I might not be able to get any of these special foods at all, if something can't be worked out.

4. During the program, things may change or happen which require a different procedure from that already described. If that happens, the doctor, his associates and assistants are allowed to do whatever they think is necessary to correct the problem. I will be told if significant changes in my long range treatment plan are made.

5. I have been taught how to care for my venous catheter and, if I have questions or problems, I should call the doctor or come to the Hospital or doctor's office.

Witness　　　　Patient's Signature

Physician's Signature　　　　Date　　Time　　A.M. P.M.

Because the above patient is a minor,_____ years of age, or is unable to sign for the following reasons:____________________, the above consent is given on behalf of the patient by:

Witness　　　　Closest Relative or Guardian

Date　　Time　　A.M. P.M.　　　　Relationship

Figure 22-1. Home nutritional support consent form.

ations. Whereas a typical home nutritional support patient may utilize approximately $40,000 of solutions and supplies per year, the same patient when hospitalized, might incur charges in excess of $75,000 to $100,000 annually. The financial advantages to the patient and the community are dramatic. Increasing pressure by third party payers, PSRO, and the other organizations to reduce hospitalization and shorten lengths of hospital stay will most likely further stimulate the development of home nutritional support services. The Health Care Financing Administration is presently considering demonstration projects that will further evaluate the cost effectiveness of such programs. Parallels with the growth of home renal dialysis programs are often made.

An institution that develops an acknowledged degree of expertise in this area may emerge as a regional center. This may lead to an influx of patient referrals from surrounding institutions. The provision of services that are truly life-sustaining and lifesaving and that enable patients to function in their home environment have obvious public relations benefits. Specific financial advantages need to be determined through detailed financial analysis.

WHICH HOSPITALS SHOULD DEVELOP A PROGRAM?

Because the decision to provide home nutritional support services requires a substantial commitment of institutional resources, a hospital must systematically evaluate a number of different factors to insure program feasibility and longevity. The evaluation which should be made can be structured through a series of questions.

Is There Sufficient Patient Need?

The hospital should initiate its evaluation of patient need through review of medical records, utilization statistics, pharmacy records, and other information. If a hospital already has a large number of inpatients on a nutritional support program, it is likely that a group of potential home program candidates exists. As an example, the Western Pennsylvania Hospital is a 600-bed institution with an ongoing in-house venous nutritional program consisting of 20 patients per day. Over the course of one year, 10 patients have been declared candidates for participation in the HNSP. A multidisciplinary review of in-hospital support patients on a case-by-case basis by physicians, nurses, pharmacists, social workers, and home care professionals will indicate the need for home nutritional support. *A hospital should not attempt to provide home nutritional support until a well-developed in-hospital nutritional support program is established.*

Is the Service Available Elsewhere?

Through discussions with hospital administrators, Health System Agency officials, local third party payers, and others in the commmunity, it should not be difficult to identify already existing providers of home nutritional support. Because the provision of these services is a relatively recent development, it is difficult to determine the optimum number of providers per 100,000 people in the community. Variations in a hospital's case mix and variations in the way home nutritional support services are actually provided affect the "appropriate" number of institutional providers that should maintain programs. The potential regionalization of home nutritional programs and shared service arrangements are concepts that will likely receive greater attention in the future.

Are Sufficient Staff Resources Available?

As previously indicated, an HNSP includes a variety of health care professionals and support personnel. The administrator must determine if the appropriate staff resources are available in nursing, pharmacy, social service, dietary, materials handling, and other hospital departments. If they are not readily available, can they be recruited? Do other nearby hospitals have some of the expertise on their staffs?

Will the Hospital Medical Staff Support the Program?

In the development of a clinical program, medical staff leadership and interest are essential. A physician must be identified who is both qualified and interested in directing a home nutritional support service. The director of an HNSP coordinates the efforts of a nutritional support team and assists other physicians in their use of the program for their patients. The number of patients on nutritional support, institutional involvement with education, and the level of nutritional research in progress all help determine the need for part-time or full-time medical direction and the levels of physician compensation required.

Is the Program Financially Feasible?

In order to answer this question, a detailed analysis of program expenses and revenues must be completed. This analysis requires a series of assumptions about how the services will be provided, by whom, and in what quantity. Also required is a thorough understanding of third-party payer commitments to cover the cost of these services, on both an inpatient and outpatient basis. While major medical plans cover a portion of a patient's expenses, deductible and co-insurance provisions may still result in a significant financial burden for the patient, and a resulting potential bad debt for the provider. At the present time, third-party coverage for home nutritional support services varies by insurance carrier.

A hospital's financial commitment to an HNSP can be reduced through the use of a proprietary company. Many of these companies are owned and operated by pharmaceutical houses that manufacture the solutions and related supplies and equipment. These companies will help to train patients prior to discharge, will deliver solutions and supplies to the home (or to a pharmacy for solution mixing), and will supply and maintain the I.V. pump and other necessary hardware. As the number of patients on home therapy increases, these companies are expanding their range of services and providing better staff and patient educational materials. When a hospital identifies a potential home patient, the company is notified, so that an evaluation of the patient's third party insurance coverage or ability to pay can be initiated. If a hospital chooses to use an outside company rather than provide all services, it may face a moral dilemma. The inability of these companies to accept all referred patients (due to financial considerations) may conflict with the hospital's practice of providing service to all patients regardless of the ability to pay. Careful consideration must be given to the establishment of limits on the amount of nonreimbursed home care that will be provided by the hospital. Due to the present uncertainty about reimbursement and concerns about delivery logistics, the Western Pennsylvania Hospital has decided to refer home nutritional support patients to an outside company. The hospital and the patient's physicians closely monitor the quality of service being provided by the outside company. Ultimate responsibility for overall patient care remains with the hospital and the referring physician. To that end, the hospital should develop a special informed consent form (Figure 22-1).

HOSPITAL DEPARTMENTS TO BE INVOLVED IN THE PROVISION OF NUTRITIONAL SUPPORT SERVICES

The establishment of a nutritional support service on an inpatient and/or outpatient basis requires a multidisciplinary commitment of health care specialists (Figure 22-2). Program support and coordination is required from physicians, nursing, pharmacy, social service, home care, materials management, clinical laboratory, and dietary departments and hospital administrators. Obviously, with the number of specialists involved, it is essential that a coordinated team approach to nutritional support services be established. The director of the nutritional support service should be a physician who has a special interest in

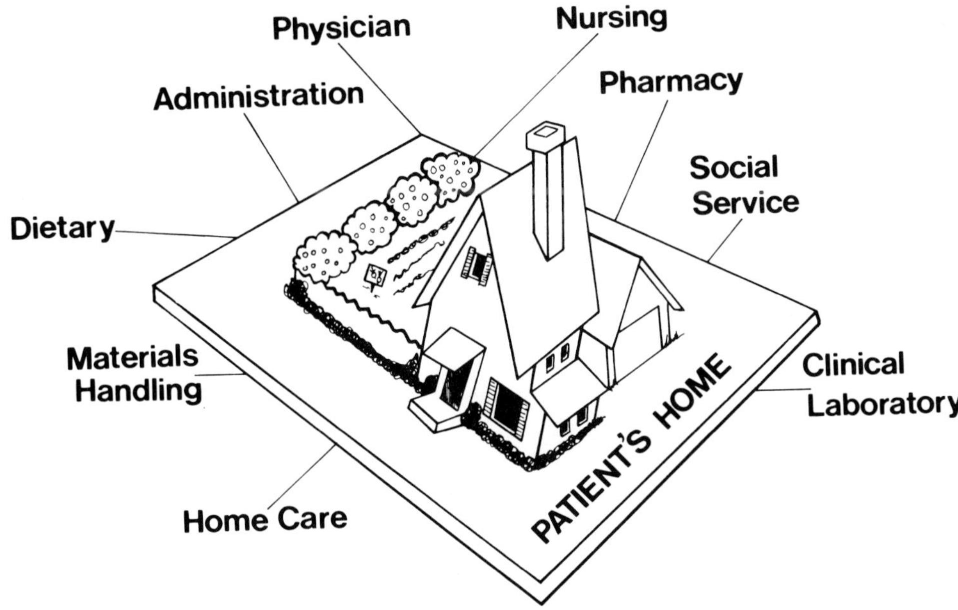

Figure 22-2. The multi-disciplinary approach to home nutritional support.

this field and who has developed a working knowledge of the concepts of nutritional support. While the physician/director might well be a specialist in any field, it is most common for a surgeon or gastroenterologist to assume this position. After seeking administrative approval and support for the establishment of a nutritional support service, the physician/director must essentially provide the day-to-day leadership in organizing the vast array of specialists who must attend the needs of the patient. An initial step is to organize a nutritional support committee comprised of members of the medical staff and associated health care specialists involved in the delivery of this service. This committee can serve as an effective means of education for both members of the medical staff and paramedical personnel. Because of the complexity of the program and the vast array of hospital specialists who play a role in effective nutritional support services, the hospital administration must fully recognize the benefits of committing a substantial number of human resources to the development of such a program. Great pains should be taken to point out that a multidisciplinary program such as this requires extreme attention to detail and the solid cooperation of all involved departments.

The Actual Team Approach

From the initial meeting of the physician/director, administration, and representatives from the various involved hospital disciplines, a team approach to organize nutritional support services should be implemented. The suggested paramedical composition of this team is as follows:

NURSING DEPARTMENT

The nursing representative to the nutritional support team should be a registered nurse with specialized training in intravenous therapy and nutritional support. In general, most hospitals do not have an individual on their staff who has gained a degree of expertise in both of these modalities. Subsequently, it is often necessary to obtain the services of a member of the nursing department who may possess a special interest in this type of therapy. Actual training can be provided both on the job (under the direction of the physician/director) and through enrollment in special continuing education courses. The American Society of Parenteral and Enteral Nutrition (ASPEN) holds a yearly symposium which includes outstanding educational programs for interested nursing personnel. We have found the use of these outside educational programs to be of extreme benefit in the educational process of the various members of our nutritional support team.

On a day-to-day basis, the nurse specialist, who in our institution is called the nutritional/metabolic support nurse (NMSN), functions in cooperation with the physician/director. This individual provides the continuity between the various interacting members of the team. In addition, this individual is also active in the patient education programs and outpatient follow-up programs which are essential to any HNSP. From an administrative point of view, adequate office provisions for this individual should be obtained in order to allow the NMSN to perform necessary administrative functions. It is also important to note that emergency situations will arise which will require the expertise of this individual. An emergency phone number should be given for these situations. In addition, an on-call beeper can be utilized to facilitate communication.

At the present time, the NMSN reports directly to the director of staff development within the nursing department. It is conceivable that a nutritional support nurse may be employed by the physician/director of the nutritional support service because of her close association with that individual and the proportion of time she spends with that individual and his patients.

PHARMACY

The pharmacist is obviously a key member of any nutritional support service. The pharmacist must be well trained in the preparation of IV admixtures and nutritional solutions. Because of the broad program decisions that must be made regarding the establishment of nutritional services, either on an inpatient and/or outpatient basis, the director of pharmacy needs to work closely with the physician/director of the nutritional support services.

The director of pharmacy should insure that adequate space is available for a mixing room to include the placement of a laminar flow hood. If a floor model horizontal laminar flow hood cannot be accommodated because of a lack of space, possible consideration can be given to a bench-model hood. It is of paramount importance that the director of pharmacy and the physician/director communicate on a daily basis so as to insure that the hospital pharmacy is able to meet the logistic demands that can accompany an ever increasing number of patients. The hospital administration must adequately support the pharmacy so that the pharmacy's resources will continue to grow in accordance with the expansion of the nutritional support services.

Most home nutritional support services are based on an outpatient admixture program. However, for certain specific reasons, our institution has chosen to begin its HNSP utilizing a hospital-based admixture program (these specific reasons are outlined in Chapter 27). This necessitates a reimbursement of compounding fees and the utilization of a reliable home delivery system. If this type of program adaptation is utilized, it will require additional communication between the hospital administration, hospital pharmacy, and the supplying companies.

DIETARY, SOCIAL SERVICE, AND HOME CARE

The additional team support rendered by the dietary, social service, and home care departments all play a vital role in a nutritional support service. The specific roles of these departments are more extensively outlined in Chapters 24 and 26, respectively.

NUTRITIONAL SUPPORT SERVICE COMPANIES

The outside companies responsible for supplying the various solutions and required hardware are important parts of the team approach. These companies support the growth of the hospital's HNSP by relieving the hospital of many legal, financial, and logistic problems. This allows the hospital to concentrate on meeting its medical and social responsibilities to the home patient. Indeed, the physician and home nutritional support service remain totally responsible for the teaching and follow-up care of the patient, while home nutritional support companies often assume responsibility for the delivery of the equipment and solutions directly to the patient's home. In addition, these companies will bear all financial risks in seeking third-party reimbursement for the solutions and equipment. As we have already pointed out, your institution may choose to utilize a hospital-based compounding program. Also, an occasional patient, for whatever reason, will be unable to mix the solutions within the home environment. Therefore, we recommend that the hospital make arrangements for an inhouse compounding program with pickup and delivery to the patient's home.

PROGRAM EVALUATION

An essential element in the development of any program is the ongoing evaluation which occurs in order to test the effectiveness of the program and whether the goals and objectives established for the program have, in fact, been met. The evaluation of a home nutritional support program should address several questions.

1. Was the projected need actually met? This would relate to both the number and the types of patients being cared for. Patient needs should also be evaluated in terms of the ongoing development of home nutritional support programs by other neighboring hospitals. The development of other programs would possibly affect the need for your hospital's program.
2. Were the required staff resources actually obtained?
3. Was the medical staff support needed for the program actually obtained?
4. Was the level of physician involvement among various members of the medical staff adequate to insure that patients requiring the service were, in fact, referred to the program?
5. Were the financial expectations of the program actually met?
6. Did the program generate the revenues that were expected?
7. Were the expenses that were projected actually incurred?
8. Was the projected bad debt experience actually realized?
9. Was the length of stay for nutritional support patients reduced due to the availability of the home program? This can be determined by comparing lengths of stay for hospitalized patients prior to the inception of the program with lengths of stay for patients following the implementation of the program.
10. Did the program actually generate the outside referrals from other institutions and physicians as expected?
11. Did the hospital, in fact, obtain a positive public relations benefit due to the implementation of the program?

The utilization of such an introspective system of program evaluation serves as a means of continually upgrading the overall service.

SUMMARY

The successful implementation of an inpatient and/or outpatient support program is based on a firm administrative commitment to this therapy. A strong commitment and continued support are necessary if such a multifaceted team approach is going to be successfully implemented. This type of program results in enhancement of the hospital's capability, which is reflected as improved medical care and service to the community.

BIBLIOGRAPHY

1. Shils, M.E.: A program for total parenteral nutrition at home. Am. J. Clin. Nutr., *28:*1429, 1975.
2. Skoutakis, V.A., et al.: Team approach to total parenteral nutrition. Amer. J. Hosp. Pharm., *32:*693, 1975.
3. Bistrian, B.R., et al.: Prevalence of Malnutrition in general medical patients. JAMA, *235*(15):1567, 1976.
4. Jeejeebhoy, K.N.: Total parenteral nutrition at home. Can. J. Surg., *19*(6):477, 1976.
5. Sorg, J.L.: A protocol for hyperalimentation in a community hospital. Amer. Surg., *42*(9):716, 1976.
6. Brown, R.S., and Grenkoski, J.: Total parenteral nutrition: A safe procedure in the small community hospital? Crit. Care Med., *5*(5):241, 1977.
7. Havill, J.H., et al.: Home parenteral nutrition. N. Z. Med. J., *86:*82, 1977.
8. Shaw, J., and Lamy, P.P.: A total parenteral nutritional program for a community hospital. Hosp. Form., *12*(9):583, 1977.
9. Powel-Tuck, J., et al.: Team approach to long-term intravenous feeding in patients with gastrointestinal disorders. Lancet, *2*(8094):825, 1978.
10. Wateska, L.P., et al.: Coordinating a total parenteral nutrition program. Am. J. Intravenous Ther., *5*(3):13, 1978.
11. Lokey, H., Hitt, D., and McMahan, J.J.: A hyperalimentation manual for the small hospital. Surg. Clin. North Amer., *59*(3):411, 1979.

Chapter 23
Medical/Surgical Indications for Hospital and Home Nutritional Support

Lester A. Dunmire, M.D.
Joseph Johnson, M.D.
Members of the Nutritional and Metabolic Support Committee of The Western Pennsylvania Hospital

The concept of vigorous nutritional support for hospitalized patients has gained a tremendous amount of acceptance within the medical community during the past 15 years. Long ago it was apparent that the poorly nourished patient often failed to respond to treatment, whether medical or surgical in nature. Particularly in surgery, the protein-deficient patient dramatically demonstrated problems with wound healing, infection, and fistulas. While physicians have always paid "lip service" to the need for metabolic support in stressed patients, it was not until Dr. Dudrick's work in the late 1960s that this therapeutic modality began to achieve practical utilization. Initially, the administration of venous nutritional support solutions was regarded as a specialized technique to be utilized by only a very few physicians. However, with the establishment of a pool of literature and the dissemination of information within training programs, these techniques have gained wide utilization among physicians in all hospital settings. At the present time, it is not uncommon for many physicians within the same institution to be utilizing this therapeutic modality either alone, or in conjunction with their hospital's nutritional support team. While it is feasible for a wide variety of hospital physicians to administer these solutions to the in-house population, this is not the most desirable system for the administration of home nutritional support solutions. *The numerous potential logistic complications, and the need for a well coordinated team approach mandate that all home nutritional support patients be placed under the direct supervision of one designated physician and the nutritional support team.*

At the present time, approximately 600 patients internationally are receiving total parenteral nutrition as outpatients. An active registry of patients is at the New York Academy of Medicine.

Published registry data from a survey conducted in 1979 reported the incidence of etiologic factors leading to the need for home total parenteral nutrition as follows:

Inflammatory bowel disease	28.6%
Bowel infarction with subsequent resection	23%
Malignancy resulting in bowel dysfunction	20.5%
Motility disorders	8.7%
General disorders	5.6%
Trauma	0.6%
Other	13%

The age distribution of this patient population was:

0 to 10 years—11%

11 to 20 years—11%
21 to 40 years—25%
41 to 60 years—38%

The indications for the initiation of this modality in each hospital will vary, depending on the hospital's patient population. In the institution that has a large referral pattern for inflammatory bowel disease, the number of patients who are kept candidates for home nutritional support will be somewhat higher than in other institutions. In institutions with a large oncology service, the percentage of patients who are started on this therapy because of mitotic pathology may be somewhat higher than the national average. In our particular institution, the vast majority of candidates consists of patients with inflammatory bowel disease and those with mitotic problems. The oncotic patients have problems with bowel dysfunction secondary to either chemotherapy or radiation therapy. While patients with inflammatory bowel disease and those with mitotic pathology may comprise the most common group of candidates, on a practical basis, any patient on in-house nutritional support may be an eventual candidate for home nutritional support.

The initiation of intravenous nutritional support is not a procedure to be undertaken lightly. Even among physicians working closely together, there may be differing opinions as to when to start actual treatment. Possibly the old adage about tracheostomies should apply to hyperalimentation—"when one thinks about it, it's time to do it." Nevertheless, the ultimate decision to start treatment depends on the patient and the underlying disease. In general, we can divide patients into three broad groups with indications for the initiation of nutritional support.

PATIENTS WHO DO NOT POSSESS AN INTACT GASTROINTESTINAL TRACT

The term intact applies not only to continuity from mouth to anus, but also to the functional integrity of the intestinal mucosa. Into this category one could place those patients with inflammatory bowel disease, fistulas, gastrointestinal tract obstruction, and malabsorption syndromes. Some specific points are relative to the various anatomic locations of gastrointestinal disease. These points may be presented in relation to the specific organ involved as follows:

Esophageal Disease

Not infrequently, nutritional problems encountered with diseases of the esophagus can best be treated by the insertion of enteral feeding tubes placed beyond the involved areas. Thus, patients with strictures and carcinoma may not require standard intravenous nutritional support. These patients may be maintained both on an in-house and outpatient basis through the placement of nasoduodenal silicone elastomer feeding tubes. Specific utilization of these tubes is discussed in Chapter 25. It should be noted, however, that fistulas, developing after surgery on the esophagus, may be an indication for the initiation of intravenous therapy.

Gastric Disease

Obstructing lesions of the pyloric area of the stomach are best managed by the initiation of intravenous nutritional support. Frequently, these patients are in extremely poor nutritional status secondary to prolonged emesis and associated diminished oral intake. Treatment of these patients should begin as soon after admission as possible and should not be delayed while diagnostic evaluation is initiated. Even after surgical intervention, venous nutritional support should be continued to maintain a state of positive nitrogen balance during the postoperative period.

Duodenal and Small Bowel Disease

Patients with small bowel disease represent the classic candidates for the initiation of venous nutritional support. Those with high-output gastrointestinal fistulas present the surgeon with a challenging management problem. Nutritional support is beneficial in providing for spontaneous closure of fistulas. Esophageal, pancreatic, lateral, and end duodenal fistulas are likely to heal in 15 to 25 days following the initiation of intravenous nutritional support. Spontaneous closure of jejunal and ileal fistulas is less likely to occur. However, a course of nutritional support renders these patients better surgical candidates and leads to a higher incidence of successful surgical management. It must be stressed that this support enhances recovery but does not always preclude the utilization of surgical intervention.

In the case of inflammatory bowel disease without concomitant fistula formation, the cause of malnutrition may be multifactored. Chronic inflammation, decreased oral intake, loss of visceral protein through diseased segments of bowel, and increased catabolism from steroids all contribute to the malnutrition so frequently seen in these patients. The rationale for the utilization of venous nutritional support is to replace nutritional deficits, allow complete bowel rest, and supply nutritional support as an adjunct to surgical and medical therapy. A 3- to 4-week course of parenteral nutrition during an acute exacerbation of transmural inflammatory disease has often led to a dramatic response and a reduction in the number of required surgical interventions. Patients who go on to develop postoperative short bowel syndromes constitute the classic group of candidates for the initiation of home nutritional support.

Colonic Disease

As a general rule, the use of intravenous nutritional support is not of tremendous value in colonic problems except for patients who present with ulcerative colitis. While patients with colonic malignancies, or those who have sustained trauma to the colon may require nutritional support, the use of elemental diets delivered into the small bowel via various types of enteral tubes is generally the technique of choice. Few patients with isolated colonic disease would be considered eventual candidates for the initiation of home nutritional support.

Pancreatic Dysfunction

Pancreatic dysfunction remains a major indication for the use of intravenous nutritional support. The classic management of pancreatitis has generally consisted of a 1 to 3 week period of bowel rest. This is the ideal situation for the initiation of intravenous nutritional support. Pancreatic damage, however, may seriously alter the patient's ability to handle the administered concentrations, and the need for insulin supplementation must be anticipated. Trauma to the pancreas generally necessitates a prolonged period of diminished oral intake and venous nutritional support may be utilized in this situation. In the case of pancreatic carcinoma, nutritional support is generally not indicated except as a means of providing subjective improvement in the patient's tolerance to either chemotherapy or radiation therapy.

PATIENTS WITH EXAGGERATED CALORIC AND/OR SPECIAL PROTEIN REQUIREMENTS

This group of patients consists of those who by virtue of their underlying pathologic state have a requirement for exogenous calories far in excess of their ability to meet this requirement by standard therapy. In addition, patients with specific metabolic problems that may be managed by amino acid manipulative therapy are also included in this category. This group of patients would include those with multiple system trauma, massive thermal injury, renal failure, and hepatic disease. In general, these patients are not candidates for any type of home nutritional support. One possible exception might be the patient with chronic renal disease who might benefit from the utilization of specialized solutions in order to achieve a reduction of blood urea nitrogen levels. Some authors advocate the administration of high-dextrose solutions in conjunction with low concentrations of essential amino acids for the management of renal failure. The absence of the nonessential amino acids facilitates the conversion of urea to the nonessential amino acids. Theoretically, this would result in a lowering of the BUN and possibly the associated morbidity and mortality of renal failure in these patients. To that end, there are both venous and enteral solutions that consist solely of essential amino acids. The amino acids are generally combined with high dextrose concentrations in order to provide final solutions with a high calorie to protein ratio. There is little evidence to suggest that these specialized solutions offer any benefit over standard amino acid solutions (containing both essential and nonessential amino acids) in combination with high concentrations of dextrose. In general, the utilization of these special solutions is limited to acute tubular necrosis, and no conclusive evidence has appeared showing their efficiency in chronic renal disease.

ONCOLOGY PATIENTS

Patients with mitotic pathology become candidates for nutritional support on the basis not only of their progression to a cachectic state, but also as an adjunct to other therapeutic maneuvers. The cachectic patient who is ravaged by both the basic disease and by progressive therapeutic intervention is often the most nutritionally neglected patient in any hospital population. Cachexia, with its attendant weakness and lethargy, is too often accepted as unavoidable. Utilization of chemotherapeutic agents and radiation therapy, with their associated propensity for gastrointestinal dysfunction, generally serves to intensify the problem. While there is no convincing objective evidence to show that the utilization of nutritional support in these patients increases survival, there is subjective evidence that this therapy does offer some patient benefits. Specifically, patients who receive nutritional support seem to tolerate their chemotherapy and radiation therapy better than those who do not receive nutritional support. We have been impressed by the improved sense of well-being and better toleration of adjunct therapy in patients who have been nutritionally supported.

In general, the problems of nausea and emesis negate the utilization of enteral feedings through small silicone tubes in this group of patients. The vast majority of these patients are dependent on some type of venous nutritional support in order to obtain a state of positive nitrogen balance. Since many of these patients have already had silicone elastomer catheters inserted into the subclavian vein for administration of chemotherapeutic agents, we have elected to use these catheters also as the route of administration for venous nutritional support solutions. Most of these patients return to the hospital on a monthly basis for subsequent chemotherapy. When the patient is admitted to the hospital for chemotherapy, the chemotherapy is administered through the subclavian catheter. The subclavian catheter is then exchanged, using the wire technique described in Chapter 19. The new catheter is then utilized as a route of administration for home nutritional support. The solutions are generally administered on a 12-hour cycle; thereby not "tieing" the patient to the pump, and allowing him to lead a more normal life. We have not experienced any incidence of catheter related sepsis, utilizing this technique.

Benefits obtained in this group of patients include the following:

1. Increased subjective tolerance of chemotherapeutic drugs and radiotherapy, providing for a more complete course of therapy.
2. Reduction of gastrointestinal side effects.
3. Decreases in surgical morbidity and mortality.
4. Probable improvements in immunocompetence and subsequent reductions in sepsis.

SUMMARY

It is important for the physician to identify possible candidates for home nutritional support as early in their hospital course as possible. With a patient who is a candidate for intravenous nutritional support, the physician should always anticipate the possible utilization of this therapeutic modality on an outpatient basis. Once the determination for home nutritional support has been made, the nutritional support team should begin to acclimate the patient to the anticipated schedule of solution administration that will be utilized following discharge. In addition, the vigorous home training program for both the patient and the designated family member should be instituted by the nutritional/metabolic support nurse. It should be noted that the absence of a designated family member is of sufficient concern so as to exclude a patient from the program. The social service and home care departments should become involved in the patient's care in order to facilitate the transition from the hospital to the home environment. The actual skills required by the patient and/or the designated family member may be outlined as follows:

1. A knowledge of the potential glucose complications and the techniques for monitoring patient response to glucose administration.
2. A knowledge of the techniques of central venous catheter care.
3. A knowledge of the potential complications of long-term central venous catheterization and the indications for immediate notification of the nutritional metabolic support specialist.
4. A knowledge of pump mechanics and the basic techniques of intervention in case of pump failure.

While these skills may appear beyond the scope of most patients, we have found that both patient and designated family members can easily master the necessary skills to facilitate home nutritional support.

BIBLIOGRAPHY

1. Aguirre, A., Fisher, J.E., and Welch, C.E.: The role of surgery and hyperalimentation in therapy of gastrointestinal-cutaneous fistulae. Ann. Surg., *180:*393, 1974.
2. Blumenkrantz, M.J., et al.: Total parenteral nutrition in the management of acute renal failure. Am. J. Clin. Nutr., *31:*1831, 1978.
3. Copeland, E.M., Daly, J.M., and Dudrick, S.J.: Intravenous hyperalimentation, bowel rest and cancer. Crit. Care Med., *8:*21, 1980.
4. Copeland, E.M., Daly, J.M., and Dudrick, S.J.: Nutrition as an adjunct to cancer treatment in the adult. Cancer Res., *37:*2451, 1977.
5. Dudrick, S.J., and Ruberg, R.L.: Principles and practice of parenteral nutrition. Gastroenterology, *61:*901, 1971.
6. Dudrick, S.J.: Rational intravenous therapy. Am. J. Hosp. Pharm., *28:*82, 1971.
7. Fleming, C.R., et al.: Home parenteral nutrition for management of the severely malnourished adult patient. Gastroenterology, *79:*11, 1980.
8. Graham, J.A.: Conservative treatment of gastrointestinal fistulas. Surg. Gynecol. Obstet., *144:* 512, 1977.
9. Jeejeebhoy, K.N., and Langer, B.: Home parenteral nutrition. CMA Journal, *122:*143, 1980.
10. MacFadyen, B.V., Dudrick, S.J., and Ruberg, R.L.: Management of gastrointestinal fistulas with parenteral hyperalimentation. Surgery, *74:*100, 1973.
11. Mullen, J.L., et al.: Ten years experience with intravenous hyperalimentation and inflammatory bowel disease. Ann. Surg., *187:*523, 1978.
12. Ota, D.M., Imbembo, A.L., and Zuidema, G.D.: Total parenteral nutrition. Surgery, *83:*503, 1978.
13. Rault, R.M.J., and Scribner, B.H.: Treatment of Crohn's disease with home parenteral nutrition. Gastroenterology, *72:*1429, 1977.
14. Reilly, J., et al.: Hyperalimentation in inflammatory bowel disease. Am. J. Surg., *131:*192, 1976.
15. Sheldon, G.F., et al.: Management of gastrointestinal fistulas. Surg. Gynecol. Obstet., *133:*385, 1971.
16. Steiger, E., and Fazio, V.W.: Total parenteral nutrition—a manual of principles and techniques. Cleveland, The Cleveland Clinic Foundation, 1976.
17. Abel, R.M., and Fischer, J.E.: Intravenous essential amino acids in the treatment of acute renal failure. Clin. Dig., *3*(1):1, 1974.
18. Bordos, D.C., and Cameron, J.L.: Successful long-term intravenous hyperalimentation in the hospital and at home. Arch. Surg., *110:*439, 1975.
19. Bozzetti, F.: Parenteral nutrition in surgical patients. Surg. Gynecol. Obstet., *142:*16, 1976.
20. Copeland, E.M., III, MacFadyen, B.V., Jr., and Dudrick, S.J.: Intravenous hyperalimentation in cancer patients. J. Surg. Res., *16:*241, 1974.
21. Copeland, E.M., III, MacFadyen, B.V., Jr., and Dudrick, S.J.: Intravenous hyperalimentation as an adjunct to cancer chemotherapy. Am. J. Surg., *129:*167, 1975.
22. Souchon, E.A., et al.: Intravenous hyperalimentation as an adjunct to cancer chemotherapy with 5-fluorouracil. J. Surg. Res., *18:*451, 1975.
23. Jeejeebhoy, K.N., et al.: Total parenteral nutrition at home: studies in patients surviving 4 months to 5 years. Gastroenterology, *71:*(6):943, 1976.
24. Copeland, E.M., and Dudrick, S.J.: Nutritional aspects of cancer. Curr. Probl. Cancer, *1*(3):1, 1976.

25. Marshall, R., II.: Hyperalimentation as a treatment of Crohn's disease. Am. J. Surg., *128*(5):652, 1974.
26. Byrne, W.J., et al.: Home total parenteral nutrition: an alternative approach to the management of children with severe chronic small bowel disease. J. Pediat. Surg., *12*(3):359, 1977.
27. Fleming, C.R., McGill, D.B., and Berkner, S.: Home parenteral nutrition as primary therapy in patients with extensive Crohn's disease of the small bowel and malnutrition. Gastroenterology, *73*(5):1077, 1977.
28. Rault, R.M.J., and Scribner, B.H.: Treatment of Crohn's disease with home parenteral nutrition. Gastroenterology, *72*(6):1249, 1977.

Chapter 24

Nutritional Assessment and Long-Term Follow-up

Lesley Eyman, R.D.
Gwen Webb, R.D.
Members of the Nutritional and Metabolic Support Committee of The Western Pennsylvania Hospital

A thorough nutritional assessment is the initial screening procedure used to diagnose and categorize malnutrition in the hospitalized patient. It serves to provide guidelines for the initiation of therapy and for subsequent modifications in that therapy. Historically, nutritional assessment has been viewed as a "luxury," and as such, its utilization has generally been restricted to large teaching institutions. In reality, nutritional assessment can and must be an integral part of any community hospital that is implementing an in-house or home nutritional program.

THE FIRST STEP

In those institutions where nutritional assessment is currently not a common procedure, the first goal of the dietitian is one of hospital education. Both the physician and nursing staffs must be familiarized with the basic concepts and techniques of nutritional assessment. Realizing the importance of this process, our dietary department sought measures not only to demonstrate their interest in this modality, but also to enlighten others as to the value of this tool in health care. Although many articles have appeared over the past decade on the "starving hospitalized patient," the actual techniques utilized to diagnose and measure the degree of protein-calorie malnutrition have not been disseminated to most community hospitals.

First, an educational program should be planned as a series of in-services for all involved personnel. In our particular situation, these in-services were widely attended and subsequently led to the establishment of a day-long seminar offered to physicians, pharmacists, nurses, and dietitians from other institutions. The goal was to generate information and encourage interest in nutritional assessment and team-based therapy. This is particularly important when one considers that many of the patients who are candidates for home nutritional support may be referred to your institution from other hospitals. Subsequently, if other hospitals develop the capabilities to adequately assess nutritional status, patient referrals can be better coordinated, and previously initiated therapy can be continued without interruption. For the specific in-service programs, outside speakers sponsored by various pharmaceutic companies, films, and actual demonstrations of anthropometric measurement techniques were utilized. Some of these companies also assisted in the development of the standard nutritional assessment charts which are not utilized within our institution. Various hospital personnel collaborated in the planning of the

THE WESTERN PENNSYLVANIA HOSPITAL

Dietary Department

NUTRITIONAL ASSESSMENT

	PARAMETERS	Patient Values	PERCENT OF STANDARD > 90% Not Depleted	60-90% Mod. Depleted	< 60% Severely Depleted
MARASMUS	% I.B.W. = [Actual Weight / IBW X 100]	%			
	Triceps Skinfold (TSF)	mm			
	Mid Arm Circumference (MAC)	cm			
	Mid Arm Muscle Circumference MAMC (cm) = MAC (cm) – (3.14 x TSF (cm))	cm			
KWASHIORKOR	24 Hour Urinary Creatinine	mg			
	Creatinine Height Index [CHI = Actual Ucr / Ideal Ucr X 100]	%			
	Albumin	g/dl			
	Lymphocyte Count [= % Lymphocyte's x WBC / 100]	mm^3			
	Transferrin [= (0.8 x TIBC) – 43]	mg/dl			
	24 Hour Urinary Urea Nitrogen	g			

SKIN TESTS* (0.1 ml)

	Reactive >5mm	Unreactive <5mm
Mumps	______	______
Candida	______	______
Varidase	______	______
Trichophytin	______	______

(*Read induration at 24 and 48 hours)

Normal ______ (2 or more positive)
Relatively Anergic ______ (one positive)
Anergic ______ (none positive)

CALORIC EXPENDITURE: BASAL ENERGY EXPENDITURE (BEE) ______ Kcal/day

Men = 66@ (13.7 x W) @ (5 x H) – (6.8 x A)
Women = 655@ (9.6 x W) @ (1.7 x H) – (4.7 x A)
W = Actual Weight in kg. H = Height in cm. A = Age in Years
Parenteral Anabolic = 1.75 x BEE Oral Anabolic = 1.5 x BEE Oral Maintenance = 1.2 x BEE

PROTEIN REQUIREMENT: ______ g/day = 1.2 = 1.5 x actual weight (kg)

DAILY INTAKE: Calories ______ Kcal/day Protein ______ g/day
Nitrogen ______ g/day

NITROGEN BALANCE: ______ g/day = Protein Intake / 6.25 – (Urinary Urea Nitrogen + 4)

NUTRITIONAL STATUS:

- ☐ Normal
- ☐ Kwashiorkor (K) (Visceral Attrition) — Depressed: ALB, Transferrin and Anergy; Preserved: TSF, MAMC, CHI. MAC)
- ☐ Marasmus (M) (Depletion Parietal Muscle & Fat) — Depressed: TSF, MAL, MAMC, CHI; Preserved: ALB, Transferrin)
- ☐ Combination M-K (Advanced PCM) — (All Parameters Depressed)

PROPOSED NUTRITIONAL THERAPY:

USUAL WEIGHT: – (kg)
IDEAL WEIGHT: – (kg)
ADMISSION WEIGHT: – (kg)
HEIGHT: – (cm)
BSA (Body Surface Area) (m^2)
DIAGNOSIS: –

Figure 24-1A. Front of standard nutritrional assessment form.

seminar. An advisory committee consisting of representatives from the nursing department, pharmacy, and medical education departments and the medical staff selected the speakers. The seminar staff included in-house participants, physicians, and dietitians. Under the guidance of the hospital's medical education department, the seminar

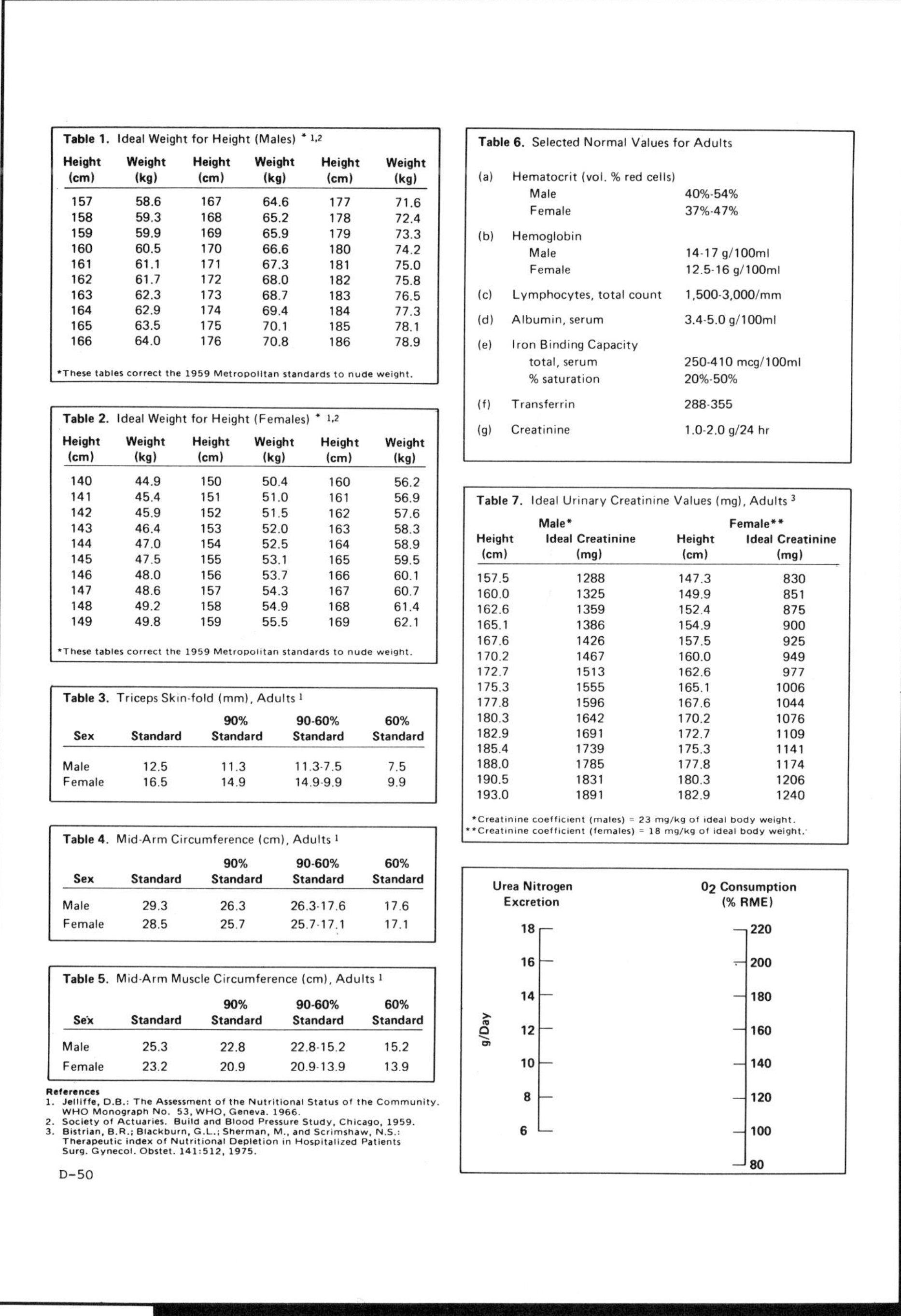

Table 1. Ideal Weight for Height (Males) * [1,2]

Height (cm)	Weight (kg)	Height (cm)	Weight (kg)	Height (cm)	Weight (kg)
157	58.6	167	64.6	177	71.6
158	59.3	168	65.2	178	72.4
159	59.9	169	65.9	179	73.3
160	60.5	170	66.6	180	74.2
161	61.1	171	67.3	181	75.0
162	61.7	172	68.0	182	75.8
163	62.3	173	68.7	183	76.5
164	62.9	174	69.4	184	77.3
165	63.5	175	70.1	185	78.1
166	64.0	176	70.8	186	78.9

*These tables correct the 1959 Metropolitan standards to nude weight.

Table 2. Ideal Weight for Height (Females) * [1,2]

Height (cm)	Weight (kg)	Height (cm)	Weight (kg)	Height (cm)	Weight (kg)
140	44.9	150	50.4	160	56.2
141	45.4	151	51.0	161	56.9
142	45.9	152	51.5	162	57.6
143	46.4	153	52.0	163	58.3
144	47.0	154	52.5	164	58.9
145	47.5	155	53.1	165	59.5
146	48.0	156	53.7	166	60.1
147	48.6	157	54.3	167	60.7
148	49.2	158	54.9	168	61.4
149	49.8	159	55.5	169	62.1

*These tables correct the 1959 Metropolitan standards to nude weight.

Table 3. Triceps Skin-fold (mm), Adults [1]

Sex	Standard	90% Standard	90-60% Standard	60% Standard
Male	12.5	11.3	11.3-7.5	7.5
Female	16.5	14.9	14.9-9.9	9.9

Table 4. Mid-Arm Circumference (cm), Adults [1]

Sex	Standard	90% Standard	90-60% Standard	60% Standard
Male	29.3	26.3	26.3-17.6	17.6
Female	28.5	25.7	25.7-17.1	17.1

Table 5. Mid-Arm Muscle Circumference (cm), Adults [1]

Sex	Standard	90% Standard	90-60% Standard	60% Standard
Male	25.3	22.8	22.8-15.2	15.2
Female	23.2	20.9	20.9-13.9	13.9

References
1. Jelliffe, D.B.: The Assessment of the Nutritional Status of the Community. WHO Monograph No. 53, WHO, Geneva. 1966.
2. Society of Actuaries. Build and Blood Pressure Study, Chicago, 1959.
3. Bistrian, B.R.; Blackburn, G.L.; Sherman, M., and Scrimshaw, N.S.: Therapeutic index of Nutritional Depletion in Hospitalized Patients Surg. Gynecol. Obstet. 141:512, 1975.

D-50

Table 6. Selected Normal Values for Adults

(a)	Hematocrit (vol. % red cells)	
	Male	40%-54%
	Female	37%-47%
(b)	Hemoglobin	
	Male	14-17 g/100ml
	Female	12.5-16 g/100ml
(c)	Lymphocytes, total count	1,500-3,000/mm
(d)	Albumin, serum	3.4-5.0 g/100ml
(e)	Iron Binding Capacity	
	total, serum	250-410 mcg/100ml
	% saturation	20%-50%
(f)	Transferrin	288-355
(g)	Creatinine	1.0-2.0 g/24 hr

Table 7. Ideal Urinary Creatinine Values (mg), Adults [3]

Male* Height (cm)	Male* Ideal Creatinine (mg)	Female** Height (cm)	Female** Ideal Creatinine (mg)
157.5	1288	147.3	830
160.0	1325	149.9	851
162.6	1359	152.4	875
165.1	1386	154.9	900
167.6	1426	157.5	925
170.2	1467	160.0	949
172.7	1513	162.6	977
175.3	1555	165.1	1006
177.8	1596	167.6	1044
180.3	1642	170.2	1076
182.9	1691	172.7	1109
185.4	1739	175.3	1141
188.0	1785	177.8	1174
190.5	1831	180.3	1206
193.0	1891	182.9	1240

*Creatinine coefficient (males) = 23 mg/kg of ideal body weight.
**Creatinine coefficient (females) = 18 mg/kg of ideal body weight.

Figure 24-1B. Back of standard nutritional assessment form.

proved to be successful as both an educational tool and promotional vehicle.

Simultaneously, the physician members of the hospital nutritional support team began an intense program of grand rounds-type presentations with the hospital's residents and medical staff. During weekly meetings, the necessary nutritional assess-

CALORIE COUNT

Name________ Room No.____ Diet________ Date________

FOOD ITEM	AMOUNT USED	(GMS) PROTEIN	CALORIES	SUPPLEMENT FEEDINGS
BREAKFAST				10 A.M.
Juice (cc)				Milkshake (cc)
Cereal (cups)				Eggnog (cc)
Egg				Sustacal (cc)
Bacon				Ensure (cc)
Toast				
Butter (pats)				OTHERS:
Jelly				
Milk - Skim				
- Whole				
Sugar (packets)				
Creamers				
Coffee or Tea				
LUNCH				2 P.M.
Soup				Milkshake (cc)
Meat Entree (oz)				Eggnog (cc)
Noodles, Rice or Potatoes				Sustacal (cc)
Cooked Vegetable				Ensure (cc)
Salad				
Fruit				OTHERS:
Dessert (Specify)				
Bread				
Jelly				
Butter (pats)				
Milk - Skim				
- Whole				
Creamers				
Sugar (packets)				
Coffee or Tea				
DINNER				8 P.M.
Soup				Milkshake (cc)
Meat entree (oz)				Eggnog (cc)
Noodles, Rice or Potatoes				Sustacal (cc)
Cooked Vegetable				Ensure (cc)
Salad				
Fruit				OTHERS:
Dessert (specify)				
Bread				
Jelly				
Butter (pats)				
Milk - Skim				
- Whole				
Creamers				
Sugar (packets)				
Coffee or Tea				
Juice				
TOTAL				

Figure 24-2A. Front of standard "Calorie Count Form."

ment forms were reviewed and refined to meet with the specific needs of our institution. Initially, the form was used as a work sheet for the dietitians; but over the ensuing months, the director of medical records successfully submitted the form to the appropriate committees for inclusion as part of the patient's permanent medical record. The specific form includes all formulas utilized and a section showing the degree of depletion and the associated clinical classifications of malnutrition (e.g., marasmus, kwashiorkor, and marasmus-kwashiorkor). The back of the sheet includes the evaluation standards for the anthropometric and laboratory values (Figure 24-1). An additional useful form is the "calorie count form." The nurses on the floor are responsible for the recording of data on this form. The back of the form provides information

SUPPLEMENT FEEDINGS	AMOUNT	PROTEIN (GRAMS)	CALORIES
DELMARK			
Vanilla Milkshake	8 oz.	8.3	229
Chocolate Milkshake	8 oz.	8.3	229
Eggnog	8 oz.	15.2	290
ROSS			
Ensure	8 oz.	9	250
Ensure Plus	8 oz.	13	355
Polycose (Liquid)	4 oz.		240
MEAD JOHNSON			
Sustacal	8 oz.	14.5	240
Sustacal Pudding	5 oz. (1 can)	6.8	240
Isocal	12 oz. (1 can)	12	375
DOYLE			
Compleat B	1 bottle (250 cc)	10	266
Meritene	8 oz.	14	240
Precision Isotonic	8 oz.	7.5	250
Citrotein	8 oz.	8	126
REGULAR			
Orange Drink	8 oz.		120
Lemonade	8 oz.		104
Ice Cream	1/2 cup	3	150
Sherbet	1/2 cup	.9	134
Custard	1/2 cup	8.8	205
Vanilla Pudding	1/2 cup	4.2	152
Tapioca	1/2 cup	6.5	174
TRAVENOL			
TPN-Regular	1 liter	28.94	850
Hypermetabolic	1 liter	44.69	850
Renal Failure	1 liter	17.8	1360
Peripheral	1 liter	28.9	170
Travasorb STD	1000 cc	30 g	1 KCal/cc
Travasorb HN	1000 cc	45 g	1 KCal/cc
Travasorb MCT	1000 cc	50 g	1 KCal/cc
	1000 cc	100 g	2 KCal/cc
CUTTER			
Intralipid	1.1 calories/ML:		
McGAW			
Amin-Aid	1000 cc	19.4 g	2 KCal/cc

Figure 24-2B. Back of standard "Calorie Count Form."

relative to the protein-calorie composition of the various supplemental, enteral, and parenteral formulas (Figure 24-2). The calorie count forms are distributed to the patient's room and 24-hour food intakes are recorded by the nursing department. This information, in terms of its calorie-protein composition, is then analyzed and recorded by the dietitian. It should be noted that an alert and interested patient can prove to be an invaluable asset in recording supplemental oral intake.

MECHANICS OF ASSESSMENT

During the initial implementation of nutritional assessment at the Western Pennsylvania Hospital, we encountered some basic logistic problems. Specifically, we found that heights and weights were not consistently recorded on the patient's chart at the time of admission. Frequently, the unit clerks and laboratory personnel became somewhat confused with respect to creatinine clearance and 24-hour urinary creatinine levels. Although 24-hour urinary creatinine levels were ordered as a routine part of the assessment, not infrequently we received values of creatinine clearance rather than urinary creatinine. With respect to the calorie count records, we encountered numerous inconsistencies in the recording of this important data. The Nursing Staff Development Office proved an invaluable form of assistance in providing the nursing department with frequent, informative memos and a vigorous in-service program. With time, these logistic and communications problems were resolved. The resolution of these problems led to the establishment of an effective nutritional assessment procedure which can be outlined as follows:

1. Upon the individual physician's written order for nutritional assessment, or upon the receipt of a nutritional support team consult, one dietitian will respond.

2. The dietitian reviews the chart and obtains available data such as height, weight, age, admitting diagnosis, and applicable laboratory values (e.g., serum albumin, transferrin levels).

3. The patient is interviewed and a dietary history is obtained. This dietary history includes information relating to the patient's usual weight, dietary habits, activity level, bowel habits, and any existing dietary problems.

4. The dietitian performs a *series* of anthropometric measurements and then *averages* the data to arrive at final values.

5. The information gathered is then recorded by the dietitian in the progress note, with a specific request for any additional laboratory tests that are needed to complete the assessment.

6. The nursing service is notified of the initiation of collection of a 24-hour urine specimen for urinary urea nitrogen and urinary creatinine. A 24-hour calorie count is scheduled to coincide with the time period during which the urine specimen is collected.

7. When all test results are obtained, the assessment form is completed and filed in the "Consultation Section" of the chart. Additional compiled results and subsequent recommendations are recorded in the progress notes.

While the literature indicates the importance of skin testing as part of the assessment of the visceral protein compartment, this modality has not been utilized in our institution on a routine basis. When skin testing is indicated, these procedures are generally performed by a physician and the results are recorded in the progress notes for utilization by the dietary department.

During the course of therapy, a reassessment is done on a regular basis. Reassessment of visceral protein is usually done once a week, whereas a complete reassessment is performed every other week in order to obtain information indicative of the need for therapeutic adjustments.

THE DIETITIAN AND HOME TPN

With the standardization and successful implementation of these procedures on a routine basis for in-house nutritional support, the dietary department may then turn its attention to the development of its role in the HNSP. In essence the dietary department has two potential roles in the HNSP:

1. To assist in the implementation of the "home schedule" on an in-patient basis prior to discharge.
2. To provide for follow-up nutritional assessments.

The following case study is provided to illustrate these functions.

"Mrs. T." is a 44-year-old female who presented at an outlying hospital with a 20-year history of Crohn's disease. At the time of her admission to the primary hospital, she presented with persistent abdominal pain, nausea, emesis, and an 18-pound weight loss over a 2-month period of time. Initial management at the primary hospital consisted of bowel rest, steroid administration, and intravenous fluid support. Over a 3-week period of time, the patient failed to display a resolution of her symptom complex and was subsequently transferred to the Western Pennsylvania Hospital. Upon arrival, a nutritional assessment was initiated (Figure 24-3). This data was indicative of a continuing catabolic

THE WESTERN PENNSYLVANIA HOSPITAL

Dietary Department

NUTRITIONAL ASSESSMENT

1-17-81

	PARAMETERS	Patient Values	> 90% Not Depleted	60-90% Mod. Depleted	< 60% Severely Depleted
MARASMUS	% I.B.W. = [Actual Weight / IBW x 100]	61 %		✓	
	Triceps Skinfold (TSF)	10 mm		✓	
	Mid Arm Circumference (MAC)	18 cm		✓	
	Mid Arm Muscle Circumference MAMC (cm) = MAC (cm) – (3.14 x TSF (cm))	14.9 cm		✓	
KWASHIORKOR	24 Hour Urinary Creatinine	480 mg			✓
	Creatinine Height Index [CHI = Actual Ucr / Ideal Ucr x 100]	52 %			✓
	Albumin	3.5 g/dl	✓		
	Lymphocyte Count [= % Lymphocyte's x WBC / 100]	4,900 mm³	✓		
	Transferrin [= (0.8 x TIBC) – 43]	~ mg/dl	~	~	~
	24 Hour Urinary Urea Nitrogen	14.45 g			

SKIN TESTS* (0.1 ml)

	Reactive >5mm	Unreactive <5mm
Mumps		
Candida		
Varidase		
Trichophytin		

(*Read induration at 24 and 48 hours)

Normal _____ (2 or more positive)
Relatively Anergic _____ (one positive)
Anergic _____ (none positive)

CALORIC EXPENDITURE: BASAL ENERGY EXPENDITURE (BEE) 1042 Kcal/day

Men = 66@ (13.7 x W) @ (5 x H) – (6.8 x A)
Women = 655@ (9.6 x W) @ (1.7 x H) – (4.7 x A)
W = Actual Weight in kg. H = Height in cm. A = Age in Years
Parenteral Anabolic = 1.75 x BEE → 1823 Kcal/day
Oral Anabolic = 1.5 x BEE Oral Maintenance = 1.2 x BEE

PROTEIN REQUIREMENT: 82.5 g/day = 1.2 – 1.5 x ~~actual~~ ideal weight (kg)
DAILY INTAKE: Calories 1378 Kcal/day Protein 106 g/day Nitrogen 17 g/day
NITROGEN BALANCE: ⊖ 1.45 g/day = Protein Intake / 6.25 – (Urinary Urea Nitrogen + 4)

USUAL WEIGHT: – 50.45 (kg)
IDEAL WEIGHT: – 55 (kg)
~~ADMISSION~~ Actual WEIGHT: – 34 (kg)
HEIGHT: – 157.5 (cm)
BSA (Body Surface Area) (m²) age: 44
DIAGNOSIS: – Crohn's disease

NUTRITIONAL STATUS:

- ☐ Normal
- ☐ Kwashiorkor (K) (Visceral Attrition) (Depressed: ALB, Transferrin and Anergy; Preserved: TSF, MAMC, CHI, MAC)
- ☑ Marasmus (M) (Depletion Parietal Muscle & Fat) (Depressed: TSF, MAL, MAMC, CHI; Preserved: ALB, Transferrin)
- ☐ Combination M-K (Advanced PCM) (All Parameters Depressed)

PROPOSED NUTRITIONAL THERAPY:

Figure 24-3. "Mrs. T's" Initial Assessment.

state clinically classified as a marasmus type of malnutrition.

A silicone elastomer catheter was percutaneously inserted into the right subclavian vein, and total parenteral nutrition was instituted, using a 50% dextrose and 8.5% amino acid solution with a standard electrolyte profile. The patient was maintained on a strict npo status and subsequent reassessments were performed over the ensuing weeks to assess the effect of therapy. During the third week of hospitalization, the patient's clinical status and a subsequent radiographic evaluation revealed the presence of an incomplete small bowel obstruction with stricture formation. The patient subsequently underwent abdominal exploration, subtotal small bowel resection, and anastomosis. Postoperatively, the patient was maintained on a vigorous parenteral nutritional support program, which was again monitored by nutritional assessments (Figure 24-4).

Because of the patient's underlying disease, the recent surgery, and the present inability to maintain adequate protein and caloric intake by mouth, the

THE WESTERN PENNSYLVANIA HOSPITAL

Dietary Department

NUTRITIONAL ASSESSMENT

2-17-81

	PARAMETERS	Patient Values	> 90% Not Depleted	60-90% Mod. Depleted	< 60% Severely Depleted
MARASMUS	% I.B.W. = [Actual Weight / IBW X 100]	85 %		✓	
	Triceps Skinfold (TSF)	15.5 mm	✓		
	Mid Arm Circumference (MAC)	22.4 cm		✓	
	Mid Arm Muscle Circumference MAMC (cm) = MAC (cm) – [3.14 x TSF (cm)]	17.4 cm		✓	
KWASHIORKOR	24 Hour Urinary Creatinine	530 mg			✓
	Creatinine Height Index [CHI = Actual Ucr / Ideal Ucr X 100]	57 %			✓
	Albumin	2.4 g/dl		✓	
	Lymphocyte Count [= % Lymphocyte's x WBC / 100]	252 mm³			✓
	Transferrin [= (0.8 x TIBC) – 43]	312 mg/dl	✓		
	24 Hour Urinary Urea Nitrogen	10.33 g			

SKIN TESTS* (0.1ml)

	Reactive >5mm	Unreactive <5mm
Mumps		
Candida		
Varidase		
Trichophytin		

(*Read induration at 24 and 48 hours)

Normal ______ (2 or more positive)
Relatively Anergic ______ (one positive)
Anergic ______ (none positive)

CALORIC EXPENDITURE: BASAL ENERGY EXPENDITURE (BEE) 1165 Kcal/day

Men = 66@ (13.7 x W) @ (5 x H) – (6.8 x A)
Women = 655@ (9.6 x W) @ (1.7 x H) – (4.7 x A)
W = Actual Weight in kg. H = Height in cm. A = Age in Years

Parenteral Anabolic = 1.75 x BEE → 2039 Kcal/day; Oral Anabolic = 1.5 x BEE; Oral Maintenance = 1.2 x BEE

PROTEIN REQUIREMENT: 82.5 g/day = 1.2 = 1.5 x ~~actual~~ ideal weight (kg)
DAILY INTAKE: Calories 2550 Kcal/day Protein 134.9 g/day Nitrogen 21.4 g/day
NITROGEN BALANCE: (+) 7.07 g/day = Protein Intake / 6.25 – (Urinary Urea Nitrogen + 4)

USUAL WEIGHT: – 50.45 (kg)
IDEAL WEIGHT: – 55 (kg)
~~ADMISSION~~ Actual WEIGHT: – 46.8 (kg)
HEIGHT: – 157.5 (cm)
BSA (Body Surface Area) (m²) age: 44
DIAGNOSIS: – Crohn's disease

NUTRITIONAL STATUS:

- ☐ Normal
- ☐ Kwashiorkor (K) (Visceral Attrition) (Depressed: ALB, Transferrin and Anergy; Preserved: TSF, MAMC, CHI, MAC)
- ☐ Marasmus (M) (Depletion Parietal Muscle & Fat) (Depressed: TSF, MAL, MAMC, CHI; Preserved: ALB, Transferrin)
- ☐ Combination M-K (Advanced PCM) (All Parameters Depressed)

PROPOSED NUTRITIONAL THERAPY:

Figure 24-4. "Mrs. T's" postoperative assessment.

patient was considered a candidate for home nutritional support. A social service evaluation was obtained, and numerous discussions between the team members and the patient's family were instituted. It was decided that the patient should be started on a 12-hour cycle of solution administration. The nutritional support team adjusted the patient's fluid administration to coincide with an evening cycle (8 P.M. to 8 A.M.). The patient was maintained on this cycle for a 2-week period, and a nutritional assessment was again performed to assure the maintenance of an anabolic state (Figure 24-5). After adequate in-

THE WESTERN PENNSYLVANIA HOSPITAL

Dietary Department

NUTRITIONAL ASSESSMENT

3-12-81

	PARAMETERS		PERCENT OF STANDARD		
		Patient Values	> 90% Not Depleted	60-90% Mod. Depleted	< 60% Severely Depleted
MARASMUS	% I.B.W. = [Actual Weight / IBW X 100]	86.7 %		✓	
	Triceps Skinfold (TSF)	14 mm		✓	
	Mid Arm Circumference (MAC)	23.1 cm		✓	
	Mid Arm Muscle Circumference MAMC (cm) = MAC (cm) – (3.14 x TSF (cm))	18.7 cm		✓	
KWASHIORKOR	24 Hour Urinary Creatinine	640 mg		✓	
	Creatinine Height Index [CHI = Actual Ucr / Ideal Ucr X 100]	70 %		✓	
	Albumin	3.1 g/dl		✓	
	Lymphocyte Count [= % Lymphocyte's x WBC / 100]	1104 mm^3		✓	
	Transferrin [= (0.8 x TIBC) – 43]	271 mg/dl	✓		
	24 Hour Urinary Urea Nitrogen	11.57 g			

SKIN TESTS* (0.1ml)

	Reactive >5mm	Unreactive <5mm
Mumps	______	______
Candida	______	______
Varidase	______	______
Trichophytin	______	______

(*Read induration at 24 and 48 hours)

Normal ______ (2 or more positive)
Relatively Anergic ______ (one positive)
Anergic ______ (none positive)

CALORIC EXPENDITURE: BASAL ENERGY EXPENDITURE (BEE) 1174 Kcal/day

Men = 66@ (13.7 x W) @ (5 x H) – (6.8 x A)
Women = 655@ (9.6 x W) @ (1.7 x H) – (4.7 x A)
W = Actual Weight in kg. H = Height in cm. A = Age in Years

(Parenteral Anabolic = 1.75 x BEE) → 2055 Kcal/day; Oral Anabolic = 1.5 x BEE; Oral Maintenance = 1.2 x BEE

PROTEIN REQUIREMENT: 82.5 g/day = 1.2 – 1.5 x ~~actual~~ ideal weight (kg)

DAILY INTAKE: Calories 3176 Kcal/day Protein 140 g/day Nitrogen 22.4 g/day

NITROGEN BALANCE: (+) 6.83 g/day = Protein Intake / 6.25 – (Urinary Urea Nitrogen + 4)

USUAL WEIGHT: – 50.45 (kg)
IDEAL WEIGHT: – 55 (kg)
~~ADMISSION~~ Actual WEIGHT: – 47.7 (kg)
HEIGHT: – 157.5 (cm)
age: 44
BSA (m^2) (Body Surface Area)
DIAGNOSIS: – Crohn's disease

NUTRITIONAL STATUS:

- ☐ Normal
- ☐ Kwashiorkor (K) (Visceral Attrition) — Depressed: ALB, Transferrin and Anergy; Preserved: TSF, MAMC, CHI, MAC)
- ☐ Marasmus (M) (Depletion Parietal Muscle & Fat) — Depressed: TSF, MAL, MAMC, CHI; Preserved: ALB, Transferrin)
- ☐ Combination M-K (Advanced PCM) — (All Parameters Depressed)

PROPOSED NUTRITIONAL THERAPY:

Figure 24-5. "Mrs. T's" pre-discharge assessment.

VALUES BASED ON 1000 CC

PRODUCT	KCAL per cc	CHO	PRO	FAT	NA (MG.)	K(MEQ.)	CA	P (MG.)	LACTOSE 9/1.	CAL to NIT. RATIO	MOSM KG
SUSTACAL	1	138	60	23	920	53	1000	920	0	104:1	625
ENSURE	1	145	37	37	740	32.56	530	530	0	178:1	450
ENSURE PLUS	1.5	200	55	53	1060	48.7	630	630	0	171:1	600
MERITENE	1	110	57.6	32	880	40.8	1200	1200	54.0	104:1	505
ISOCAL	1	130	34.2	44	530	34	630	530	0	192:1	300
TRAVASORB STD	1	190	30	13	900	30	500	500	0	230:1	450
TRAVASORB HN	1	175	45	13	900	30	500	500	0	155:1	450
TRAVASORB MCT	1	126	49	33	350	44	500	500	0	135:1	250
TRAVASORB MCT IN CONCENTRATED FORM	2	250	99	66	700	88	1000	1000	0	135:1	475

SUSTACAL PUDDING	5 ounce can - 240 KCal, 6.8 gms Pro, 32 gms Carb., 9.5 gms Fat, NA 100 mg (Choc) Van - 120 mg, P 290 mg, Lactose 9.7 mg/5 oz., K 290 mg, CA 220 mg
CITROTEIN:	1/4 cup powder in 6 ounces water - 7.67 gms Protein, 23.3 gms Carb., 33 gms Fat, 130 mg NA, 126 KCal
POLYCOSE:	1 tablespoon provides 32 KCal, 7.52 gms Carbohydrates, 9.76 mg NA, .64 mg. Potassium
AMIN-AID:	340 cc (1 packet + 250 cc water) provides 118 gm Carb., 22 gm Fat, .8 gm Total Nitrogen, 700 KCal (670 Non-Protein KCal), 6.35 gm Amino Acids, .25 gm Histidine, 2 mEg of NA, K, Ca & Mg.

Figure 24-6. Dietary formulary for oral and enteral support.

house training, the patient was discharged on this treatment program. The patient is being followed by the dietary department and the nutritional support service on a regular basis, and repeat nutritional assessments are obtained throughout the home course.

It is the dietary department's responsibility to continually assess the status of all patients on home nutritional support and to recommend appropriate changes in therapy as indicated. It is paramount that the patient maintain an anabolic state despite a change in activity level and environment.

ENTERAL MODALITIES

The use of oral supplements and standard enteral feedings (through the nasoduodenal route) on an outpatient basis is an additional responsibility of the dietary department. This necessitated that the dietary department develop an acceptable formulary of solutions based on composition and ease of utilization (Figure 24-6). Carbohydrates, which comprise the main source of calories in most formulas, may appear as glucose, sucrose, starches, dextrins, and glucose oligosaccharides. Amino acids may be provided as intact protein, protein isolates, hydrolyzed protein, short-chain peptides or purified free amino acids. Fat sources may be present in long-chain or medium-chain configurations. Medium-chain triglycerides have proved effective in the patient with compromised gastrointestinal absorption, because they are absorbed through the intestinal epithelium directly into the portal system as free fatty acids. Most of the commercial formulas contain vitamins or minerals equal to or in excess of the Recommended Dietary Allowances. Dietitians should have a practical knowledge of a formula's vitamin and mineral composition. Osmolality is an additional important feature to be considered. A product that is isosmolar with body fluids (300 mOsm/kg) is ideal, while formulas with a higher osmolality should be initially diluted and then gradually advanced in rate and concentration.

While osmolality is important in terms of patient tolerance, viscosity is a prime determinant of flow rates through various administration systems. These products encompass a wide range of viscosities, and not all solutions flow at sufficient rates through the newer, small-diameter, flexible silicone feeding tubes. In order to compensate for this, manufacturers advocate the administration of solutions in conjunction with pumps. Although this is acceptable for nasoduodenal tubes, it is not recommended if the tube has not passed beyond the pylorus. Despite the use of mercury-weighted tubes, not all tubes will pass through the pylorus, and thus, some solutions will have to be administered via the nasogastric route. These should not be administered by pumps but should rather flow by gravity. Our hospital formulary is designed to utilize solutions with a low enough viscosity to permit flow through the feeding tubes we have elected to utilize (Figure 24-6).

SUMMARY

Through involvement in both the venous and enteral modalities, the dietitian thus serves as an active member of the Nutritional Support Team. This involvement encompasses both inpatient and outpatient programs and ensures the utilization of a carefully planned treatment protocol. It also serves as a means of assessing the adequacy of therapy and patient tolerance.

BIBLIOGRAPHY

1. Krausi, M.V., and Mahan, L.K.: Food, Nutrition and Diet Therapy, 6th Ed. Philadelphia, W.B. Saunders, 1979.
2. Schneider, H.A., Anderson, C.E., and Caureen, D.B.: Nutritional Support of Medical Practice. New York, Harper and Row, 1977.
3. Wilmore, D.: The Metabolic Management of the Critically Ill. New York, Plenum Medical Bank Co., 1977.
4. Grant, A.: Nutritional Assessment Guidelines, 2nd Ed. Cutter Medical, 1979.
5. Bistrian, B.R.: Nutritional assessment and therapy of protein caloric malnutrition in the hospital. J. Am. Diet. Assoc., *71:*393, 1977.
6. Mullen, J., et al.: Implication of malnutrition in the surgical patient. Arch. Surg., *114:*121, 1979.
7. Blackburn, G.L., Maini, B.S., and Pierce, E.C.: Nutrition in the critically ill patient. Anesth., *47:*181, 1977.

8. Flatt, J.P., and Blackburn, G.L.: The metabolic fuel regulatory system: implication for protein-sparing therapy during caloric depreciation. Am. J. Clin Nutr., *27:*175, 1974.
9. Vazquez, R. M., and Kanunski, M. V.: A Manual of Nutritional and Metabolic Support. Cutter Labs, 1978.
10. Blackburn, G. L., et al.: Manual for Nutritional Assessment of the Hospitalized Patient. Nutritional Support Service, New England Deaconess Hosp., Harvard Medical School, Boston, Mass. 02215.
11. Blackburn, G.L., et al.: Nutritional and metabolic assessment of the hospitalized patient. JPEN, *1:*11, 1977.
12. Vanway, C.W., III, Meng, H.C., and Sandstead, H.H.: Nitrogen balance in postoperative patients receiving parenteral nutrition. Arch. Surg., *110:* 272, 1975.
13. Shils, M.E., Bloch, A.S., and Chernoff, R.: Liquid Formulas for Oral and Tube Feeding, 2nd Ed. New York, Memorial Sloan-Kettering Cancer Center, 1977.
14. Long, J.M., Wilmore, D.W., and Pruitt, B.A.: Comparison of carbohydrate and fat as caloric sources. Surg. Forum, *26:*108, 1975.
15. Blackburn, G.L., et al.: Nutrition and metabolic assessment of the hospitalized patient. JPEN, *1:*1, 1977.
16. Mackenzie, T., Blackburn, G. L., and Flatt, J.P.: Clinical assessment of nutritional status using nitrogen balance. Fed. Prog., *33:*683, 1974.
17. Clark, R.G., and Rowlands, B.J.: Nitrogen balance in parenteral nutrition. Arch. Surg., *110:* 1256, 1975.
18. Freeman, J.B., Egan, M.C., and Millis, B.J.: The Elemental Diet. Surg. Gynecol. Obstet., *142*(6): 925, 1976.
19. Shils, M.E.: Enteral nutrition by tube. Cancer Res., *37*(7):2432, 1977.

Chapter 25

Vascular Access, Catheter Care, and Nursing Implications

Frank Breggar, M.D.
Paul Kim, M.D.
Maureen DeCourcy, R.N.
Angela Cavalier, R.N.
Members of The Nutritional and Metabolic Support Committee of The Western Pennsylvania Hospital

Vascular access for outpatient nutritional support has historically been the "weak link" in this form of therapy. Until recently, there has not been a viable alternative to administration through surgically implanted venous catheters. Now, there is a simpler and apparently equally secure means of venous catheterization in this group of patients.

VASCULAR ACCESS

The administration of total parenteral nutritional support solutions necessitates cannulization of the central venous circulation. These solutions are hyperosmolar in nature, and therefore, require administration through a vessel with a high flow rate, so as to decrease the propensity for phlebitis and/or thrombus formation. Whereas these potential complications of infusion are primarily an effect of high osmolarity, their incidence is also directly affected by the choice of catheter material. Ideally, a catheter should be inert, supple, and possess surface characteristics that impede thrombus formation. Catheters composed of silicone elastomer do possess these characteristics. The utilization of other "plastic catheters" (e.g., polyvinyl chloride, polytetrafluoroethylene) should be avoided not only as routes of administration for nutritional support solutions, but also for elective central vein catheterization for any other reason. The use of silicone elastomer catheters provides for a lower incidence of both insertion and infusion complications. Clinically, this is reflected as increased catheter "stay times."

Classically, patients who receive venous nutritional support solutions for prolonged periods of time have undergone the surgical placement of Hickman Broviac catheters. These catheters consist of a silicone elastomer intravenous portion with a Teflon-reinforced proximal segment. The proximal end of the catheter has a standard Leurlock connector. A Dacron cuff is attached to the mid portion of the proximal catheter (subcutaneous), which is utilized to stimulate fibrous tissue formation. This type of catheter is outstanding for the administration of both long-term in-house and outpatient nutritional support solutions. However, it requires surgical placement and does not lend itself to catheter exchange should that procedure be required for any reason. Rather than these catheters, we have elected to use a modification of the Centrasil placement technique for all our in-house and home nutritional support patients. In addition, we are using the same catheter system to obtain long-term venous access in the oncology patient who is receiving multiple courses of chemotherapy. The catheter system consists of the catheter, a 16-gauge 4-inch connector tubing with Leurlock connectors, slide clamp, and latex injection port (Figure 25-1). This system is based on the experience at M.D. Anderson Hospital in which 1700 oncology patients have been maintained for long periods of time on an outpatient basis, using this type of catheter arrangement. We have simply adapted it for use in our HNSP. The technique of insertion varies from the standard one used in placing this particular catheter. Insertion may be performed in the patient's room or in a special room equipped for catheter insertion. The procedure need not be performed in the operating room. The insertion procedure is as follows:

1. With the bed or table in the Trendelenburg position, a rolled blanket is placed under the patient at the scapular level to facilitate posterior movement of the shoulder and head. The head is directed to the left.
2. The skin is defatted with 10% acetone solution.
3. The physician performing the insertion puts on sterile gloves.
4. The skin is prepped with Betadine solution (× 3).
5. The area is draped with sterile towels.
6. The skin is infiltrated, using 1% lidocaine (without epinephrine), to achieve local anesthesia. In the case of the infraclavicular approach to the subclavian vein, the skin at the site of the junction of the medial third and lateral third of the clavicle is the point of insertion. It is important to note that central venous catheterization should always be performed on the right, when possible, in order to avoid injuries to the thoracic duct.
7. The subclavian vein is localized using a 3 ml syringe and a 22-gauge, 1½-inch needle. The needle is inserted at a 30-degree angle from the chest wall at approximately the junction between the medial and lateral third of the clavicle. "Hugging" the inferior aspect of the clavicle and aiming for

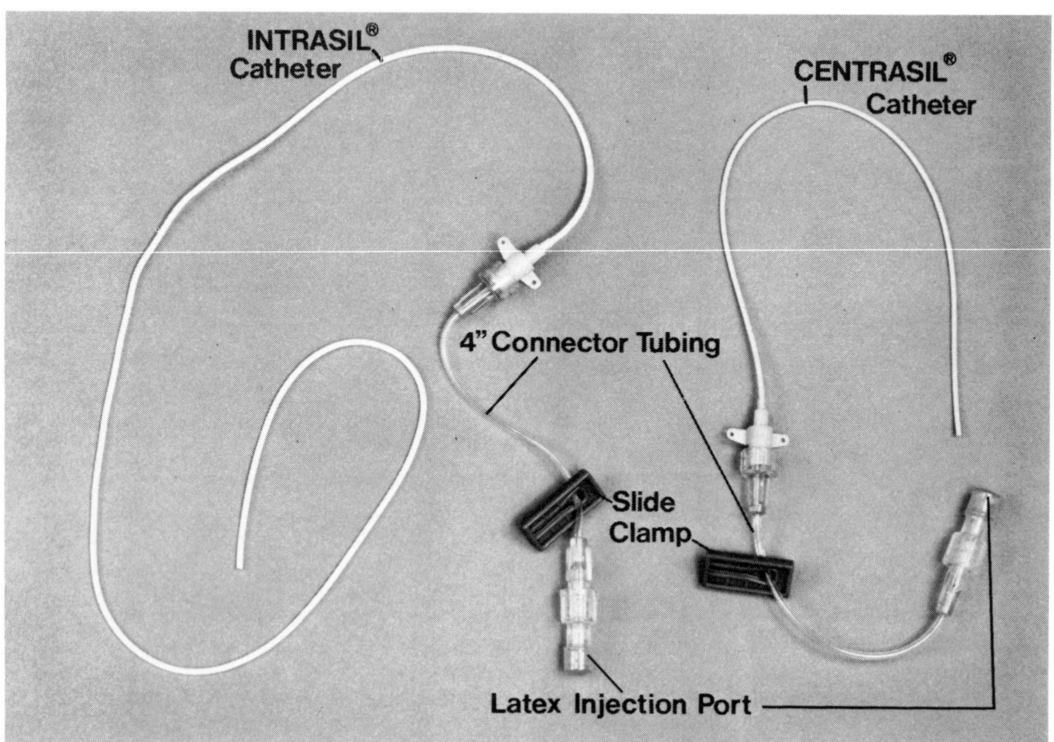

Figure 25-1. The catheter system.

the sternal notch, the needle is slowly advanced, occasionally aspirating, until venous blood is obtained.

8. After localization, the needle is removed and the Centrasil Teflon catheter introducer with its needle are inserted along the same tract. When the blood return is obtained, the Teflon sheath is advanced and the needle is removed. At this point, the procedure for insertion differs from that typical for the Centrasil catheter.

9. An .025 cardiovascular J-wire is inserted through the introducer, after having instructed the patient to perform the Valsalva maneuver. This wire is 145 cm in length. In actual practice, one does not need a J-wire of such length, but that is the only size of this wire commercially available. Arrangements are being made with a particular company to secure a similar gauge J-wire in a shorter length. Only about 25 cm of the J-wire is introduced through the Teflon sheath.

10. The Teflon sheath is then withdrawn over the J-wire.

11. The silicone elastomer catheter, which has been pretrimmed to compensate for the added length that would have been required had the introducer system been completely utilized, is then threaded over the J-wire to the site of insertion.

12. The silicone catheter and the J-wire are "squeezed together" and advanced together as a total unit.

13. When the silicone catheter has been advanced all the way to its hub, the patient is asked to perform the Valsalva maneuver and the J-wire is removed from the catheter.

14. A syringe is attached to the hub to check for adequate blood return.

15. The Centrasil catheter hub is then secured to the skin. The suturing technique involves one suture placed around the reinforced point where the silicone elastomer is attached to the hub. "Stay" sutures are placed through the eye holes on the catheter wings. It is important that these sutures be placed in a cephalad fashion in order to decrease piston motion (Figure 25-2). Prolene is the suture material of choice because it leads to less skin reaction.

16. The preflushed IV tubing with its 4-inch connector tubing is then attached to the catheter hub. The IV bag is lowered below the level of the bed in order to again demonstrate adequate blood return.

17. The insertion site is dressed according to the dressing protocol (see section on nursing implications).

18. The chest is auscultated, and an x-ray is obtained for documentation of placement.

The silicone elastomer has a strong affinity for particulate matter, the adherence of which to the catheter might well increase the incidence of phlebitis. Therefore, it is important to wear well-rinsed sterile gloves. The catheter itself is supplied from the manufacturer with a pair of powderless gloves. Even when using these gloves, we advocate that they be rinsed with sterile saline in order to assure low particulate matter.

In some patients, particularly those with oncotic problems and subsequent thrombocytopenia, percutaneous catheterization of the subclavian vein may be deemed too hazardous. In this group of patients, long-term central venous catheterization can be obtained by a basilic vein approach. Again, a silicone elastomer catheter is utilized and may be placed either percutaneously or by a cut-down approach. The catheter itself is a 55.9 cm 16-gauge silicone elastomer catheter (Figure 25-1). It is supplied in a drum cartridge with an attached slotted needle (Intrasil). In those patients where percutaneous access to the basilic or cephalic systems has not been destroyed by previous procedures or by chemotherapy, this drum catheter may be utilized. Unfortunately, in most oncology patients, the superficial basilic or cephalic systems have already been thrombosed secondary to previous catheterization and the administration of chemotherapeutic agents. In this group of patients, we have utilized a cut-down approach to the basilic vein, with the site of exposure being approximately 5 cm above

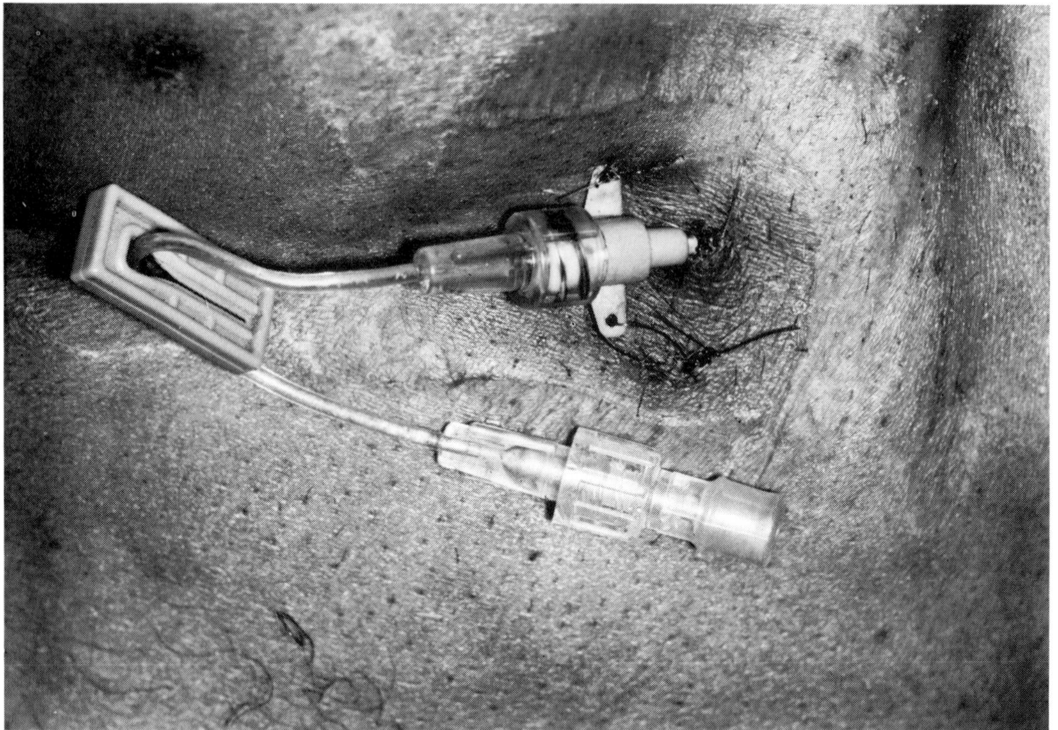

Figure 25-2. Suture technique.

the elbow. Specifically, the cut-down site is along the medial aspect of the upper arm just over the palpable pulse. The basilic vein arises from the ulnar surface of the hand and progresses to occupy an anteromedial position at the antecubital fossa. The vein then leaves its subcutaneous position at the junction of the middle and lower third of the upper arm and penetrates the deep fascia. Shortly after perforating the deep fascia, it joins the venae comitantes at the lower border of the teres major to form the axillary vein. It must be remembered that the median nerve and the brachial artery are in close proximity to the basilic vein. When the basilic vein has been identified, the catheter is delivered to the venotomy site by a separate stab wound. It should be noted that this catheter is too long for most patients, and therefore, should be pretrimmed prior to insertion. Again, the propensity for phlebitis can be limited by the use of prewashed sterile gloves. Following the insertion, a chest x-ray must again be obtained in order to document proper positioning. This insertion site is dressed in exactly the same manner as the subclavian site. The techniques of catheter care are presented later in this section.

The use of both these catheter systems also has the advantage of affording the opportunity to perform a catheter exchange (over a .025-gauge J-wire) without the need for a second needle cannulization of the vessel. The catheter system is simple in its composition and appears to offer the same increased stay time and decreased venous complications that are afforded by the more elaborate catheter systems. In addition, this simple system does not require surgical placement, thus eliminating the expensive utilization of operating time and personnel.

NURSING IMPLICATIONS AND CATHETER CARE

A coordinated HNSP provides complete and comprehensive care for the patient in need of long-term therapy. The nutritional/metabolic support nurse (NMSN) is an integral part of this team approach. With the advent of our HNSP, and in view of our rapidly expanding in-house program, it became quickly evident that a registered nurse who possessed a thorough knowledge of this modality would need to be available on a 24-hour basis. In our institution, this individual is an active part of the nutritional support team and provides continuity of care and coordination between the numerous involved departments. In addition, this team specialist works closely with the patient and the family members in order to facilitate the transition from in-house to home therapy.

In developing a job description for this specialist, it is necessary to outline primary responsibilities. These responsibilities may be summarized as follows:

1. Coordinate the in-house nutritional support program.
2. Assist in the placement of all nutritional support lines and enteral feeding tubes.
3. Reduce the incidence of associated catheter complications by providing for the maintenance of the catheter dressing.
4. Initiate and direct patient and family training.
5. Provide the coordination and follow-up of the outpatient program through the establishment of an outpatient clinic for the care of central lines and subsequent nutritional assessments.

Historically, the role of a nutritional and metabolic support nurse was based on the high incidence of catheter related complications that occurred when numerous individuals within an institution were caring for intravenous catheters. During the past 10 years, numerous articles have appeared in the literature that illustrate a decrease in associated catheter complications when one individual is charged with the responsibility of caring for the catheter and the catheter dressing. In addition, the use of one individual to conduct training programs for the care of outpatient venous lines provides continual reassurance and stability for the patient and the patient's family. Identification with one particular individual eliminates many of the stresses and fears that may accompany the patient who is discharged from the institution with a permanent indwelling line.

When a patient becomes a candidate for in-house nutritional support and a subsequent candidate for home nutritional support, the first member of the team he is exposed to is the NMSN. This individual conducts an initial interview with the patient and the patient's family in order to assess their ability to deal with this therapy on an outpatient basis. Social service is also involved in this evaluation, and the recommendations of both individuals are important parts of the ultimate decision as to whether therapy should be continued on an outpatient basis.

Once the decision has been made to initiate the in-house and subsequent home nutritional support therapy, the nutritional support nurse then coordinates the nutritional assessment performed by the dietary department. In addition, the techniques of catheter placement and subsequent care are briefly explained to the patient, and the patient is given an information pamphlet which will answer many of the common questions they may have pertaining to this modality. Twenty-four hours later, the catheter is actually inserted, with the physician performing the insertion assisted by the NMSN. Following the insertion of the catheter, this individual then becomes solely responsible for the care of the catheter site and the dressing. In order to facilitate this procedure and provide continuity on an outpatient basis, we have elected to develop our own catheter care dressing kit. This dressing kit (assembled by the Clinipad Corporation) is used by the nutritional support nurse for in-house dressing changes and is then used by the family for outpatient dressing changes. The contents of this kit are as follows:

1. Two pairs of sterile gloves.
2. One alcohol-impregnated swab.
3. Two Betadine-solution-impregnated swabs.

4. One tincture-of-benzoin-impregnated swab.
5. One packet of Betadine ointment.
6. One 2 × 2 inch all-gauze two-ply sponge.

All of these components are packaged in a sterile "tub" and wrapper. In addition to this kit, we also use a special outer dressing. This dressing consists of Op-Site (Acme) which is in essence a semipermeable material that provides an occlusive dressing. Its particular characteristics allow the patient to shower with the material in place, and to go from 4 days to 1 week without the need for an additional dressing change (Figure 25-3). We use two different sizes of Op-Site, depending on the site of catheter insertion. If a percutaneous infraclavicular approach to the subclavian vein is utilized, we use a small 6 × 8.5 cm piece to facilitate coverage. On the other hand, if the antecubital fossa is utilized as the site of insertion, a larger 10 × 14 cm piece of Op-Site is utilized.

The technique of dressing change is as follows:

1. The dressing kit is opened and the first pair of sterile gloves is applied prior to the initiation of the dressing change. The old dressing is then removed and discarded along with the first pair of gloves.

2. The second pair of gloves is then put on. (This second pair of gloves is prewashed because of the affinity of silicone for particulate matter and the attendant increased incidence of phlebitis.) Each individual swab packet is then opened and handed to the patient without touching the patient's ungloved hand. The 2 × 2 inch sponge is prepared by placing a small amount of Betadine ointment in the center of the gauze.

Note: At this point we establish a "clean hand" and a "dirty hand" concept. We made the dominant hand the "clean hand." We have found this method enables the family members and patient to complete the dressing without difficulty while implementing aseptic technique. Each swab is then individually removed from the packet being held in the patient's hand. The "clean hand" is used to aseptically remove the swab from the packet the patient is holding.

3. Using a circular motion, the catheter

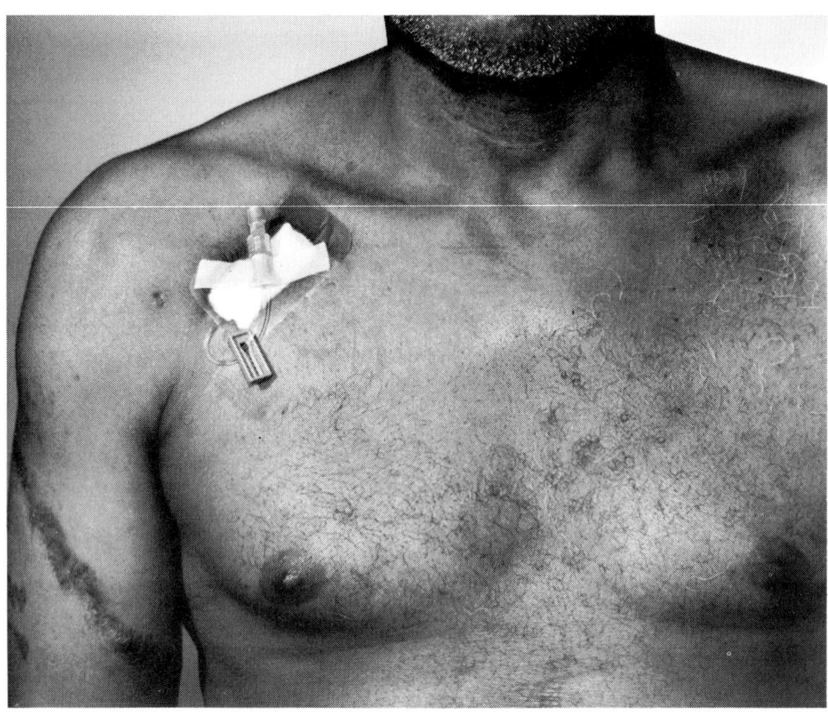

Figure 25-3. The completed dressing.

insertion site and surrounding skin are then cleaned with the alcohol-impregnated swab. The cleaning procedure is started at the point of catheter insertion and worked outward in a circular fashion.

Note: Many family members are hesitant to apply a firm steady circular motion. Fear of hurting a loved one is uppermost in their mind. Reassurance from the nurse must be given frequently at this time.

4. This procedure is repeated using the Betadine-impregnated swabs.
5. The benzoin-impregnated swab is then used to protect the surface of the skin and to enhance adhesiveness.
6. The 2 × 2 inch gauze with its applied Betadine ointment is placed over the catheter insertion site.
7. The gloves are removed.
8. The Op-Site dressing is applied to the area.

Note: Several practice sessions are usually required prior to allowing a family member to apply the Op-Site dressing to the catheter insertion site.

Patient positioning during the dressing change is an important consideration. With the insertion site in the subclavian area, the patient should be in the supine position, with his head rotated away from the site of insertion. This technique of changing dressings is reviewed numerous times with the designated member of the patient's family. In general, the patient's family is able to master these techniques within 5 days. The greatest difficulty encountered is generally centered around the process of gloving. Over-sized gloves are used to make this task simpler. In those cases where the patient is doing the dressing change alone, the training program uses a mirror technique, which affords the patient the opportunity to learn and perform the dressing changes without assistance.

The physical layout of the patient's home environment is an extremely important consideration in determining the best location for completing the dressing change procedure. Patients and family members are reminded to select a place without distractions such as televisions or telephones. The dressing change is not time-consuming, but it does require some degree of concentration. A schedule is generally devised for providing bi-weekly or weekly dressing changes. It is emphasized, for the sake of continuity, that these procedures should be performed on the same day, during the same period. The home care nurse can be an important adjunct to this therapy. Specifically, a home care nurse can provide additional information as to the physical layout of the patient's home, and also can be utilized to supervise family members on an outpatient basis.

A record sheet is given to the patient. The patient and the designated family member are instructed that this sheet is to be filled out at the time of each dressing change. Details such as temperature, skin condition, and stability of suture materials are recorded in the appropriate columns (Figure 25-4). This record is brought to the outpatient clinic and reviewed on each visit.

The components of the catheter system (4-inch connector tubing, heparin injection port) become the direct responsibility not only of the patient but also the NMSN. The 4-inch connector tubing is changed on a monthly basis when the patient returns to the outpatient catheter care clinic. The heparin injection port is changed every 2 weeks and can be done by the designated family member. It is important to emphasize that the blue slide clamp should be utilized to prevent air embolus during this procedure. Because the blue slide may show through clothing, some patients have requested a change in color. The manufacturer is currently planning to produce the clamp in a clear plastic.

After the patient and the designated family member have become familiar with the principles of catheter care and dressing changes, they are instructed in the technique of catheter heparinization. Maintenance of the central line is dependent on daily heparinization. A routine daily time is selected for the instillation of heparin on an outpatient basis. The family members are instructed to adhere to this procedure on a

NAME: ______ W.P.H.#: ______

TYPE CATHETER: CENTRASIL INSERTION DATE: 10/8/80 DR.: ______

Date/Time	Heparin Injection	CAP Change	Dressing Change	Temperature	Comments
1/16/81	+	−	+	97.8	INSERTION SITE LOOKS GOOD
1/17/81	+	−	−	97.2	
1/18/81	+	−	−	97.6	
1/19/81	+	−	−	97.6	
1/20/81	+	+	+	97.2	SITE LOOKS GOOD
1/21/81	+	−	−	97.4	
1/22/81	+	−	−	97.2	
1/23/81	+	−	−	97.4	
1/24/81	+	−	+	97.6	ONE SUTURE MISSING - REPLACED BY PHYSICIAN
1/25/81	+	−	−	97.6	
1/26/81	+	−	−	97.4	
1/27/81	+	−	−	97.6	
1/28/81	+	−	+	97.6	INSERTION SITE LOOKS GOOD SUTURES SECURE
1/29/81	+	−	−	97.4	

Figure 25-4. Dressing Change Record Sheet

daily basis following discharge. The necessary components for daily heparinization are as follows:

1. Tubex syringe
2. Wyeth Heparin cartridge containing 10 units of heparin per ml (1 ml cartridge)
3. Destruc-Clip
4. Alcohol wipe

A step-by-step demonstration of the use of these components is performed several times with the designated family member. It is emphasized that the injection of heparin should not be performed on a "power push" basis, because of the propensity for catheter rupture. Family members are also instructed that the inability to smoothly instill the heparin is an indication of possible catheter thrombus formation. The NMSN should be notified of this immediately. The patient and designated family member also undergo training relative to pump care and urine reductions.

All of these techniques are presented in the educational format, utilizing a standard slide presentation. This slide presentation can be done in either the patient's room or in the office of the NMSN. The use of this slide presentation and frequent, repetitious training sessions usually leads to family competence with respect to line-care within 5 days. The family and the patient are continually assured that the nurse or a representative member of the Nutritional Support Team will be available to them on a 24-hour basis should any problems arise. It is important to be sure that the paging system within your hospital is coordinated to this effort so as to facilitate communication during "off hours."

BIBLIOGRAPHY

1. Baker, D.I.: Hyperalimentation at home. Am. J. Nurs., *74*(10):1862, 1974
2. Broviac, J.W., and Scribner, B.H.: Prolonged parenteral nutrition in the home. Surg. Gynecol. Obstet., *139:*24, 1974.
3. Broviac, J.W., Cole, J.J., and Scribner, B.H.: A silicone rubber atrial catheter for prolonged parenteral alimentation. Surg. Gynecol. Obstet., *136:* 602, 1973.
4. Hoshal, V.L., Jr.: Total intravenous nutrition with peripherally inserted silicone elastomer central venous catheters. Arch. Surg., *110:*644, 1975.
5. Ivey, M., et al.: Long-term parenteral nutrition in the home. Am. J. Hosp. Pharm., *32:*1032, 1975.
6. Ryan, J.A., Jr., et al.: Catheter complication in total parenteral nutrition. A prospective study of 200 consecutive patients. N. Engl. J. Med., *290:* 757, 1974.
7. Riella, M.C., and Scribner, B.H.: Five years' experience with a right atrial catheter for prolonged parenteral nutrition at home. Surg. Gynecol. Obstet., *143:*205, 1976.
8. Heimbach, D.M., and Ivey, T.D.: Technique for placement of a permanent home hyperalimentation catheter. Surg. Gynecol. Obstet., *143:*634, 1976.
9. Macdonald, A.S., Master, S.K.P., and Moffitt, E.A.: A comparative study of peripherally inserted silicone catheters for parenteral nutrition. Can. Anaesth. Soc. J., *24*(2):263, 1977.
10. Amos, A.: Parenteral nutrition-2: The nurse's role. Nurs. Times, *72*(30):1153, 1976.
11. Mullen, J.L., Oleaga, J., and Ring, E.J.: Catheter migration during home hyperalimentation. JAMA, *238*(18):1946, 1977.
12. Blackett, R.L., et al.: A prospective study of subclavian vein catheters used exclusively for the purpose of intravenous feeding. Brit. J. Surg., *65*(6): 393, 1978.
13. Steward, R.D., and Sanislow, C.A.: Silastic intravenous catheter. N. Engl. J. Med., *265:*1283, 1967.
14. Baker, D.I.: Hyperalimentation at home. Am. J. Nurs., *74*(10):1826, 1974.
15. Bordos, D.C., and Camero, J.L.: Successful long-term intravenous hyperalimentation in the hospital and at home. Arch. Surg., *110:*439, 1975.
16. Calley, R.R., and Phillips, K.: Helping with hyperalimentation. Nursing 76, *3:*6, 1973.
17. Calley, R.R., and Wilson, J.: Meeting patient's nutritional needs with hyperalimentation. Nursing 79, May-Sept., 1979.
18. Goldfarb, I.W., Slater, H., and Cavalier, A.: Infusion therapy catheter—A Patient Handbook. Western Pennsylvania Hospital, Pittsburgh, PA.
19. Goldfarb, I.W., and Yates, A.P.: Total Parenteral Nutrition—Concepts and Methods. Synapse Publications, Pittsburgh, PA; 1978.
20. Lawson, M., Bottino, J.C., and McCredie, K.B.: Long-term intravenous therapy—A new approach. Am. J. Nurs., *79:*1100, 1979.

Chapter 26

The Role of the Social Service and Home Care Departments

Ethel Gandy, R.N.
Joyce Grater, G.S.W.
Members of The Nutritional and Metabolic Support Committee of The Western Pennsylvania Hospital

A structured Home Nutritional Support Program (HNSP) enables the patient to continue necessary therapy in the comfort of his own home as opposed to an extended hospital stay. It also serves to diminish the frequency of the repeated, psychologically stressful admissions that are so common for these patients. The transition from in-house therapy to home therapy carries with it specific sociomedical implications for both the patient and his extended family. It is generally acknowledged that an illness in one family member causes stressful repercussions in the whole family unit. The family suffers the illness from its own emotional perspective. Hopefully, early social service intervention for assessment and prenutritional-support counseling helps to reduce the stresses to a more manageable level for the patient and the family. The patient and family are certain to have many questions and fears that go far beyond the scope of medicine (e.g., the effect upon sexual activity, peer group perception). Especially in the case of oncology patients, home nutritional support may produce particularly fearful fantasies (e.g., increased dependence, further deterioration of self-image).

Family relationships may be subject to significant changes when the patient is discharged on an HNSP. It is helpful to consider in what stage of the life cycle the family exists. Are there very young or adolescent children at home? How will relationships change with them? By seeing the family as a unit prior to the initiation of home nutritional support, the social worker can evaluate the family strengths and weaknesses and determine the need for, and eventual direction of subsequent counseling.

Because of the cost of this therapeutic modality, one of the family's major concerns may be that of employment and future compensation. If the patient provided a needed source of income to the family and is now no longer able to provide this, the family may suffer additional economic stress. Moreover, the inability to return to work may carry with it decreased or even discontinued work benefits, including hospital insurance coverage. Some patients may be covered by their insurance only as an inpatient, but not have any, or at best, limited coverage for home care services.

Another important consideration that could be problematic in terms of home care follow-up and specific pharmacy delivery systems is that of the patient's geographic residence. Patients at the Western Pennsylvania Hospital are representative of the Tri-State area (Ohio, West Virginia, and Pennsylvania) with home care coverage limited to a small region within the hospital's surrounding county. Although most counties do have either visiting nurse agencies or available public health nursing services, many of these agencies will not feel comfortable following patients on an HNSP. Also, the patient and his family may feel some anxiety at being so far away from the "parent hospital." The 24-hour availability (through a beeper system) of the nutritional/metabolic support nurse can serve to alleviate some of these concerns.

The social worker also plays an important role in helping these patients articulate concerns and questions relative to their therapy. The patient and the patient's family may be so overwhelmed by the concept of home nutritional support in addition to the underlying medical condition, that they may encounter problems in formulating questions and concerns. The instructing nurse and the social worker should work together to make certain that the patient and family are adequately informed about the hospital's program. In addition, continuity in dealing with the same social worker and nutritional support nurse builds a degree of rapport and camaraderie that helps to alleviate some of the difficulties in communication.

It is also important to realize that these patients may need to develop a new sense of personal well-being. The patient, particularly, may have to adjust to diminished gratification and satisfaction in many areas of life. Affected areas may include participation in family activities, sexual relationships, and diminished work roles. Both patient and family must learn to cope with a new reality. It is at this time that the patient and family need maximum support, because it is a time of tremendous change.

Although the medical, surgical, and nursing components are certainly the core of the Western Pennsylvania Hospital's HNSP, there are still the far-reaching emotional complications inherent in home nutritional support that must be treated along with the underlying medical condition. Patients and their families must be psychologically prepared and educated in a sensitive manner to the stresses they will encounter if home nutritional support is to be a truly comprehensive program that meets both physical and emotional needs.

Following discharge, the emotional support initiated in the hospital must be continued. This continuity may be provided by the home care program run by the hospital's home care department. Follow-up visits maximize continuity of care and help to provide the support that the patient and family require during the transitional phase from hospital to home. The home care department provides coordinated planning, evaluation, and follow-up care to patients who are essentially home bound and are in need of intermittent skilled services. These services are provided under the medical supervision of the physician/director of the nutritional support team. It is essential that the home care nurses be familiar not only with the common problems encountered with solution administration and day-to-day catheter care. This information is best obtained through the use of an in-service program run by the nutritional/metabolic support nurse and the program social worker. We feel that it is important for the home care nurse to be available during initiation and completion of the in-house nutritional support program. This not only serves to familiarize the patient and the patient's family with this individual, but also serves to further familiarize the home care nurse with this treatment modality. Once the patient has been discharged, the home care nurse may function as an extension of the nutritional support team. In this sense, the nurse provides a "safeguard" by being available to routinely review the patient's progress at home and to inspect not only the maintenance of hardware equipment but also the central venous line.

SUMMARY

The social service department and home care department provide necessary pre-discharge nutritional support planning and follow-up care once this therapy has been instituted. Respresentatives of both departments should become involved in the patient's treatment program as soon as possible. In reality, they provide necessary information as to the feasibility of continuing this therapy on an outpatient basis. In addition, their follow-up evaluation provides useful information which may dictate necessary changes in the treatment program.

BIBLIOGRAPHY

1. The family as our patient. Journal of Family Practice, *1*(1):70, 1974.
2. Family tasks and reactions in the crisis of death. Social Casework, *July:*398, 1973.
3. Intervention at times of transition: Sources and forms of help. Journal of Contemporary Social Work, *May:*259, 1980.
4. Pre-dialysis counseling. Perspectives, *2:*(2):24, 1978.
5. Role of the family in rehabilitation. Social Casework, *November:*544, 1972.
6. The family interview: Helping patient and family cope with metastatic disease. Geriatrics, *29:*83, 1974.

Chapter 27

Pharmaceutic Logistics

Monica Obsheatz, R.Pharm.
James Sandala, R.Pharm.
Members of The Nutritional and Metabolic Support Committee of The Western Pennsylvania Hospital

The pharmacy plays an integral role in the successful implementation of an HNSP. This program at the Western Pennsylvania Hospital was the direct outgrowth of a comprehensive in-house parenteral nutritional program that had been in operation for the preceding 5 years. *It must be emphasized that it is not feasible to develop an outpatient program without first successfully implementing an in-house nutritional support program.* In order to better understand our home care admixture protocol, it is first necessary to explain the mechanics of our in-hospital nutritional support program. This is of importance because all patients who are candidates for home nutritional support are at some point in their therapy receiving nutritional support on an inpatient basis. A rigorous pharmacy protocol facilitates a smooth transition from hospital to home therapy.

PHARMACY FLOOR PLAN

The size and physical layout of any sterile admixture room is dependent on the space and area available to the pharmaceutic department. Ideally, the physical layout should be arranged in such a fashion as to provide for the orderly process of transforming the physician's written order into the delivery of the actual solution. The floor plan from our institution is presented in Figure 27-1 and is offered as an illustrative example of the layout of a sterile admixture room. It is important that the mix room be as far as possible from the areas of high traffic flow and as separate as possible from the other routine pharmaceutic activities. Obviously, the room must be kept as clean as possible and void of all contaminated supplies and refuse. Individuals working within the room should be restricted not only from food and beverage consumption but also from smoking. Adequate lighting, both overhead and at the level of the work counter, is essential to competent mixing. Traffic into and out of the room must be kept to a bare minimum. In order to accomplish this, all supplies should be stocked before the compounding procedures are begun each day and after they are finished. This insures a low level of particulate airborne matter from contaminating the room during compounding. Similarly, all paper work should be done prior to the initiation of the mixing processs and should be kept as far away as possible from the actual compounding area. Facilities for hand washing, gloving, and gowning should be available within or nearby the work area.

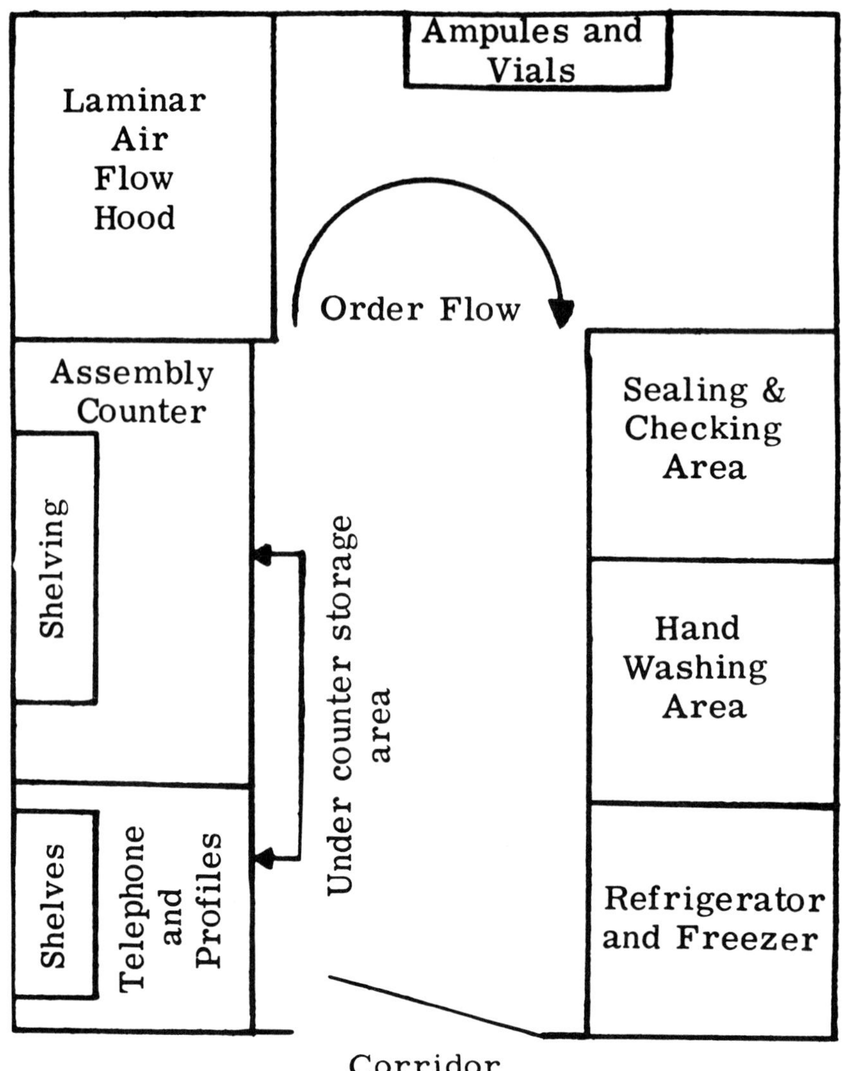

Figure 27-1. Floor plan of pharmacy nutritional support workroom.

EQUIPMENT REQUIREMENTS

After having designed the floor plan for the sterile admixture room, the next step is to obtain the equipment necessary for the compounding procedures. The following is a suggested list of some of the basic equipment that is required.

1. Laminar air flow hood (horizontal)
2. Adequate counter space
3. Refrigerator-freezer
4. Adequate storage shelving
5. Adequate ceiling and counter lighting
6. Sink and wash area
7. Compatibility reference material
8. Delivery cart
9. Waste containers
10. Filing cabinets
11. Telephone
12. Typewriter

Additional supplies that are required and must be stored in the sterile admixture room itself include the following:

1. Various constituents of the venous solutions
   a. Amino acid solutions (3.5%, 5.5%, 8.5%)

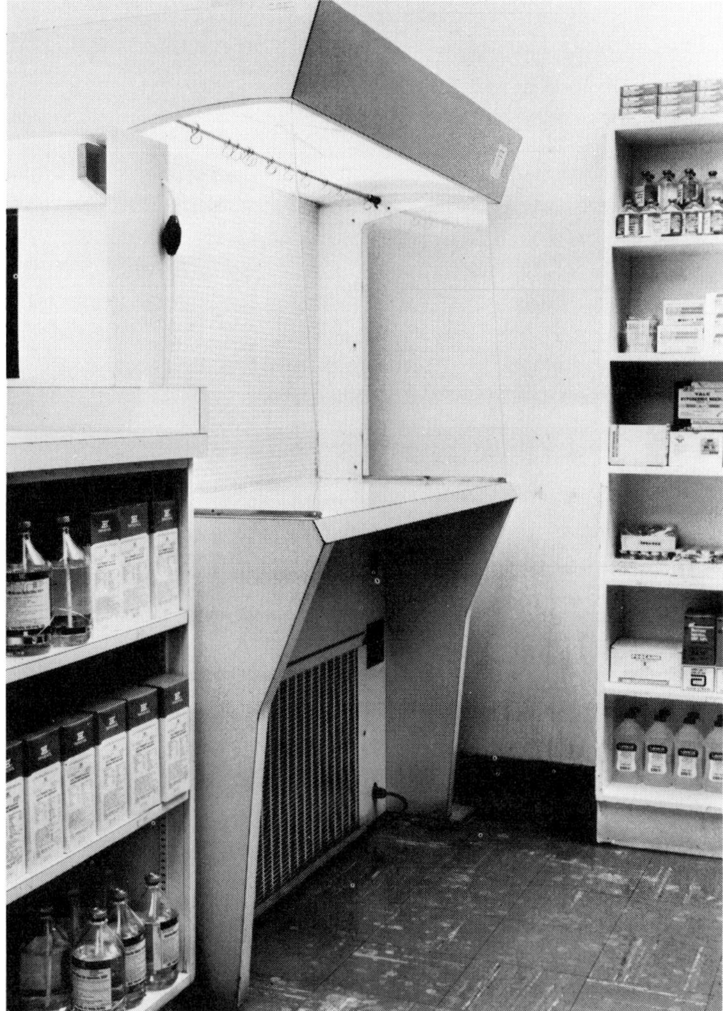

Figure 27-2. The laminar flow hood and supplies.

   b. Dextrose solutions (5%, 10%, 20%, 30%, 50%, 70%)
   c. Sterile water
   d. Vacuum containers, Viaflex bags, and various transfer sets
2. Electrolyte additives
3. Vitamin additives
4. Heparin
5. Gloves, masks, gowns
6. Needles and syringes of various standard sizes, including 5 micron filter needle and 0.22 micron filter unit
7. 70% isopropyl alcohol and other bactericidal cleaning agents (Betadine, Hibiclens)
8. Hand washing material (Betadine scrub)
9. Labels, order forms, patient profiles
10. Alcohol swabs and towels

These supplies will obviously vary with each institution's specific needs and habits and are presented merely as a sample of recommended equipment.

MONITORING SAFEGUARDS

Having established a floor plan and stocked the sterile admixture room with the basic requirements, it will be necessary throughout the course of the utilization of these facilities to periodically monitor the effectiveness of the system safeguards. The laminar flow hood is probably the most important piece of equipment (Figure 27-2). It must be kept in peak working order at all times. Checks on the HEPA (high efficiency particulate air) filter and air flow pattern should be conducted on a regular basis by a reputable servicing agent (at least every 6 months). The prefilters should also be changed routinely (approximately every 1 to 2 months) to maintain proper air flow and insure the efficiency of the HEPA filter. In addition, it is recommended that random samples of mixed TPN solutions be checked intermittently to provide solid evidence of the maintenance of sound aseptic technique. The specific methods of doing this can be set up by the hospital's infection control committee. A random sampling is done on approximately 10% of the TPN solutions compounded, utilizing the millipore Addi-chek quality control system and the hospital bacteriology laboratory. By utilizing two systems, we can screen most types of microbial contamination. With the first thoughts of sending a patient home on solutions, we realized the importance of microbial screening procedures on solutions that were stored for 3, 7, and 30 days under refrigeration. Thus far, none of the samples have shown microbial growth. However, we do limit our supply to a 4-day period.

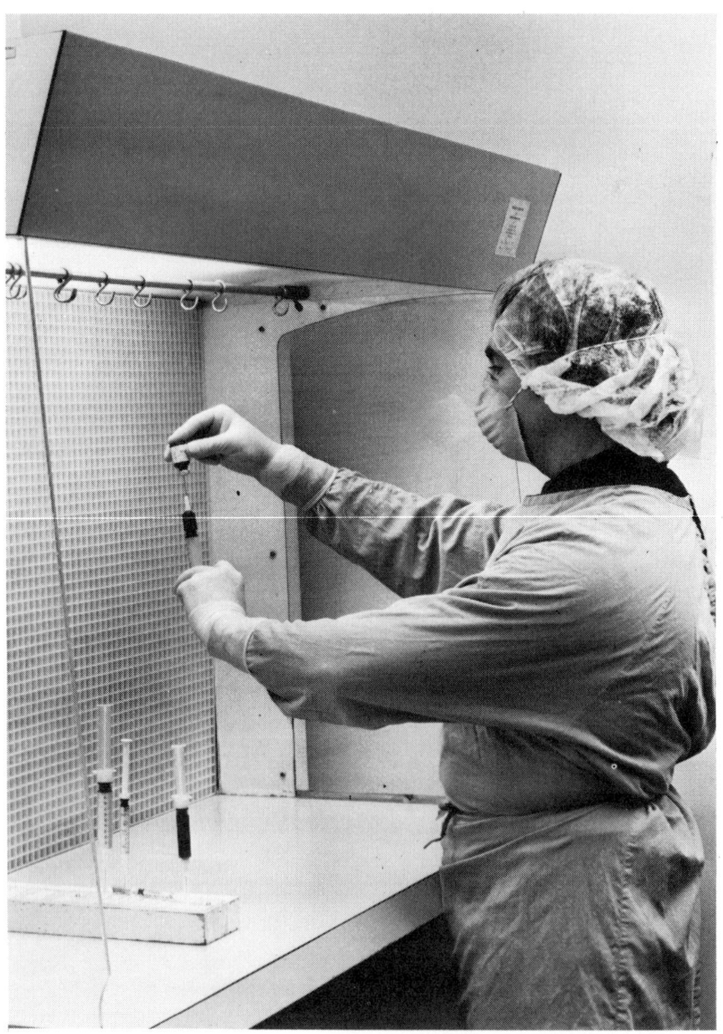

Figure 27-3. The aseptic mixing technique.

Environmental sampling procedures should be initiated within the sterile admixture room on a periodic basis. This can be easily accomplished by the use of settling plates obtained from the bacteriology laboratory. These plates are periodically placed in various parts of the room and in the laminar flow hood itself to insure that the procedures are being conducted in a clean environment. During the actual preparation of these sample cultures and during the mixing procedure, the person conducting the test should be following aseptic technique. This includes the use of a surgical mask, cap, gown and sterile surgical gloves (Figure 27-3).

An additional safeguard is the routine culturing of the tubing and 0.22 micron filter from all patients with a central line. The IV nursing team collects the bag tubing and filter from all central line patients on Friday of each week. The equipment is taken to the hospital bacteriology laboratory for culture studies. The lab results are sent to the floors and become a permanent part of the chart.

IMPLEMENTATION OF PHYSICIAN'S ORDERS

Having established the physical layout of the sterile admixture room, the pharmacist will quickly be confronted with the TPN orders. A simplified but all inclusive order sheet should be adopted by the institution through a joint effort of both the medical and pharmaceutic departments (Figure 27-4). When the physician writes the orders, the first link in the chain involves the nursing personnel and unit clerk on the floor. The nurse at this point must cosign the parenteral nutrition order sheet and then send two duplicates to the pharmacy with a pharmacy charge slip. (Note: The order sheet consists of three contact back sheets, thus providing three copies). The front sheet of the order form stays with the patient's chart at all times as part of the permanent record. It is important that the unit clerks deliver the order sheets as quickly as possible to insure that the pharmacist will not be rushed in performing the compounding procedure. This has been one of our most common logistic problems. For this reason, the members of the medical staff are encouraged to write the orders as early in the morning as possible. Should the physician, during his daily rounds, decide to taper and discontinue any of the solutions, it is the nurse's responsibility to inform the pharmacy promptly.

Once the order is received in the pharmacy, the pharmacist interprets and checks the order sheet to insure that there are no errors in the ordering sequence or time sequence. Each patient's bags are sequentially numbered and each solution has a specified time and rate of administration. In addition, the pharmacist must check for incompatibilities and other mixture discrepancies. It is the responsibility of the pharmacist to contact the physician if there are any problems and recommend alternative electrolyte additives, so that the necessary medications can be added without any inherent solution incompatibilities. A prime example of this is the incompatibility that exists between potassium phosphate and calcium above a certain concentration (precipitation often occurs if more than 40 mEq potassium phosphate are mixed with 9 mEq calcium). While the pharmacist is thoroughly checking the orders, the pharmacy technician begins to prepare the bag labels according to the physician's written order sheet (Figure 27-5). The labels are printed so as to coincide with the original order sheet. This minimizes the chance for mislabeling the solution and also provides us with a means of double checking the orders. In addition, we have elected to color code each of our labels to signify whether a peripheral (blue) or central (red) solution is being administered. This is of particular advantage to the nursing department, enabling the floor nurse to identify at a glance the mode (central vs. peripheral) of solution administration.

Following the completion of these steps, the pharmacy technician or pharmacist then

The Western Pennsylvania Hospital
PARENTERAL NUTRITION ORDERS

DATE: ____________________

PHYSICIAN SIGNATURE: ____________________

NURSE SIGNATURE: ____________________

T.P.N. LITERS REQUIRED [ ] PER 24 HRS. BAG NOS. [ ] [ ] [ ] [ ] ADMINISTRATION RATE [ ] MLS PER HR

[ ] **1. REGULAR TPN FORMULA**
Subclavian catheter use only
D_{25} + Crystalline Amino Acids 2.75%, 250g Dextrose, 850 Non-Protein Carbohydrate Cal. 27.5g Amino Acids, 28.94g Protein Equiv., 4.63gN, Cal/N-184/1, (1687mOsm)

[ ] **2. HYPERMETABOLIC TPN FORMULA**
Subclavian catheter use only
D_{25} + Crystalline Amino Acids 4.25%, 250g Dextrose, 850 Non-Protein Carbohydrate Cal. 42.5g Amino Acids, 44.69g Protein Equiv. 7.15g N. Cal/N-118.9/1, 1842 mOsm.

[ ] **3. RENAL FAILURE FORMULA (Without Electrolytes)**
Subclavian catheter use only
D_{40} + Crystalline Amino Acids 1.7% Per 1000ML
400g Dextrose, 1360 Non Protein Carbohydrate Cal. 17g Amino Acids, 17.88g Protein equivalent, 2.86g-N, Cal/N ratio 475/1,2190 mOsm

[ ] **4. PERIPHERAL FORMULA**
For use with intralipid
D_5 + Amino Acids 2.75% – 50g Dextrose, 170 non protein Carbohydrate Cal. 27.5g Amino Acids, 28.94g Protein Equivalent, 4.63g N, Cal/N – 36.7/1, 687mOsm.

[ ] **STANDARD FORMULA**
CONCENTRATION PER LITER

SODIUM	35 mEq/L	
POTASSIUM	30 mEq/L	
MAGNESIUM	5 mEq/L	
	2.75%	4.25%
ACETATE	50 mEq	65 mEq
CHLORIDE	35 mEq/L	
PHOSPHATE	30 mEq/L	
ZINC	3 mg/L	
CALCIUM GLUCONATE	10 cc (bottle #1 only)	
M.V.I.	5 cc (bottle #1 only)	
FOLIC ACID	1 mg (bottle #1 only)	

[ ] ADDITIONAL ELECTROLYTES; OR IF PRE-ADDED ELECTROLYTES **NOT** ACCEPTABLE, **CHECK** BOX, AND INDICATE CONCENTRATIONS DESIRED **PER LITER**

		FOR PHARMACIST USE ONLY
SODIUM CHLORIDE	[ ] mEq	[ ] ml
POTASSIUM CHLORIDE	[ ] mEq	[ ] ml
POTASSIUM PHOSPHATE	[ ] mEq	[ ] ml
MAGNESIUM SULFATE	[ ] mEq	[ ] ml
CALCIUM GLUCONATE (Bottle #1 only)	[ ] cc	[ ] ml
ZINC	[ ] mg	[ ] ml
REGULAR INSULIN	[ ] units	[ ] ml
SODIUM ACETATE	[ ] mEq	[ ] ml
M.V.I. (bottle #1 only)	[ ] cc	[ ] ml
FOLIC ACID (bottle #1 only)	[ ] mg	[ ] ml
HEPARIN SODIUM USP (1000 units/ml)	[ ] ml	[ ] ml
____________	[ ]	[ ] ml
____________	[ ]	[ ] ml

Figure 27-4. Standard venous nutritional support order sheet.

prepares the "Patient Profile." This provides the pharmacy with an accurate record of the patient's specific solution requirements; the date and time the solution was prepared and by whom; the starting time for each solution; the rate of administration (in ml per hour); and when the next order is due. A sample profile form is presented in Figure 27-6. Modifications of this form, to include the various additives and results of such laboratory parameters as the BUN, serum protein, albumin, and electrolytes, may be adopted to suit each institution's needs. Having completed the necessary paper work, the solution is prepared by the pharmacy technician.

In this institution, the total parenteral nutrition solutions are dispensed in 1 L polyvinylchloride (Viaflex) bags. We do not use any of the pre-packaged kits but prefer to combine the protein and caloric source into a Viaflex bag by gravity flow. The pharmacist checks the TPN label against the physician's order sheet and assembles the materials required for the formulation. The amino acid and dextrose solutions are exam-

WEST PENN HOSP TPN RECORDS

BOTTLE NO.______ROOM NO.__________

NAME________________________________

TIMES_______________________________

DATE____________RATE____________

_______gtts/min._______________cc/hr.

SOLUTION:

_______cc________% Amino Acid Sol

_______cc________% Dextrose

_______cc Sterile Water

ADDITIVES:

_______ccNaCl_____Meq's

_______ccKcl______Meq's

_______ccKPhos_____Meq's

_______ccMag So4_____Mgm's

_______ccCa Gluconate______Amp

_______ccZinc_____Mgm's

_______ccReg Insulin______U

_______ccNa Acetate________Meq's

_______ccMVI_____ Amp

_______ccHeparin____U

_______cc

_______ccApprox. Total Volume

CENTRAL

Figure 27-5. Solution label.

ined against the lighted black and white backgrounds to check for visible particulate matter (Figure 27-7). After inspection for particulate matter, the bottles are marked with a black wax pencil so the technician knows the volume of each solution that is required for the formulation. The glass containers come from the manufacturer with overfills and this marking technique eliminates the propensity for overfill. The necessary additives are then prepared under the laminar hood by the technician and are assembled on the "syringe board" to be checked by the pharmacist. The glass bottles of amino acids and dextrose solutions are wiped with 70% isopropyl alcohol prior to being placed in the laminar hood. While the amino acid and dextrose solutions are filling into the bag via gravity flow (Figure 27-8), the additives are prefiltered by injection through a system consisting of an injection cap locked into a 5 micron filter needle which is placed into the flash ball of the transfer tubing. When completed, excess air is removed from the bag and the bag is then taken from the laminar hood to the

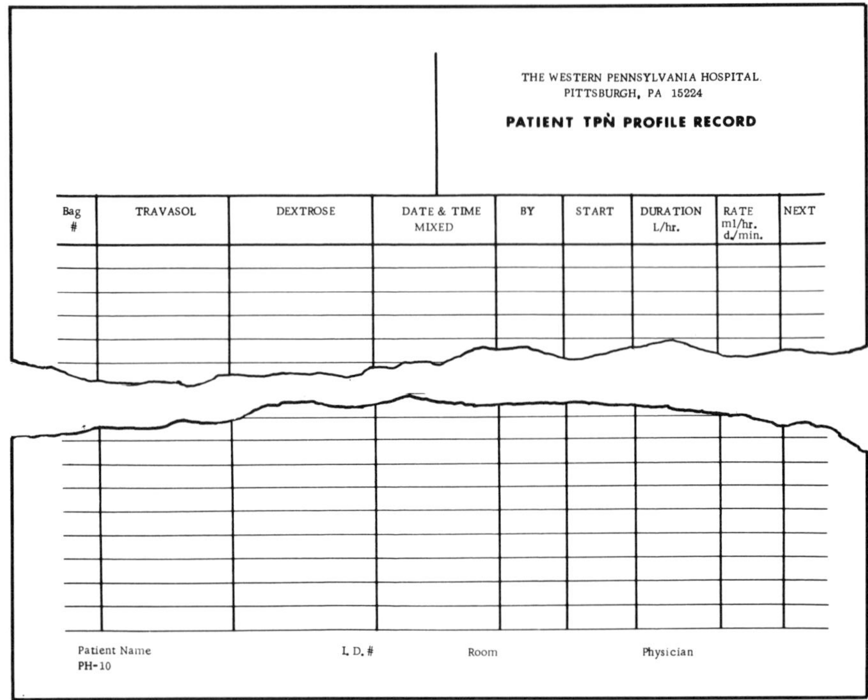

THE WESTERN PENNSYLVANIA HOSPITAL
PITTSBURGH, PA 15224

PATIENT TPN PROFILE RECORD

Bag #	TRAVASOL	DEXTROSE	DATE & TIME MIXED	BY	START	DURATION L/hr.	RATE ml/hr. d/min.	NEXT

Patient Name I. D. # Room Physician
PH-10

Figure 27-6. Patient profile.

Hematron for heat sealing of the tubing. Each TPN solution is labeled, inspected for visible particulate matter against the lighted black and white backgrounds, and stored in the refrigerator. A separate expiration date label is placed on each bag above the solution label. With the increased usage of the amino acid solutions with pre-added electrolyte profiles and the development of the 1 L underfilled dextrose bags (500 ml dextrose), the pharmacy compounding time has been significantly reduced. This decrease in time cost-justifies the use of the newer products.

The solutions are now ready for distribution and at this time are taken from the pharmacy to the nursing IV team office along with the third copy of the physician's original order sheet as a final check. In the IV office, the solutions are again stored under refrigeration (not exceeding 24-hours) until they are due for administration. It is no longer necessary for solutions to be removed from the refrigerator approximately 1 hour prior to the specified time of administration. Recent evidence suggests that sufficient warming occurs more rapidly (5 to 10 minutes) when a bag is removed directly from the refrigerator and "hung" (i.e., run through IV tubing) than when it is allowed to warm as a unit volume of 1 L. To ensure that the wrong solution is not "hung" at the wrong time, the pharmacy labels all bags in sequential numerical order, and the starting time of each particular bag is specified on each label.

During the administration of the solution, it is advised that the solution be infused through an in-line filter as a final safeguard for the patient. We use 0.22 micron air-eliminating filters on a routine basis. Also, in an effort to maintain exact flow rates and flow times, all solutions must be administered by means of an intravenous pump. This ensures that each solution will be administered over the correct time sequence.

The final link in the pharmaceutic chain involves the restocking of the sterile admixture room. We recommend that this be done on a daily basis in order to maintain an adequate and proper stock level, and also to eliminate the need for leaving this area dur-

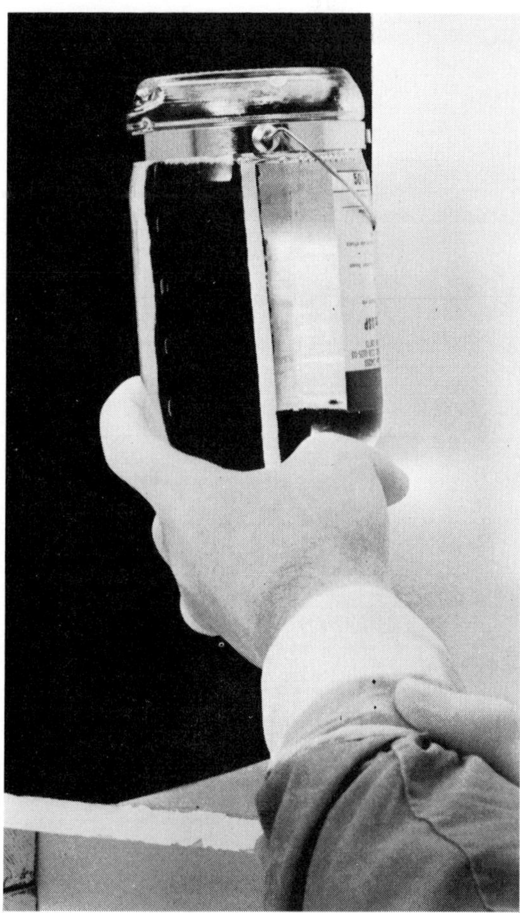

Figure 27-7. The use of lighted black and white backgrounds to check for particulate material.

ing the compounding phase. A minimal amount of cardboard containers should be brought into and stored in the room to reduce particulates in the air. The less traffic through the sterile admixture room the greater the chance of maintaining stable air conditions and the clean environment that are so necessary within this area.

EXTENDED ROLE OF THE HOSPITAL PHARMACIST

It is vital for the pharmacist to establish a maximum degree of communication between himself and the physician involved in the administration of these solutions. An open line of communication between the hospital pharmacist and the nutritional/metabolic support nurse provides a means of quickly solving logistic problems that may occur (e.g., incomplete physician's orders, late orders, variations in the time schedules). The pharmacist must also develop an open line of communication with the floor nurses so that he can ensure that the physician's orders are properly implemented. In addition, it is essential that the pharmacist develop a rapport with the patient, especially if the patient is being considered as a candidate for the HNSP. In order to accomplish this, the pharmacist should routinely make rounds with the nutritional support team. In our institution, the pharmacist routinely sees each of the patients on Monday, Wednesday, and Friday to check the following:

1. Significant changes in the overall medical condition.
2. Weight gain.
3. Laboratory parameters (BUN, serum protein, serum albumin, electrolytes, etc.).
4. Correct rate of infusion and maintenance of an appropriate time schedule. The pharmacist should also be willing to answer the patient's questions regarding the specialized solutions. By working with the nursing units, the pharmacist makes himself readily available to communicate with the patients, thus facilitating the transition to the home support program.

SPECIAL CONSIDERATIONS FOR A HOME NUTRITIONAL SUPPORT PROGRAM

With a successfully functioning in-hospital nutritional support program, the development of an HNSP becomes a relatively natural extension. However, many logistic aspects should be considered and certain administrative questions should be addressed by the hospital pharmacist. Some of these questions may be summarized as follows:

1. Will the hospital elect to allow the patient to compound the solution at home

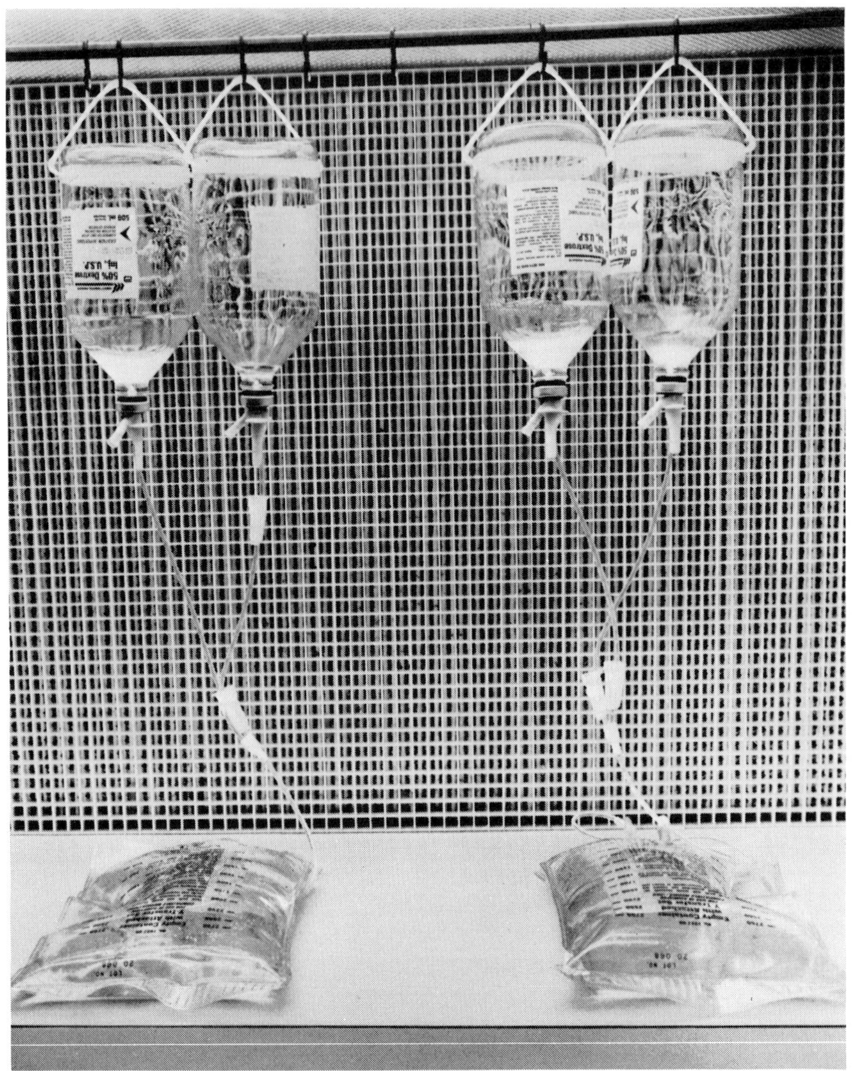

Figure 27-8. The gravity fill system.

or continue to utilize the hospital's compounding program?

2. What will be the back-up delivery system for solutions compounded in the hospital?
3. Will the hospital be responsible for sterility testing?
4. When an in-house compounding program is utilized, will there be a reimbursement fee provided by the pharmaceutic companies?

Naturally, many of these problems can be eliminated if the patient is mixing these solutions at home or if the supplier is providing a pharmacy mix and delivery system. However, the Western Pennsylvania Hospital elected to begin their program with an in-house compounding approach with subsequent delivery to the patient's home. In order to maintain quality control, scrutiny of the patient, with respect to overall mental and physical capabilities, and the availability of extended family members, will identify patients who may be candidates for home mixing programs. While our initial concerns were best alleviated by assuming the mixing responsibility, we are planning to gradually switch some of our patients to a home mixing program. There are several training manuals and visual aids available from the solution suppliers which will help the pharmacist and the nutritional/metabolic support nurse train the patient to prepare these solutions at home.

In some cases, the hospital pharmacy will elect to continue to provide the patient with solutions that have been mixed in the hospital pharmacy. Subsequently, a delivery system must be established between the pharmacy and the patient's home. Several methods can be used. The first way is to make a member of the patient's family responsible for obtaining these solutions from the institution. A family member can pick up the solutions from the pharmacy any time after 12 noon on designated days (generally two days per week—Tuesday/Friday or Monday/Thursday). A second method is to set up a special common carrier delivery service through the company obtaining reimbursement for the home care patient. In either case, the family member or delivery driver must sign a log book which verifies the receipt of these solutions from the hospital pharmacy. In one case, a special circumstance existed where it was necessary for a home care nurse to visit the patient on a weekly basis. Arrangements were made through the social service department for the visiting nurse to pick up the hospital-compounded solutions from the pharmacy just prior to her visit to the patient's home.

Once the physician has identified a patient who is a candidate for home nutritional support, the pharmacy should be notified as soon as possible. The physician and pharmacist should define as early as possible the type of venous nutritional support formula which will best meet the patient's need. This formula should be started several weeks prior to the patient's discharge in order to ensure adequacy. If the patient is going to be placed on an evening cycle schedule (e.g., 8 P.M. to 8 A.M.), the solution should be prepared in a 3 L bag during the last few weeks of the patient's hospital stay. In general, these 12-hour cyclic schedules involve the administration of 2 L of solution. Thus, the use of a 3 L bag obviates the patient or a member of the patient's family having to change bags during mid-cycle. Familiarizing the patient with the system on an inpatient basis enables the patient and the patient's designated family member to develop the skills necessary to utilize the system on an outpatient basis. Since M.V.I. concentrate is only stable in solution for 24-hours, it should be placed in solutions the patient will be able to use that same day (assuming an in-hospital compounding program). The physician and pharmacist may, however, elect to train the patient to make additions to the solution prior to the administration of the solution at home. This would facilitate the more frequent administration of M.V.I. concentrate and other special additives to the patient.

The hospital pharmacy must also consider the number of days of solution they will provide to the patient at any one time (again assuming an in-house compounding program). Is a 1-day supply practical? What about a 3- or 4-day supply? Is a 7-day supply safe? These are very important questions which must be carefully studied. As part of our routine sterility testing, we included solutions that had been stored for longer periods of time under refrigeration. The storage time of these solutions ranged from 3 to 30 days. Solutions were then evaluated by the following two methods:

1. The millipore Addi-check system.
2. Evaluation by the hospital bacteriology laboratory.

All tests thus far have been negative, and our sterility studies continue to be an ongoing part of our pharmacy practice. However, we have elected to limit storage of mixed solutions to 4 days. The pharmacy places home nutritional support patients on a biweekly delivery schedule (Mondays/Thursdays, Tuesdays/Fridays). In order to obtain reimbursement for the pharmacy's compounding efforts, a monthly bill is submitted from the pharmacy to the company supplying the compounding solutions. This bill is based on the outpatient solution prescription written by the physician prior to discharge (Figure 27-9). The company provides the pharmacy with a 1-month supply of all materials required to compound solutions for each home nutritional support patient. This has created a significant storage problem, as the number of home nutritional support patients has grown. It may be necessary for us to obtain special facilities or to reconsider our initial approach to the pharmacy compounding program.

Continual evaluation of the pharmacy resources is necessary to ensure that the pharmacy's capabilities keep up with the overall growth of the program. In this way, the pharmacy can continue to function as a solid base for program expansion.

SPECIAL CONSIDERATIONS

Three separate patient situations will be presented to illustrate some of the special problems we have encountered, using different equipment and different compounding techniques.

Patient One

This patient is receiving solution on a 12-hour cycle. The final concentration of dextrose is usually 25%, with a final protein concentration of 4.25%. Two liters of solution are contained in a 3 L bag (Figure 27-10). This bag is an efficient gravity-fill system. Additives can be injected into the amino acid or dextrose solution prior to transfer to the bag or injected through the medication port on the bag itself. We have not encountered any difficulties in the mixing procedure or patient utilization of this system and rely upon it as our modality of choice.

Patient Two

This patient was initially sponsored by a company that supplied the hospital with pre-mix kits, which resulted in having the

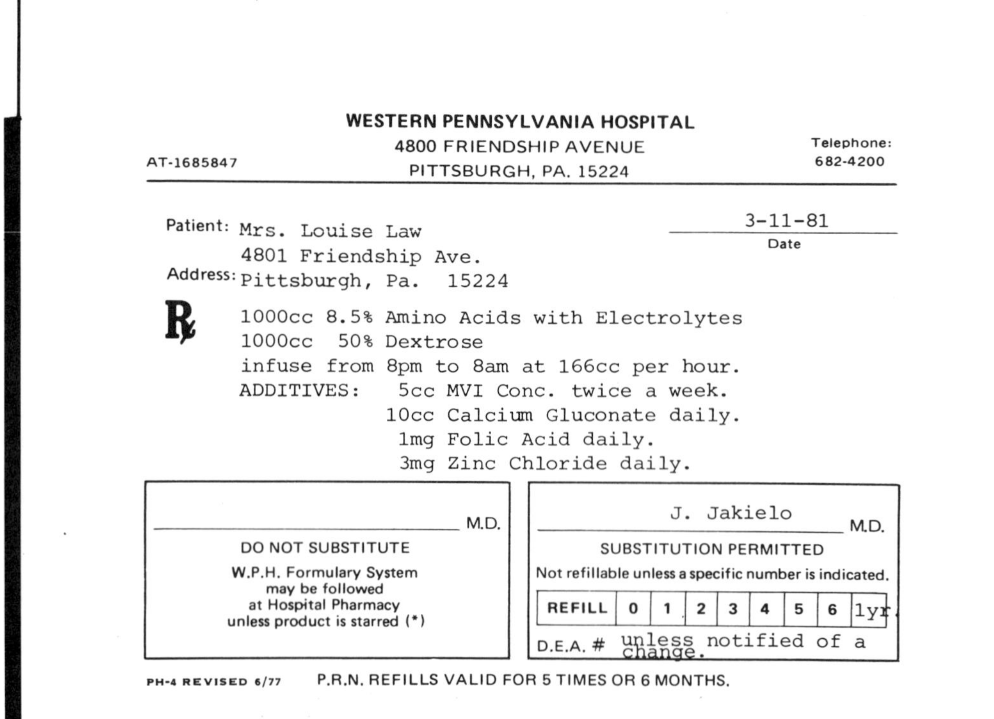

WESTERN PENNSYLVANIA HOSPITAL
4800 FRIENDSHIP AVENUE
PITTSBURGH, PA. 15224

AT-1685847

Telephone: 682-4200

Patient: Mrs. Louise Law
4801 Friendship Ave.
Address: Pittsburgh, Pa. 15224

3-11-81
Date

℞ 1000cc 8.5% Amino Acids with Electrolytes
1000cc 50% Dextrose
infuse from 8pm to 8am at 166cc per hour.
ADDITIVES: 5cc MVI Conc. twice a week.
10cc Calcium Gluconate daily.
1mg Folic Acid daily.
3mg Zinc Chloride daily.

________ M.D.
DO NOT SUBSTITUTE
W.P.H. Formulary System may be followed at Hospital Pharmacy unless product is starred (*)

J. Jakielo M.D.
SUBSTITUTION PERMITTED
Not refillable unless a specific number is indicated.

REFILL	0	1	2	3	4	5	6	1yr

D.E.A. # unless notified of a change.

PH-4 REVISED 6/77 P.R.N. REFILLS VALID FOR 5 TIMES OR 6 MONTHS.

Figure 27-9. A home support prescription.

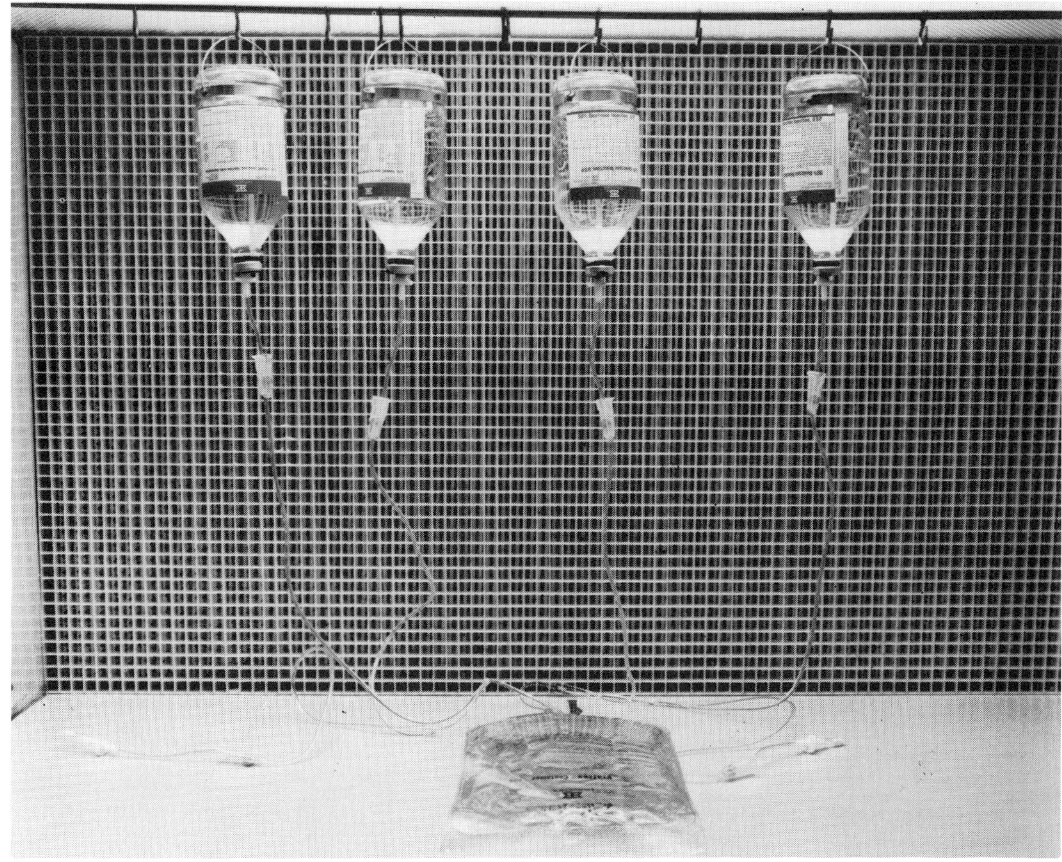

Figure 27-10. The Viaflex 3 liter bag system.

solution in 1 L glass vacuum containers. Since our patients are trained to utilize the 3 L bag in the hospital, it was necessary for us to transfer the solution to bags. Initially, we tried to utilize 3 L empty blood plastic containers for this transfer but this proved to be unsuccessful. It required "spiking" of the glass bottle and the use of transfer tubing which had been separately vented. Coring frequently occurred and the transfer was exceedingly slow. The bags were also more awkward for the patient to handle. Subsequently, we were supplied with a 3 L bag with vented transfer tubing which worked somewhat better. The additives were injected into the medication port of the tubing while the amino acid solution was transferred into the dextrose bottle. Then the two 1 L solutions can be transferred into a 3 L bag.

Patient Three

This patient is somewhat special because he receives continuous infusion therapy utilizing the Cormed pump and vest. This necessitates the use of two 500 ml bags every 8 hours. Although it is possible to underfill 1 L bags with 500 ml of the solution, this does not comfortably fit into the vest unit. In addition, we had some difficulty in maintaining proper flow rates with larger bags. Another means of preparing 500 ml bags had to be designed. Since the 500 ml bag does not have transfer tubing attached to it, an 18 gauge needle attached to an injection cap was inserted into the medication port. Multiple 50 ml injections were made into this injection cap to provide the proper amount of solution. The preparation of six 500 ml bags for a single day's supply was a very tedious and time-consuming task. Our present technique is to remove the rubber medication port from the 500 ml bag and spike this port with a transfer tubing set. The other part of this set is used to spike the amino acid solution and the dextrose solution. Additives are injected into the amino acid solution or dextrose solution prior to transfer. The tubing is crimped three times with a Hematron system just below the flash ball to seal the transfer tubing. By sealing below the flash ball, we have provided a medication additive site if needed. This patient is receiving insulin in his bags, which means the pharmacy has to prepare this solution every 2 days in order to maintain stability.

FUTURE PLANNING

If the home nutritional support program in our institution continues to grow at its projected rate, the in-house compounding approach will have to be reevaluated. In our opinion, the hospital would have three possible options:

1. Establish a comprehensive patient compounding training program under the direct supervision of the hospital pharmacist and in conjunction with the solution supplier.
2. Establish a separate pharmacy home nutritional support staff with their own facilities so as to continue the inhouse and outpatient compounding programs.
3. Utilize a separate company mixing center.

These options are continually discussed within the nutritional and metabolic support committee meetings. At this time, we are leaning toward a combination of the first and second options and are still reluctant to be exclusively dependent on only one outside or sole capability.

As a result of our ongoing sterility studies, it may prove beneficial to compound the solutions once a week instead of twice a week. The pharmacy could prepare the stock solution and the patient could add the necessary additives. This would alleviate much of the burden being placed on the pharmacy staff and act as a transitional step in converting the patient to a complete home mixing program.

SUMMARY

Developing an HNSP was not a difficult task with the full cooperation of the nutritional and metabolic support committee and the hospital administration. For the pharmacy, it was a direct outgrowth of an efficient and competent in-house nutritional support program. Even when solution compounding is performed by an outside company or by the patients themselves, the hospital pharmacist still remains an active component of the outpatient program. He provides the necessary critical evaluation to ensure that the program is safe and effective.

BIBLIOGRAPHY

1. National Coordinating Committee on Large Volume Parenteral: Recommended methods for compounding intravenous admixtures in hospitals. Am. J. Hosp. Pharm., *32:*261, 1975.
2. NCCLVP: Recommendations to pharmacists for solving problems with large-volume parenterals. Am. J. Hosp. Pharm., *33:*231, 1976.
3. Pipp, T.: Special Series for Infusion 1980: Recommendations of the NCCU infusion. *4*(1):5, 1980.
4. NCCLVP: Recommended guideline for quality assurance in hospital centralized intravenous admixture services. Am. J. Hosp. Phar., *37:*645, 1980.
5. Rapp, R.P., Bivens, B., and Deluca, P.P.: In-line filtration of IV fluids and drugs. Am. J. IV Therapy, *2:*18, 1975.
6. Avis, K.E.: Chemicals and Particulate Matter. *In* Symposium on Total Parenteral Nutrition. Chicago, American Medical Association, 1972.
7. Burke, A.: Preparation, Including Incompatabilities and Instability. *In* Symposium on Total Parenteral Nutrition. Chicago, American Medical Association, 1972.
8. Goldman, D.A., Martin, W.T., and Worthington, J.W.: Growth of bacteria and fungi in total parenteral nutrition solutions. Am. J. Surg., *126:*314, 1973.
9. Hull, R.L.: Use of trace elements in intravenous hyperalimentation solutions. Am J. Hosp. Pharm., *31:*759, 1974.
10. Kaminski, M.V., et al.: Electrolyte compatibility in a synthetic amino acid hyperalimentation solution. Am. J. Hosp. Pharm., *31:*244, 1974.
11. Rowlands, D.A., Wilkinson, W.R., and Yosnimura, N.H.: Storage stability of mixed hyperalimentation solutions. Am. J. Hosp. Pharm., *30:*436, 1973.

12. Ivey, M., et al.: Long-term parenteral nutrition in the home. Am. J. Hosp. Pharm., *32*(10):1032, 1975.
13. Kaminski, M.V., et al.: Parenteral hyperalimentation—a quality of care survey and review. Am. J. Hosp. Pharm., *31*(3):228, 1974.
14. Bergman, H.D.: Incompatabilities in large volume parenteral. Drug Intel. Clin. Pharm., *11:*345, 1977.
15. Deluca, P.P., et al.: Filtration and infusion phlebitis: A double-blind prospective study. Am. J. Hosp. Pharm., *32:*1001, 1975.
16. Doris, G.G., et al.: Inflammatory potential of foreign particles in parenteral drugs. Anesth. Analg., *56:*422, 1977.
17. Maki, D.G.: Final filters. Hosp. Infect. Control, *3:*22, 1976.
18. Miller, R.C., and Grogan, J.B.: Efficacy of inline bacterial filters in reducing contamination of intravenous nutritional solutions. Am. J. Surg., *130:*585, 1975.
19. Burke, W.A.: Prototype format for developing parenteral hyperalimentation (H-A) protocol. Department of Pharmacy, Wilmington Medical Center, Wilmington, Delaware. Manuscript. No Date.
20. Goldman, D.A., and Maki, D.G.: Contamination of fluid for parenteral nutrition. N. Engl. J. Med., *290:*1437, 1974.
21. Hanson, A.J., Nighswander, R.M., and Verhulst, J.H.: Monitoring of intravenous solutions. A study to determine the incidence of bacterial and fungal contamination in I.V. solutions and their administration sets, with patient safety the primary concern. Hosp. Form. Manag., *8*(1):17, 1973.
22. Kleinman, L.M., et al.: Stability of solutions of essential amino acids. Am. J. Hosp. Phar., *30:* 1054, 1973.
23. Laegeler, W.L., Tio, J.M., and Blake, M.I.: Stability of certain amino acids in a parenteral nutritional solution. Am. J. Hosp. Pharm., *31:*776, 1974.
24. Sauve, F.: The pharmacist and a nutritional intravenous therapy program. Am. J. Hosp. Pharm., *28:*106, 1971.
25. Tsallas, G., and Baun, D.C.: Home care total parenteral alimentation. Am. J. Hosp. Pharm., *29:* 840, 1972.
26. Scheutz, D.H., and King, J.C.: Compatibility and stability of electrolytes, vitamins and antibiotics in combination with 8% amino acid solution. Am J. Hosp. Pharm., *35*(1):33, 1978.
27. Hauer, E.C., and Kaminski, M.V., Jr.: Trace metal profile of parenteral nutrition solutions. Am. J. Clin. Nutr., *31*(2):264, 1978.
28. Schneider, P.: The pharmacist's role in inpatient and home care hyperalimentation programs. Hosp. Pharm., *13*(2):71, 1978.
29. Lowry, S.F., et al.: Parenteral vitamin requirements during intravenous feeding. Am. J. Clin. Nutr., *31*(12):2149, 1978.
30. Wolman, S.L., et al.: Zinc in total parenteral nutritions: requirements and metabolic effects. Gastroenterology, *76*(3):458, 1979.
31. Kishi, H., et al.: Thiamin and pyridoxine requirements during intravenous hyperalimentation. Am. J. Clin. Nutr., *32*(2):332, 1979.
32. Allinson, R.: Plasma trace elements during total parenteral nutrition. JPEN, *2*(1):35, 1978.
33. Greenlaw, C.W.: Pharmacist as team leader for total parenteral nutrition therapy. Am. J Hosp. Pharm., *36*(5):648, 1979.

Chapter 28

Techniques of Administration

I. William Goldfarb, M.D.
Harvey Slater, M.D.
Members of The Nutritional and Metabolic Support Committee of The Western Pennsylvania Hospital

Regardless of the type of system utilized (venous or enteral), the principles of administration are essentially the same. The initiation of inpatient therapy is based on a gradual process of increasing volumes and concentrations until the desired therapeutic magnitude is reached. This step-by-step therapeutic increase is an effort to reduce the incidence of associated complications. When the patient who has been successfully maintained on inpatient therapy is deemed a candidate for home nutritional support, specific alterations in the administrative regimen often must be made. The actual techniques of in-house administration and the subsequent transition maneuvers are outlined in this chapter for each specific type of therapy.

VENOUS MODALITIES

After the completion of the nutritional assessment and the placement of a central line, the patient is gradually started on a course of venous nutritional support. Because of the high dextrose concentration (D_{50}), it is generally not feasible to initiate therapy using the volumes of solution that are ultimately desired. Instead, the therapy is initiatd with smaller volumes of base solutions and increased over a 72-hour period as follows:

Day one: 1000 ml of the base solution (500 ml of D_{50} plus 500 ml of 8.5% protein hydrolysate) is administered over 24 hours. The patient's urine reductions and serum glucose are closely monitored (reductions, q 6 hr; serum glucose, q 12 hr). If there is no evidence of glycosuria or hyperglycemia, the rate of administration is increased.

Day Two: 1000 ml of the base solution (500 ml D_{50} plus 500 ml 8.5% protein hydrolysate) is administered over two 12-hour periods. Again, the patient's urine reductions and serum glucose are followed. If there is no evidence of glycosuria or hyperglycemia, the rate of administration is increased.

Day Three: 1000 ml of base solution (500 ml D_{50} plus 500 ml 8.5% protein hydrolysate) is administred every 8 hours. Urine reductions and serum glucose are again followed to detect the presence of glycosuria or hyperglycemia. The literature abounds with articles detailing the need for trace element supplementation in venous nutritional support solutions. On a practical basis, we have been using zinc, (3 mg per L) as the sole additive for the vast majority of our in-house patients. In the patient who is on prolonged in-house venous nutritional support or in the patient who is on home nutritional support, we do advocate the addition of other trace element solutions. Specifically, we have utilized a 1 ml additive which consists of zinc, chromium, manganese, selenium, and copper. Clinically relevant trace element deficiencies, with the exception of zinc, are exceedingly rare in patients maintained on venous nutritional support for a short period of time. In patients in whom venous nutritional support is extended and in those patients with significant malabsorption states or the need for continuous home nutritional support, the other trace elements should be added to the solution.

Potential Metabolic Complications

Should the patient manifest a hyperglycemic response (greater than 250 mg/dl) or glycosuria with attendant free-water loss of sufficient magnitude to precipitate hyperosmolar nonketotic coma, then adjustments in the concentration of administered dextrose and/or insulin supplementation must be made. Specifically, we begin by adding five units of regular insulin to each bag of solution. The patient's serum glucose and urine reductions are again monitored. If this does not correct the error of glucose metabolism, then gradual increases in insulin supplementation are made. In rare cases, we have had to utilize continuous insulin infusion by a separate route of venous administration. One may also elect to decrease the concentration of glucose in the solution (e.g., 250 ml D_{50} plus 250 ml sterile water plus 500 ml 8.5% protein hydrolysate) in order to negate this error of glucose metabolism. Even in those patients who require this type of manipulation, gradual tolerance may well develop that will eliminate the need for the continuation of these maneuvers over a long period of time. It should be noted that any patient who has tolerated solution administration and then developed an error of glucose metabolism may well be reflecting an underlying septic problem. These patients should be thoroughly evaluated for a source of sepsis, and appropriate adjustments in solution administration should be simultaneously performed.

In addition to errors of glucose metabolism, patients may also display errors of protein metabolism. Specifically, patients may develop hyperchloremic metabolic acidosis which will be manifested as a decrease in serum CO_2 content and associated hyperchloremia. This error of protein metabolism may be managed by the addition of sodium acetate to the solution (sodium acetate will be converted to bicarbonate and act as a buffer). In addition, one may decrease the concentration of protein administration (500 ml D_{50} plus 250 ml 8.5% protein plus 250 ml sterile water) in much the same way as the error of glucose metabolism was managed. In addition to hyperchloremic metabolic acidosis, one may also encounter hyperammonemia, as a result of the incomplete metabolism of the glycine contained in the solution. Some evidence indicates that a relative deficiency of arginine may also serve as an etiologic factor in the development of this particular complication. The propensity for these and other basic biochemical complications and additional technical complications can be limited by the utilization of standard supplemental orders (Figure 28-1).

Once the patient has been discharged, continued monitoring is required on a regular basis. Ketodiastix are given the patient during his hospitalization. A review of the need for urine reductions along with a demonstration of the use of the Ketodiastix is given to the patient and the designated family member. As this "skill" is acquired easily, it is usually the first step reviewed during the home instruction program. Patients are given a flow sheet to keep at home and to record the results of their urine reductions (Figure 28-2). This sheet is brought with them to the outpatient nutritional support clinic. The patients are also instructed to notify the nutritional/metabolic support nurse of a sudden change in reductions.

THE WESTERN PENNSYLVANIA HOSPITAL
Pittsburgh, Pa. 15224
BNDD-AT-16858 47

PHYSICIANS ORDERS

Red Indicates Physicians Copy in Place

DATE		USE BALL POINT PEN
		TOTAL PARENTERAL NUTRITION
	1.	Obtain a portable chest x-ray to confirm position of catheter and to rule out pneumothorax.
	2.	Run D_5W at keep vein open rate till position of catheter is confirmed and then begin TPN.
	3.	No blood drawing, routine IV's or antibiotics through the central line.
	4.	Do not increase or decrease pump rate of infusion unless ordered by M.D.
	5.	Vital signs with BP Q 4h × 24h. Notify M.D. for Temp. greater than or equal to 38.0° or hypotension.
	6.	Daily weights.
	7.	Strict intake and output
	8.	Dressings per nutritional support nurse.
	9.	Change IV tubing and filter daily.
	10.	Notify M.D. and obtain Blood C + S for temp. greater than or equal to 38.0 °C, or for shaking chills.
	11.	Baseline Laboratory Studies: CBC with diff., Lytes, Creatinine, SMA-12, Protime.
	12.	Blood Sugar, BUN, Lytes: QAMx3 every Tues., Thurs., and Sat.
	13.	SMA-12, TIBC: Every Tuesday.
	14.	CBC with diff., Protime: every Thursday.
	15.	24 Hour urine for creatinine and urea nitrogen: Every Monday.
	16.	Nutritional assessment Q 2 weeks per Dietary Department.
	17.	Urine Reductions Q6h--if 4+ get stat blood sugar and notify M.D.
		Coverage 4+ .... units of CZI subcut
		3+ .... "
		2+ .... "
	18.	Vitamin B_{12} 500 mcg. IM every other Monday.
	19.	Aquamephyton 20 mg. IM every Monday.
	20.	INTRALIPID 500 cc IV over 6 hours every Wednesday via Periph. IV.

Figure 28-1. Standard supplemental orders.

Transition Period and Pump Selection

Solution administration on an outpatient basis is dependent on the use of some type of pump mechanism. There are numerous pumps on the market which can be utilized for solution administration. In general, it is best to utilize pump equipment that is standard in your own hospital so as to have an adequate backup system should the patient's home pump fail. The physician and nutritional/metabolic support nurse should be familiar with the numerous pumps available. They should also continue to update their knowledge so as to be aware of pump developments and improvements.

At the present time, we are utilizing two separate delivery systems for home nutritional support:

1. *Volumetric pumps (Travenol infusion pump or IVAC 530 pump).* This system is used for patients who are on home nutritional support over a 12-hour infusion cycle.
2. *The Cormed pump.* This system is used in conjunction with a vest for those few patients who require continuous 24-hour support.

Although the hospital does stock pumps, we have decided, by separate arrangement with our home care supplier, to have two full sets of equipment available in the hospital for home nutritional support patients. Therefore, a patient who will be discharged on the HNSP will be trained in the hospital on the exact machine that he will be utilizing at home. When the patient is discharged with the equipment, the supplier then sends a replacement set of equipment to the institution so as to insure continual in-hospital

URINE REDUCTION

	Mon.	Tues.	Wed.	Thurs.	Fri.	Sat.	Sun.	Mon.	Tues.	Wed.	Thurs.	Fri.	Sat.	Sun.
DATE														
6 A.M.														
12 P.M.														
6 P.M.														
12 A.M.														
	Mon.	Tues.	Wed.	Thurs.	Fri.	Sat.	Sun.	Mon.	Tues.	Wed.	Thurs.	Fri.	Sat.	Sun.
DATE														
6 A.M.														
12 P.M.														
6 P.M.														
12 A.M.														
	Mon.	Tues.	Wed.	Thurs.	Fri.	Sat.	Sun.	Mon.	Tues.	Wed.	Thurs.	Fri.	Sat.	Sun.
DATE														
6 A.M.														
12 P.M.														
6 P.M.														
12 A.M.														

Figure 28-2. Home urine reduction chart.

stock of two complete home sets. The use of the pump and all necessary accompanying components is reviewed with both the patient and the designated family member numerous times during the comprehensive training program.

Assuming that the patient has received an appropriate course of inpatient therapy without any of the more common metabolic complications we have discussed, one may then prepare to make the transition to outpatient care. At this point, the physician must decide whether the patient is a candidate for continuous 24-hour infusion or whether a 12-hour schedule of administration will be used. In general, only those patients with severe short bowel syndromes or malabsorption states are truly candidates for continual 24-hour administration. The vast majority of patients will best be served by a 12-hour administration schedule. The techniques for the conversion to both of these schedules are outlined in the following:

12-HOUR SCHEDULE

This group of patients will generally receive 2 L of the basic total parenteral nutritional solution over a 12-hour period. Most patients prefer to receive their therapy during the evening and night hours. This enables the patients to be completely ambulatory and independent of their home during the daylight hours. Most of our patients receive their solutions during the period from 8 P.M. to 8 A.M. A 3 L Viaflex bag containing 2 L of the solution bag (e.g., 1000 ml D_{50} plus 1000 ml 8.5% protein hydrolysate with electrolytes) is utilized to facilitate administration. This 3 L bag negates the need for the patient to awaken midway through the therapy in order to change bags. We instruct the patients to set their initial pump flow rates at 180 ml per hour. This will provide for the infusion of 1800 ml over a 10-hour period. At the end of 10 hours, the patient is instructed to turn the rate of administration down to 100 ml per hour for the remaining 2 hours. This enables the patient to taper the glucose administration and thus, it is hoped, decreases the propensity for any hypoglycemic rebound that may occur after complete termination of the treatment cycle. The exact techniques of pump care and postinfusion line care are thoroughly taught to the patient and the patient's designated family member prior to discharge. We actually utilize this system for at least 1-week prior to patient discharge. The patient and the designated family member are asked to be available in the hospital on a few occasions in order to demonstrate their ability to initiate and terminate this therapy without any additional help.

24-HOUR SCHEDULE

In those rare patients who are candidates for continuous administration of nutritional support solutions, the Cormed pump and vest system offers a degree of freedom that they would not have with any of the standard pump systems. The utilization of this system requires a somewhat longer degree of in-hospital training prior to discharge, as compared to the training period required for the 12-hour administration schedule. In addition, the patient must be trained in the technique of bag exchange, since this system requires that procedure to be performed every 8 hours. The system utilizes

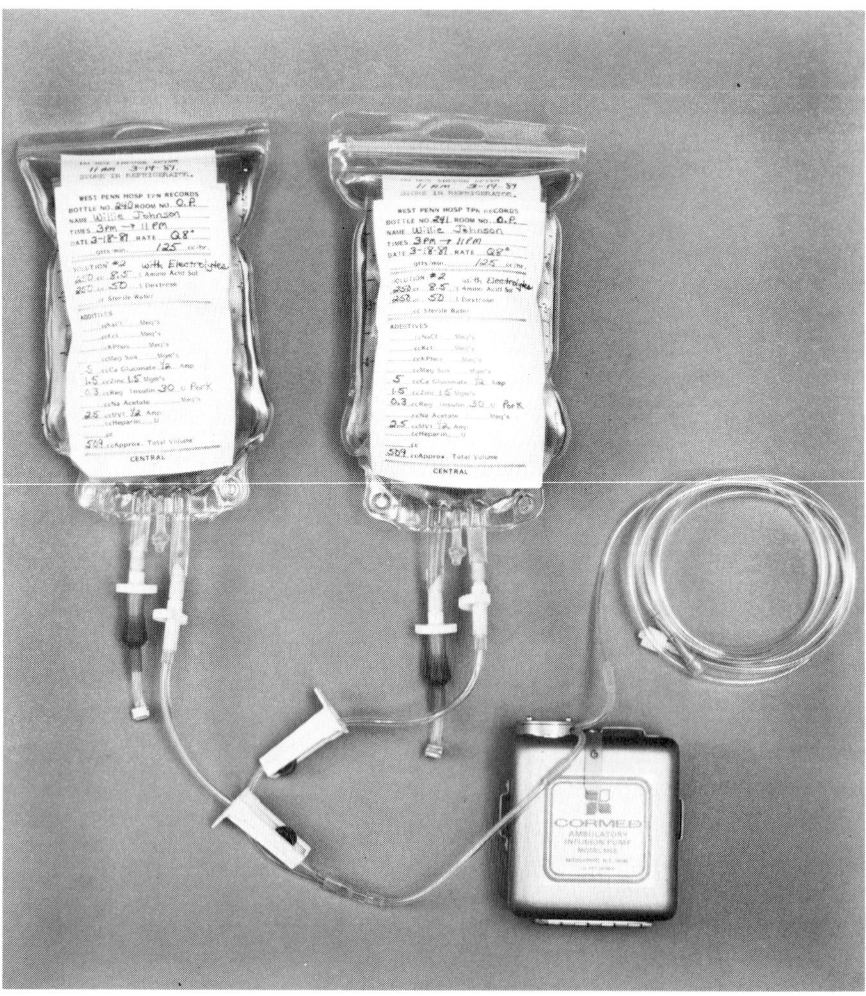

Figure 28-3. The Cormed pump with an 8-hour (1 L) supply of solution.

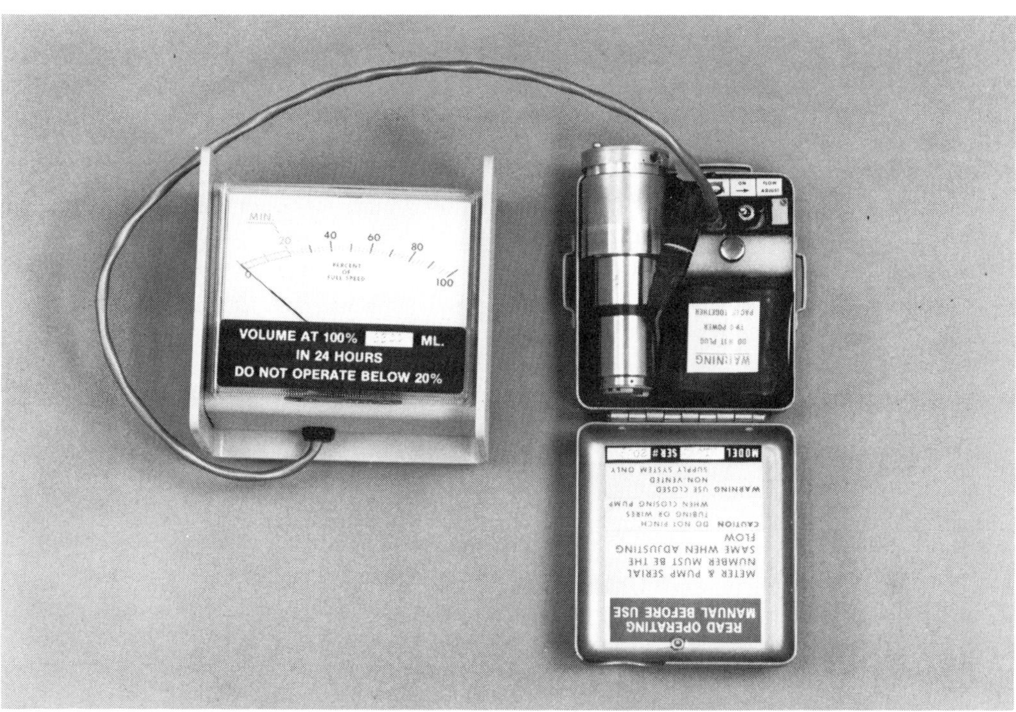

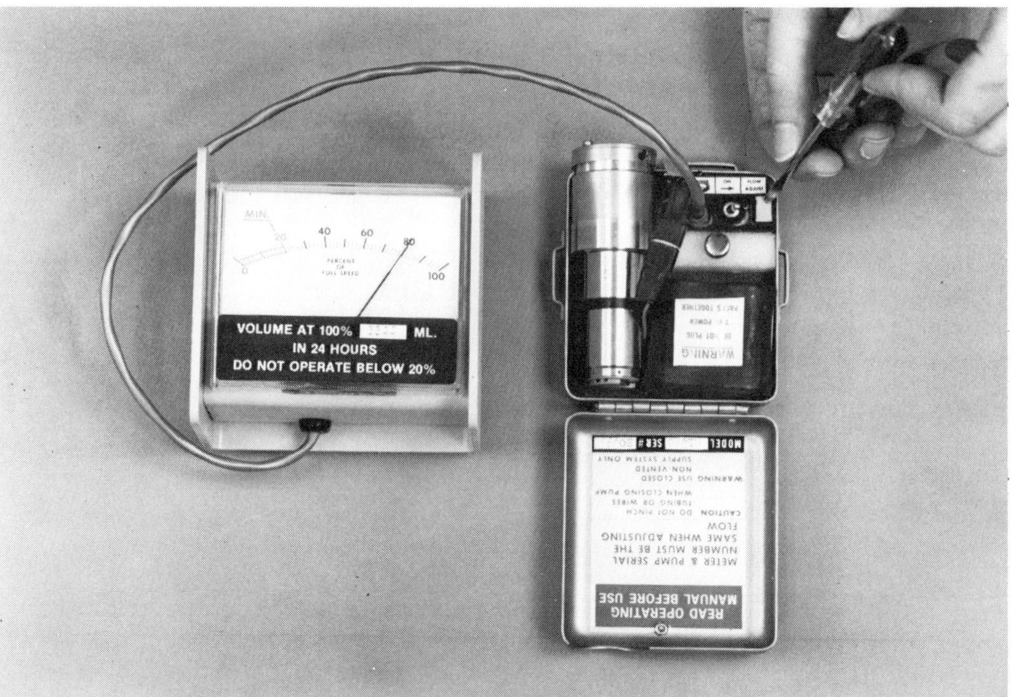

Figure 28-4. Flow-rate calibration of the Cormed pump.

500 ml plastic bags and provides for the administration of a total 1000 ml volume every 8-hours (Figure 28-3). The patient must become proficient in pump flow-rate calibration and maintenance. Flow-rate calibration is dependent on the use of a "volume meter" which is specifically calibrated to that patient's particular pump (Figure 28-4). Changes in patient positioning, particularly during sleep, may significantly effect flow and frequently cause the shift of fluid volumes from one bag to the other. In addition, the bag and tubing apparatus is predisposed to some kinking problems proximal to the pump mechanism. We have encountered difficulties with this in a few instances, and have had to resort to the use of "splint-type devices" proximal to the pump mechanism. The patient must be familiar with all of these potential problems and must also know the appropriate maneuvers to correct these problems should they arise. One important negative aspect of the Cormed pump mechanism is the absence of an alarm system. This requires that the patient continually check the equipment to ensure that no mechanical problems have developed. Newer pump mechanisms with appropriate alarm systems may soon be available.

In addition to these mechanical problems, many patients find the vest itself to be cumbersome and uncomfortable (Figure 28-5). The positioning of the nutritional support bags may pose a particular problem for the female patient. The vest material itself is somewhat uncomfortable, and a few patients have complained of a "scratching sensation."

Because of the problems we have encountered utilizing the standard vest system, we

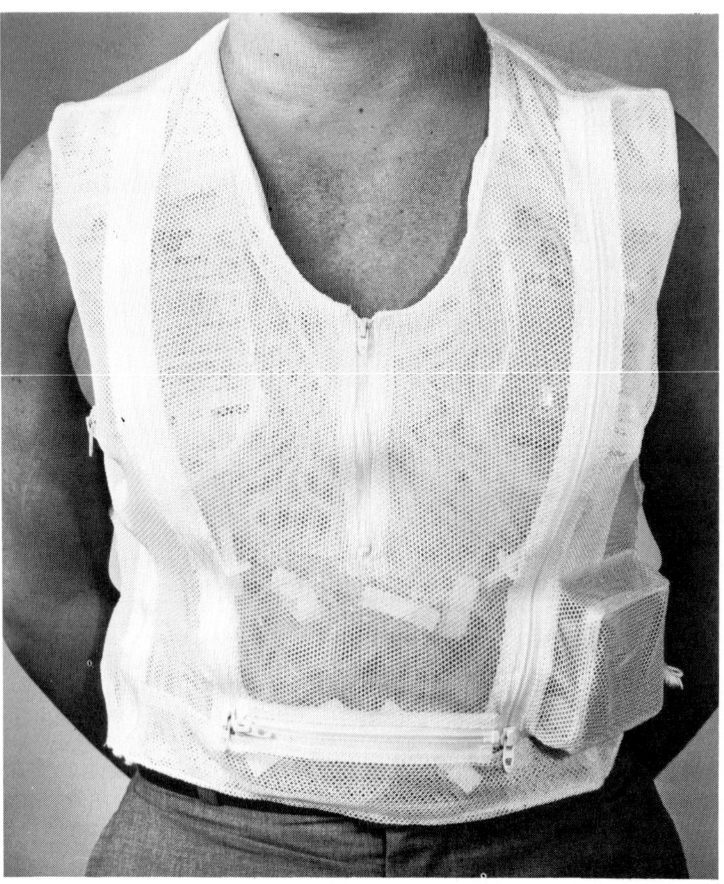

Figure 28-5. The complete vest and pump system.

have elected to custom design a new system, "the Shimko Vest." Specifically, this consists of a custom-fitted and designed vest which is made from a 100% preshrunk cotton material. This provides for patient comfort both in terms of decreased skin irritation and evaporative cooling. In addition, we have also been able to eliminate the use of zippers and most of the inherent tubing problems by using a specifically modified approach. In essence, this custom-fitted vest seems to provide for greater patient comfort and ease of utilization (Figure 28-6).

While the Cormed pump and vest system is designed to be used with the classic Hickman-Broviac catheters, we have had no difficulty in adapting this equipment for use with the Centrasil catheter. In one case, we have even utilized this system with an Intrasil catheter placed through the antecubital fossa.

Regardless of which pump system is utilized, the hospital should make arrangements with the home care provider to invoice and supply the patient with the necessary hardware on a regular basis. Following discharge, all of the long-term necessary supplies are shipped from the supplier directly to the patient's home. Supply requirements are updated by phone invoicing between the supplier and the patient. The following is a list of standard supplies needed for the maintenance of home nutritional support.

1. Volumetric pump system.
2. IV administration set with in-line 0.22 micron air-eliminating filter.
3. Home nutritional support dressing kit (components are listed in Chapter 25).
4. Op-Site dressing.
5. 25 gauge, ¾ inch needles (these small

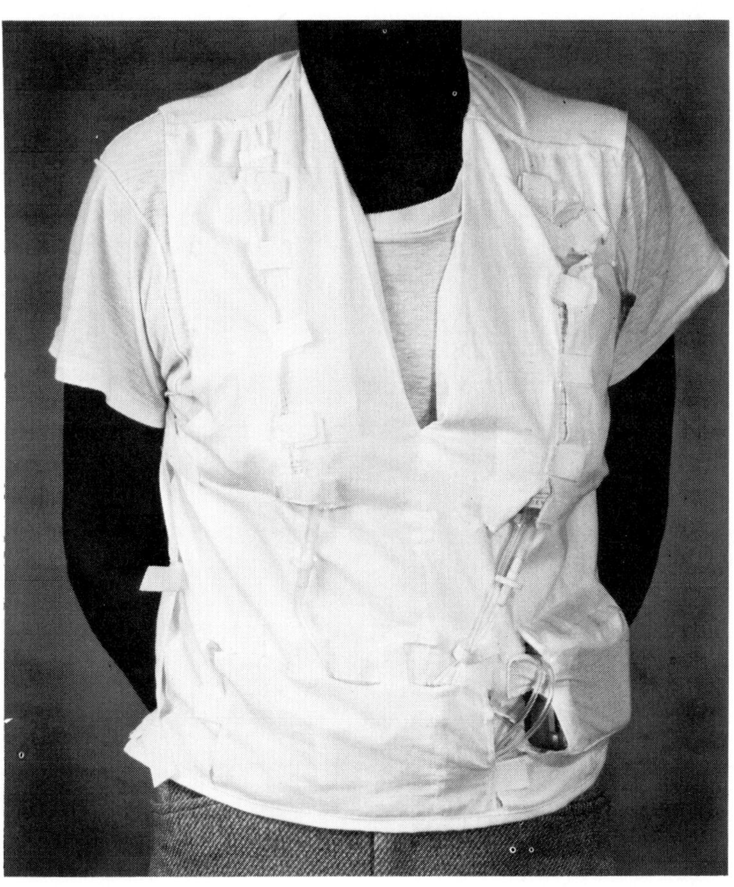

Figure 28-6. The Shimko Vest.

needles are utilized so as to avoid puncturing the 4-inch, 16 gauge connector tubing when the needle is inserted through the injection port).

6. Wyeth Tubex syringe.
7. Wyeth Heparin cartridges (10 units per ml).
8. Quest latex injection ports.
9. Quest 4-inch connector tubing.
10. Ketodiastix.
11. Thermometer.
12. Destruclip (for destruction of needles).
13. Alcohol wipes.
14. Patient record sheets to record observations at time of dressing change.

ENTERAL MODALITIES

During the past few years, a significant number of patients have become candidates for home nutritional support using the enteral modality. Specifically, these patients are maintained in positive nitrogen balance through the use of elemental solutions administered through silicone elastomer, nasogastric, or nasoduodenal feeding tubes. Some patients have elected to reinsert their tubes on a daily basis for utilization of a 12-hour administration cycle, while other patients have preferred to have their tubes remain in place 24 hours a day. Regardless of which system is utilized, we would advocate that only small bore, soft, flexible feeding tubes be used. Specifically, we restrict our utilization to 8 Fr silicone tubes. We have preferred to utilize weighted tubes in an effort to facilitate passage of the distal end of the tube beyond the pylorus. Passage of the distal end of the tube beyond the pylorus. In order to achieve passage beyond the pylorus in a high percentage of patients, reduces the propensity for reflux esophagitis and subsequent aspiration. We do not advocate the administration of any solution by pump mechanism when the distal end of the feeding tube has not passed beyond the pylorus. In order to achieve passage beyond the pylorus in a high percentage of patients, we have used mercury-weighted or silicone-weighted tubes. We prefer to utilize the 6 or 8 Fr Duo-Tube with either a mercury- or silicone-weighted tip. The use of the silicone-weighted tip eliminates mercury disposal problems. This tube is relatively easy to insert, provides patient comfort, and facilitates passage of the distal end of the tube beyond the pylorus. We restrict our utilization of elemental solutions to those with a low enough viscosity to facilitate passage through these smaller feeding tubes without the necessity for a pump mechanism. Although we have chosen to stock 10 enteral solutions, we do have a specific preference. We have been using Travasorb in the vast majority of our patients receiving enteral supplementation. We have encountered a lower incidence of both flow complications and diarrhea with the use of this product. In addition, once we have worked the patient up to the full volume and concentration, we have then been able to switch to the utilization of Travasorb-MCT in its concentrated form. This enables us to double our caloric intake while maintaining the same volume of solution administration.

Once the tube has been inserted, the position of the distal end of the tube is always confirmed by abdominal x-ray. The tube itself is secured on the cheek through the use of a small Op-Site dressing. This dressing has proved extremely comfortable for the patients, and seems to more adequately secure the smaller flexible feeding tubes than does the standard taping procedure.

Once the position of a tube has been confirmed by x-ray, solution administration is initiated, utilizing gradually increasing rates and concentrations. The specific protocol that we follow is as follows:

Day One: 60 ml of half-strength solution q 1 hour.

Day Two: 100 ml of half-strength solution q 1 hour.

Day Three: 100 ml of ¾-strength solution q 1 hour.

Day Four: 100 ml of full-strength solution q 1 hour.

Day Five: 125 ml of full-strength solution q 1 hour.

In the small percentage of patients in whom the distal end of the tube has not passed beyond the pylorus, the nursing department is instructed to aspirate on the tube every 4 hours to ensure adequate gastric emptying. It is extremely difficult to aspirate on any tube smaller than an 8 Fr diameter, as the tube will collapse and not provide for the adequate evaluation of gastric emptying. However, when 8 Fr tubes are utilized, aspiration can usually be performed.

One of the more common problems encountered with the utilization of these solutions is the onset of diarrhea. The use of a gradually increasing program of administration rates and concentrations may serve to allow the patient's gastrointestinal tract to become better adapted to these solutions. However, in a small percentage of patients, diarrhea may prove to be a persistent problem. In those cases, we have elected to add Lomotil to the solution. The use of formulas consisting of medium-chain triglycerides seems to have resulted in a lower incidence of diarrhea in both our in-house and home populations. If diarrhea persists despite the use of specialized formulas or the addition of antispasmodics, the physician should taper the solution to a lower concentration.

SUMMARY

While we have attempted to outline these techniques and some of the potential problems, we realize that other practitioners at other institutions may have additional means of avoiding or dealing with the problems we have encountered. Similarly, we are sure there are some problems that we have not encountered that have been encountered in other institutions. Suffice it to say that no description is an adequate substitute for practical experience. Each patient becomes an academic building block for the overall program. The problems encountered with one patient generally do not become problems for future patients. As with any other field of medicine, practical experience leads to proficiency and an overall improvement in susbsequent patient care.

BIBLIOGRAPHY

1. Dudrick, S.J., et al.: Parenteral hyperalimentation. Metabolic problems and solutions. Ann. Surg., *176:*259, 1972.
2. Heird, W.C., et al.: Metabolic acidosis resulting from intravenous alimentation mixtures containing synthetic amino acids. N. Engl. J. Med., *287:* 943, 1972.
3. Hull, R.K.: Use of trace elements in intravenous hyperalimentation solutions. Am. J. Hosp. Pharm., *31:*759, 1974.
4. Kaminski, M.V., Jr.: Enteral hyperalimentation. Surg. Gynecol. Obstet., *143:*12, 1976.
5. Mitty, W.F., Nealon, T.F., Jr., and Grossi, C.: Use of elemental diets in surgical cases. Am. J. Gastroenterol., *65*(4):297, 1976.
6. Dobbie, R.P., and Hoffmeister, J.A.: Continuous pump-tube enteric hyperalimentation. Surg. Gynecol. Obstet., *143*(2):273, 1976.
7. Avery, G.B.: Nasoduodenal vs. nasogastric feeding. Pediatrics, *60*(4):550, 1977.
8. Barrocas, A.: ABC's of tube feeding. J. LA. State Med. Soc., *130*(4):83, 1978.
9. Kaminsky, M.V.: Enteral hyperalimentation. Surg. Gynecol. Obstet., *143:*12, 1976.
10. Page, C.P., Ryan, J.A., and Haff, R.C.: Continual catheter administration of an elemental diet. Surg. Gynecol. Obstet., *142:*184, 1976.
11. Shils, M.E., Bloch, A.S., and Chernoff, R.: Liquid formulas for oral and tube feeding. JPEN, *1:*89, 1977.

Index

Numerals in *italics* indicate figures; "t" following a page number indicates tabular material.